TOWARD
EDUCATION
FOR
HEALTH
PROFESSIONS

Harper Series in Social Work,
Werner W. Boehm,
Series Editor

TOWARD EDUCATION FOR HEALTH PROFESSIONS

Jeanette Regensburg

Harper & Row, Publishers
New York,   Hagerstown,   San Francisco,   London

Sponsoring Editor: *Dale Tharp*
Project Editor: *Renée E. Beach*
Designer: *Michel Craig*
Production Supervisor: *Marion Palen*
Compositor: *TriStar Graphics*
Printer and Binder: *The Maple Press Company*

TOWARD EDUCATION FOR HEALTH PROFESSIONS

Library of Congress Cataloging in Publication Data

Regensburg, Jeanette
    Toward education for health professions.

    (Harper series in social work)
    Includes index.
        1. Medical social work. I. Title. [DNLM:
1. Health occupations—Education. 2. Social work.
3. Patients. 4. Hospitals W18 R334t]
HV687.R43   362.1   78-15966
ISBN 0-06-045357-5

CONTENTS

FOREWORD

A few years ago when Harper and Row established a textbook series on
social welfare we hoped to stimulate books that would serve both the
burgeoning undergraduate population and the graduate group of social work
students. In so doing, we have been guided by the best judgments we could
muster about the path to follow both at a given point and in the foreseeable
future. Thus, we are trying to create books that reflect both what is in the
profession and what might be. Obviously, as we go on, we shall find that at
times we hew too close to tradition and at other times we venture too far
from it.

We welcome Dr. Regensburg's book to the Harper series on social work.
It arrives at a time of heightened awareness of and increased attention to the
health needs of our population. There are indications that we are on the verge
of important developments in policy for health care programs. As these
developments move from the drawing board to realization, it is essential to
emphasize the significance of psychosocial factors in the development of
practice in health care programs. Therein lies the contribution of this book; a
contribution which makes it useful not only for students of medicine as was
initially envisaged but also for students in other professions concerned with
assessment of need, provision, and evaluation of health care services.

This book is based on data obtained from social work practitioners in
the five hospitals affiliated with The Mount Sinai Medical Center in New
York City. Social work has a long and honorable tradition of concern, in
education, practice, and research, with the mutuality between individual
capacity and social resources, their match and mismatch, their scope and
range, their adequacy and inadequacy. An analysis of hospital based social
work practice which, by definition, is carried on in a multidisciplinary and
multiprofessional setting, thus furnishes an excellent and appropriate base for
culling out concepts and principles relevant to health care.

The presentation and analysis of these practice data and the formulation of concepts and principles which flow from them, in my view, constitute Dr. Regensburg's contribution. Dr. Regensburg concludes this treatise with an assessment of social work practice today and a delineation of the direction in which it might move tomorrow. This is a felicitous ending because the author, in the concluding chapter, manages to draw on rich experience as a practitioner, teacher, and researcher. In so doing, she succeeds in joining mellow wisdom with disciplined appraisal, two traits which her friends and colleagues have long admired.

I see this book as a milestone in Dr. Regensburg's distinguished career in social work. Many years ago, when I was a student at Tulane University, Dr. Regensburg was my teacher and faculty advisor. Over the years, we have become close associates and I had the benefit of her professional acumen when she staffed the Commission on Social Work Education of the National Association of Social Workers from 1966 to 1969 which I chaired. It gives me both pleasure and satisfaction to lend a hand in launching a work which reflects the fruits of Dr. Regensburg's competence and wisdom in such a remarkable fashion.

Werner W. Boehm

Preface

This book is offered to students who are preparing to enter the health and health-related professions and vocations. Ours is an era of heightened awareness of the significance of the biopsychosocial factors in health and illness. It is an awareness shared by practitioners and educators in the health care field and by an increasingly informed and assertive consumer-public.

Accordingly, this book illuminates the ways in which biological, psychological, and social forces influence one another and affect the social-health status of individuals and family groups; it illustrates the impacts of illness and disability on patients, on their relatives and friends, and on the givers-of-service; and, finally, the book describes and assesses a range of social and medical resources in our voluntary and mandated systems of services, which either are, are not, or should be provided in selected areas of health care.

The data presented in this book not only are pertinent to each of the several professions and vocations engaged in health care but also are potentially enabling to the development of increasingly effective interprofessional and interdisciplinary education and practice in the health care field.

Social work traditionally has been deeply rooted in knowledge and skills concerned with human relationships, with the interaction between human beings and their environment, and with human ability to adapt to and cope with the pressures and demands of the environment.

It is not surprising, then, that the origins of this book lie in a study of social work practice made by the writer for the faculty of the Division of Social Work, Department of Community Medicine, The Mount Sinai School of Medicine, City University of New York. The study was generously financed by the Auxiliary Board of The Mount Sinai Hospital, from the fall of 1969 to the summer of 1974. The source of the funding was the Joseph Klingenstein Fund, named for its donor. Mr. Klingenstein and the members of the Auxiliary Board have been devoted supporters of the Social Service Department over many years and are greatly appreciated contributors to this text.

The primary sources for this book were 69 social workers selected from among the members of the departments of social work services established in the five hospitals affiliated with The Mount Sinai School of Medicine. They were The Mount Sinai Hospital, The Beth Israel Hospital of the Beth Israel Medical Center (New York City), The Veterans Administration Hospital (Bronx, N.Y.), The Hospital for Joint Diseases and Medical Center (New York City), and the City Hospital Center at Elmhurst (Queens, N.Y.). The social workers interviewed by the writer included the directors of these five social service departments and the ten other faculty members of the Division of Social Work.

Throughout the book are medical-social histories that are recorded in considerable detail. Their use was authorized in releases signed by either the patients or the spouses of deceased patients. The understanding was that identifiable data would be as disguised as possible and that the histories would be used for educational purposes only.

Like many texts this one has limitations. Some of them are due to the purpose and focus of the book, while other limitations reflect the nature of the social workers' experience and of our health care systems. For example, a few selected and documented illnesses and disabilities serve as paradigms on the assumption that knowledge gained in one context can be applied to similar or comparable contexts; the social work practice was hospital based and almost entirely hospital bound; payment for medical care was solely on a fee-for-service basis (except in the Veterans Administration Hospital); the medical care described lacks programs for primary care and for the promotion and maintenance of health, and, as a final illustration of limiting conditions, there is the unresolved problem of determining criteria for optimal deployment of social work staff within and outside the boundaries of the hospitals that employ them.

It is hoped that the ideas offered in the book and the manner in which they are presented will spur inquiries into unexplored territory, generate new ideas, and in general promote the look forward that is needed to cope with the uncertainties of expanding knowledge, galloping technologies, and a changing society.

Jeanette Regensburg, Ph.D.
June 1977

Acknowledgments

It is with keen appeciation that I acknowledge my debt to all those who participated in and facilitated the study of hospital-based social work practice which furnished the raw material for this book. My thanks go particularly to the social workers in direct service who generously made their experience available, and to the anonymous patients, their relatives, and their close associates, who, in the end, are the primary instructors of students and practitioners in the field of health care.

I renew my most sincere thanks to all the members of the Auxiliary Board of The Mount Sinai Hospital and in particular to Mrs. Jack R. Aron and Mrs. Seymour Klein, the two presidents of the Auxiliary Board during the conducting of the study, for their sustaining interest and financial support.

My gratitude is hereby expressed to the lasting influence of the late Doris Siegel, who, when the study began, was the first Edith J. Baerwald Professor of Community Medicine (Social Work) and the first Chairman of the Division of Social Work, Department of Community Medicine, The Mount Sinai School of Medicine, City University of New York.

My thanks go also to the then members of the faculty of the Division of Social Work, all of whom participated in the study and encouraged the writing of this book: Helen Rehr (Chairman), Jerry B. Alford, Mrs. Barbara Berkman, Margaret Dennis, Mrs. Hannah Lipsky, Helen Lokshin, Sidney Malter, Milton Nobel, Janice Paneth, Elaine Rosenfeld, Mrs. Ruth Seltzer, Herman Shepard, Mrs. Elinor Stevens, Mrs. Marilyn Wilson, and Alma T. Young. I called freely on these colleagues for consultation on matters related to their special expertness, and their responses were invaluable.

I am most deeply indebted to the members of the Advisory Committee to the original study—Mrs. Bess Dana, Associate Professor and Director, Education Unit, Department of Community Medicine, The Mount Sinai School of Medicine; Helen Lokshin, Director, Social Service Department, Mount Sinai Services, City Hospital Service at Elmhurst (Queens, N.Y.); Helen Rehr, D.S.W.,

Director, Social Service Department, and Edith J. Baerwald, Professor of Community Medicine (Social Work), Department of Community Medicine, The Mount Sinai School of Medicine—for their unfailing interest, the acuity of their criticism, and their availability whenever I sought their counsel. Their professional support was continuous throughout the long period of the study and the writing of this book.

I wish to express my gratitude to Kurt W. Deuschle, M.D., Director, Chairman, and Ethel H. Wise, Professor, Department of Community Medicine of The Mount Sinai School of Medicine, whose commitment to the idea of social-health has been a sustaining force.

My acknowledgements would be incomplete without a word of thanks to Dr. Werner W. Boehm, Series Editor, who piloted me over much unfamiliar terrain, and to Community Funds, Inc., and its Advisory Committee to the Social Work Practice Fund for the grant that made technical assistance possible for the preparation of the manuscript for this text.

I take full responsibility for the way in which I have used the contributions of others and for all errors of fact, judgment, and interpretation.

Jeanette Regensburg

PART ONE
THE CONCEPTUAL BACKGROUND

Chapter 1
The Practice of Hospital-Based Social Work:

PRIMARY CONCEPTS OF VALUES AND KNOWLEDGE

A profession lays claim to a set of values, a body of knowledge, and an assemblage of skills for the practice of the profession. The profession's values direct the pursuit and application of knowledge, the development and use of skills, and the behavior of its members, individually and collectively. The concepts and generalizations described in this chapter are central to social work, which is responsible for upholding an identified set of values and for building and carrying out functions compatible with the ultimate objectives of the profession and with the proximate objectives of a specific institution or system.

As disparate ideas, many of these concepts will be familiar to members of other professions; a number of the ideas may even be recognizable components of their beliefs and practices. But for social work they constitute a cohesive whole and a point of departure for professional practice.

The primary concepts and the major functions described in this and the following chapter were formulated inductively by the writer from the specific data provided by the social workers who participated in a study of hospital-based social work practice—the study that preceded and stimulated the writing of this book.

The social workers almost never described or explained their practice in abstract terms, even when pressed to do so. The generalized ideas that follow are those that the writer could perceive clearly in the material at her disposal. They are therefore not a complete listing of social work values, but they provide a usable structure for an orderly presentation of the practice wisdom possessed by the participating social workers.

SOCIAL WORK VALUES

The values that are subtly interwoven into every aspect of a profession are by definition enduring and deeply felt beliefs. But because they are seldom made explicit, they are not always consciously at hand to inform the judgments, decisions, and choices that every professional is called upon to make.[1] One expected expression of a profession's values is a code of ethics, and social work is no exception.[2, 3] However, codes that regulate conduct change as new conditions and problems emerge with changes in society. These changes interact also with changes in the knowledge and skills of the profession.

In addition, some of the difficulties members of different professions encounter in working together in the field of health are related to differences in their value systems or to differences in the significance given to one value over another. Givers-of-service* in the health field need to note also that problems in personnel/patient relations are often due to differences in values that neither party recognizes. The onus obviously is on personnel both to identify and to bridge the differences.

For these reasons the values implicit in the practice of social work are made explicit here. They reflect the value-concepts held by citizens committed to a democratic society and therefore are not completely separable from the values of the body politic.[4] Also, the values of social work are interrelated. In a given situation, two or more values may reinforce each other or may be in conflict, and in this case the dominant value must be determined.

Finally, in all human endeavors ideals, convictions, or beliefs—whatever word is used to convey values—are sometimes affirmed in human conduct and sometimes violated. Social workers are aware of such discrepancies, contemplate them openly, and make efforts to resolve them.[5]

The primacy of the individual, or belief in the dignity and worth of the individual, permeates the practice of social work. It is a fundamental inherent human value unrelated to such specific characteristics as sex, age, color, creed, ethnic grouping, and intellectual acuity, or to social status determined by such factors as level of education, income, and type of occupation.

This value is made explicit in the patient's right to know about his or her illness and alternative modes of treatment and their probable outcomes, the right to give informed consent to recommended procedures and the right to refuse them, the rights to a confidential relationship with givers of medical care, and the rights to privacy and respect.[6, 7] Since belief in the dignity and worth of the individual does not cancel his or her obligation to society, the individual's rights are not absolute; they are qualified by the rights of others. "The common good" or "the public welfare" as a reciprocal value is embodied also in the two concepts that follow.

Holding to this value is not easy in our technological, computerized society: "It is a value against which every social work program needs to be tested. Does it promote the worth of the individual in his/her own eyes or those of the rest of society? Or does the program itself, or the way in which it is administered, devalue the individual and relegate him/her to a state of facelessness or anomie?"[8] These are questions that can be asked also about the modalities and techniques used by the various professionals in the field of health, where, for example, imbalanced concern for efficiency and financial cost or interest in the expansion of knowledge and development of techniques

* In this text *giver(s)-of-service(s)* is used to designate those individuals who give direct services in the field of health care and in health-related fields to patients, their relatives, and their significant others, and to small groups and populations. This usage reserves the term *provider(s)* for institutions and systems within which people serve and are served and which are sources of funding for the payment of services.

may lead to dehumanizing conditions of care and desensitized patterns of professional behavior.

Maximum realization of the individual is a corollary to the concept of the individual's primacy to which social work is strongly committed. This value-concept implies the individual's right to the kinds of physical, mental, and emotional sustenance and the kinds of stimuli and opportunities that permit the fullest possible development and use of his or her innate capacities. Implicit is the quality of reciprocity: Each individual's need and right to receive are coupled with his or her obligation to use what he or she receives for self-realization and the good of others.

This value is exemplified in direct services in efforts to make available the resources patients/families* need and can be helped to use in order to live and function, not at minimal levels but at their maximal realizable levels of social-health. When the social worker in indirect services uses his or her energies, or supports the efforts of others to improve systems and subsystems for the delivery of human services or to enhance programs and standards of practice, then maximum realization of the individual is again a motivating value. The full implication of this value reaches beyond the social worker's immediate responsibility toward patients/families who need his or her services into areas of activity—such as formulating policies and promoting measures to improve delivery of human services—which will assist members of large populations to attain maximum social functioning.

Maximum feasible self-determination is clearly a value that is qualified because of the reciprocal relationships among the individual, his or her family, other reference groups, and the society in which he or she lives. The social worker believes that rights are balanced by obligations and that therefore the right to self-determination has limits and boundaries which are implied in the word *feasible.* The exercise of an individual's right to decide and to make judgments and choose according to his or her preferences, wants, and desires is limited by the obligation to respect the rights of others, to avoid endangering himself or herself and others, and to add to, rather than detract from, the general social welfare. Sometimes these limits are established by moral and ethical sanctions, sometimes by law, and sometimes by the realities of life.

Maximum feasible self-determination is a forceful value-concept in many activities undertaken by social workers in the field of health care. There are persons whom the social workers must discourage from subjectively imposing their preferences upon others. There are many persons who need help to reach an accommodation between the path they would like to take and the limits set by medical, social, and physical realities; by the right of others to self-determination; or by legal authority.

These persons are patients and their relatives, their significant others, and givers-of-services. Each of them may lay claim to this value and in so doing may create a problem of balance between rights and obligations.

Social justice is a value that is fundamental to other values such as the individual's primacy, right to self-realization, and right to maximum feasible self-determination. Social justice embodies equity, fairness, impartiality, and equality of opportunity; and social workers hold these qualities to be morally good and right. Social justice has concern for the needs of *all* the citizenry, for

* For a definition of the terms *individual/family* and *patient/family,* see the section on the individual/family as an organic unit, pp. 11–13.

the maximum development of *all* persons in our society, and for the conservation and enhancement of *all* human resources.

Social justice controverts the exercise of dual standards for meeting the needs of rich and poor persons, of the handicapped and the able-bodied, and of the members of one ethnic group as opposed to another. In essence, social justice makes a stand against special privilege and for the general welfare.

The many inequities in our society make it far easier to talk about injustice than about justice. It is also easier to recommend correctives than to carry them out, if for no other reason than that a conversion from social injustice to social justice depends on the efforts of many diverse groups with varied points of view and diverse goals.

Progress toward a just society, to say nothing of achieving a just society, will not come about by verbalizing the virtues of social justice and the immorality of injustice. It requires change in the structure and governance of our institutions and in the actions of the citizenry to make such progress. Since changes of this kind usually mean that some people have to give up a portion of their "good" in order to attain a more equitable distribution for some have-nots, inertia may become a formidable resistance. At best, efforts to effect social change arouse opposition and create new problems to be overcome.

Social workers are in general agreement that many inequities exist in the field of health. "Ability to pay, skin color, political clout, personal connections, and social class are some of the prevailing considerations that influence access to care." [9]

All in all, members of our society are made familiar with social justice as much through its absence as through its presence. Social workers have a part to play, in both the voluntary and public sectors, in eliminating injustice and promoting justice as a dominant value in the human services: "The reform measures of the late 1940s and early 1950s . . . while they represented significant steps in humanizing patient care . . . did relatively little to acknowledge or correct the imbalance in the distribution of health care service or to expand the social mission of medicine." [10]

Social workers, and in particular those engaged in the field of health care, are more and more aware that responsibility for achieving conditions of social justice lies with all health and health-related professions, including their own, and with professional persons at each level of the hierarchical structures within which they work: "Trying to do the job [of pursuing social justice] alone is quixotic and romantic, because the tasks can no longer be accomplished by one person. They must be done in concert with colleagues, with other professions, with principals and interactors in other institutions, in other systems." [11, 12]

The family as a value-concept has a meaning distinct from the concept of family based in knowledge. The two meanings fuse to inform the social worker's judgments and technical skills in the performance of professional practice.

As a value-concept the family is an enduring social institution which over the centuries and in many lands has undergone notable modifications in composition, structure, and function. Despite the changes, the family has been a persistent and consistent symbol of human support throughout each individual's life cycle and from generation to generation of the kinship group.

Both the nuclear family and the extended family are included in the value-concept; at any given time in cultural history and in the idiosyncratic history of a given family, the structural and functional relations between a nuclear family and its extended family must be understood. To perceive the family as a value-concept is to recognize it as the *basic* institution for procreation, for the biopsychosocial nurturing of children and adults, for the socialization of children, and for making a place in the larger society. Add to these functions the gratification, via the family as an institution, of human needs such as those of belonging, trusting, and being trusted; giving and taking; and having a safe haven in times of trouble, and one comprehends even better the family as value-concept.[13]

Social workers in the field of health care hold firmly to the value-concept of family. It is manifested, for example, in their gathering and evaluating of data about life-and-illness situations; in their efforts to limit or control the destructive impacts of disease or disability upon family members; in the priority they give to the family as the unit of support for a patient's recovery and social rehabilitation; and in their endeavors to understand, and ability to accept, different family patterns in different social milieus.

Compassion is "pity for the suffering or distress of another, with the desire to help or spare."[14] This definition contains the two elements that form the foundation of the social worker's professional attitude toward the persons he or she serves. Starting with feelings of sympathy and concern for others in trouble and the desire to help them, social workers learn early in their careers that their feelings and emotions must be tempered and disciplined if they wish to help others. They have to have enough self-awareness and control not to be overwhelmed by pity; they must perceive the other person as a distinct entity, lest they act in their own interests rather than in the other's. Biases held by a giver-of-service against certain traits or behavior are also a source of danger to the patient/family. Social workers with firsthand observation of devastating poverty, for example, may have to fight a bias against the affluent, who have their own troubles and suffering.

In sum, compassion is the bedrock value of the social worker's ability to be of service, but it is insufficient to guarantee professional competence. Compassion must be harnessed to knowledge and skills and be kept compatible with other basic values. For instance, in the field of health care, if unrestrained pity is permitted to outweigh a patient's right to know or right to self-determination, the obvious danger is that the social worker is losing perspective and is doing something to or for patients that they are capable of doing or deciding.

Whichever way the bias goes, compassion may be subverted if dispassionate concern is displaced by either overidentification or underidentification.

CONCEPTS BASED IN KNOWLEDGE

Concepts based in knowledge reflect the values in which the profession of social work believes, provide the building blocks for the profession's body of knowledge, and are made manifest in the practitioner's actions and judgments. The following are statements of five concepts of knowledge that significantly inform the hospital-based practice of social work.

Interdependence is a fundamental quality that permeates human relations, the professions involved in the human services, and the network of institutions and systems of service which exist for the benefit of society. Interdependence implies a state of reciprocal dependence between any two parties, whether they be individual human beings interacting with each other or interacting systems of services devised to meet specific needs. Interdependence also describes the relationship among *parts* of a single system. *System* in this context applies to a person as a whole as well as to an organized profession, a social institution, or the totality of a system of services.

The significance of interdependence to the professional social worker is, in part, that "any system is conceived to be a unified whole composed of interdependent parts . . . any change in one part of the system sets off simultaneous variations throughout the whole of the system." [15] Similarly, if two systems are interdependent, a change in one will affect the other.

Interdependence is a dynamic quality capable of shifting in kind and intensity to achieve a new balance in response to the exigencies of life and the forces in society. For example, the dependence of a newborn infant upon a nurturing, protecting, loving adult is so nearly total that it is easy to overlook the reciprocal dependence of the adult who is stimulated and motivated to bestow love and care upon the infant who is the eager recipient. Under reasonably healthy conditions the original state of interdependence between the growing, developing infant and his or her nurturing adult shifts for both parties throughout the life cycle.

Critical periods which call for changes in the kind, intensity, and gratifications of interdependence are well known. Among them are the changes demanded of a married couple when their small circle of interdependence is expanded by the birth of their first child; the changes demanded of both mother and child when the child starts school; the potentially stormy period of readjustment which affects the pattern of interdependence among all family members when adolescence disturbs the equilibrium of existing relationships; and the sometimes abrupt and traumatic shift in the balance of interdependence that may come as adult children become the ones more leaned upon than leaning when their parents' capacity to cope becomes impaired.

The human life cycle is a continuous flow with one stage of experience bringing to the next the accumulated effect of what has already been lived through. This phenomenon means that a fairly large part of a person's past is an active, though not always conscious, ingredient in his or her present. The interdependent relations experienced in the past will influence how his or her balance shifts during the later periods of the life span and how he or she develops and uses relations of interdependence in situations that are crucial or new. Human needs are expressed, recognized, and responded to in give-and-take relationships. Both parties give and both parties receive; gratifications and dissatisfaction which accrue to each party and the value each puts on what is exchanged between them are paramount in an assessment of interdependent relationships.

In the field of health care the concept of interdependence is essential to understanding and evaluating people's relations in a life-and-illness situation and to determining how these relations affect and are affected by illness and disability and how they may contribute to or impede recovery and social rehabilitation.

Something needs to be said specifically about interdependence between patient and physician and among professional givers of health care. To those who think of the physician as a person of unquestioned authority, it may seem unreal to identify interdependence as a quality of the patient-physician relationship. There are times in the course of an illness when the patient is a passive recipient of care, but he or she is most often an active participant, whether it is a child or an adult. The physician has to depend on that participation in order to carry out his or her professional responsibility. The patient's ability to be an active recipient of care will vary with age and mental competence, with the nature of the illness and its treatment, with the stage of the illness, and with the system of delivering care. Thus the balance of interdependence between a patient and his or her physician will shift as the situation demands. The kinds of decisions patients must make, in particular concerning informed consent to specific medical or surgical procedures, emphasize their right to self-determination, that is, the right to a degree of independence which is concurrent and compatible with dependence on the physician for care. Since there is such a strong trend toward consumer participation in planning health-care programs and such strong advocacy of patients' rights, we can expect recognition and utilization of interdependence to become more and more significant in the field of health care.

Interdependence among professionals is a concept directly related to the quality of care. In the sense that a patient requires services from several differentiated, health-related professionals—for example, physician, surgeon, nurse, and social worker—the professionals are interdependent, each influencing and being influenced by the others. They may work in collaboration as professional equals or in a tightly structured team when concerted effort under designated leadership is needed. In either case there is interdependence, although the *balance* and areas of dependence and independence will differ. How these varieties of interdependence operate and affect the patient's family hinges on a variety of factors. Among these are the locus of action (the patient's home, the emergency service, the intensive care unit, a "regular" floor for medical care), the composition of the caring-group, what the professionals expect of one another, and how each will time his or her entry into the patient's situation.

Interdependence applies also to a range of institutions and systems of human services related to, or integral parts of, programs that provide health care. Application of the concept *should* result in more continuous and comprehensive care. It does not at present, because inter alia, programs in the field of health care are uncoordinated, there are vast gaps in available services, and the multiple systems of payments for care exert a capricious influence. Evidence of such influence exists in many communities whose facilities for health care accommodate their functions and policies to the most convenient financial arrangements offered by governmental agencies rather than to the current and predictable needs of consumers of health care.

Biopsychosocial integrity contains the idea of the wholeness, oneness, and indivisibility of every human being. The biological, psychological, and social elements exert influences upon one another which are made manifest in the person's state of being and ability to function as a social human being. This concept is, in fact, a special case of the interdependence of the parts within a system.

The equilibrium achieved by the three interacting elements differs widely among human beings in accordance with (1) differences in personal equipment, for example, intellectual capacity and biological endowment, (2) the person's developmental stage in the life cycle, and (3) the sociocultural circumstances which shape the way in which he or she lives. For example, intellectual capacity plays a part in how and when an infant masters the tasks of the first year of life; but lack of loving attention or the absence of essential foods in his or her diet may irreversibly impair both his or her intellectual and physical development and thus reduce his or her ability to function socially.

In more general terms, phenomena such as poverty, malnutrition, hunger, and too little contact with warm and giving human beings are high risk factors in the biological, intellectual, and social development of the very young everywhere.

At a different stage of life—adolescence—the bodily changes that normally take place create emotional and attitudinal upheavals and conflicts in the young person that may lead to marked behavioral changes, for example, in relationships with parents and other persons in authority; in sexual behavior, especially toward those of the opposite sex; in loss of interest in school achievement; and in a worried search for the resolution of conflict and for the integration of new and strange impulses and a new body image into a new, more stable identity.

Among the aging, too, similar phenomena occur. Grave physiological changes in the person's vascular system may affect judgment and memory and thus bring about changes in personal and family relationships, in self-image, and in the ability to be self-determining.

The phenomenon of biopsychosocial integrity is universal, but it has special importance in the field of health care. The many threats to a person's usual balance of biological, psychological, and social elements that occur in situations of life-and-illness need to be identified, and their consequences estimated, so that the social worker can determine whether and how to intervene. Biological disorder does not exist in isolation; it may impair or completely interrupt the patient's pattern of carrying out his or her responsibilities, that is, his or her social functioning. The nature of the illness and recommended treatment can precipitate emotional and attitudinal reactions ranging from fear and discouragement to hope and a fighting spirit. The patient's intellectual processes may be sharpened by the challenge to overcome obstacles or be immobilized by despair. The social worker knows that a patient's biopsychosocial equilibrium is particularly labile during the course of an illness which is marked by special threats to survival, by the need for critical decision making, by moments of great uncertainty, and the like.

The concept holds as well for the patient's relatives and other significant people in his or her natural environment, and, finally, it holds for the people engaged in giving the patient medical care. The patient's relatives may react acutely—with worry and fear, guilt and anger, and perhaps panic—to risks to the patient's life, to the financial costs of medical care, or to loss of the patient's income, among the many possible consequences of illness. The relatives may find it difficult to carry out their usual responsibilities at home or to be normally productive at work. Loss of sleep and appetite may affect their physical well-being. They may become too upset emotionally to think clearly so that their ability to make sound judgments in their own or the patient's behalf is severely impaired.

Lastly there is the applicability of the concept to individual practitioners in the health care field. Inherent in the responsibilities they carry is their obligation to keep themselves optimally intact (that is, to maintain biopsychosocial integrity at a high level) in the interests of competent performance and ethical behavior. They are constantly exposed to events and conditions that may have deep and far-reaching impacts on them as human beings and therefore on their professional behavior. Givers-of-service can be vulnerable, for example, to economic pressures; to strains and stresses in family relations; to biases and prejudices in respect to race, creed, and social status; or to fear of failure. They are motivated by desires to help, to heal, and to save, and they do not always succeed. They are capable of compassion, sympathy, and identification with people in distress, and therefore also capable of feeling overwhelmed.

Practitioners in the health care field become socialized into their respective professions, adopting and adapting to objectives, values, attitudes, and conduct which have acquired the status of acceptable and desirable standards. The ability to maintain those standards can be impaired when the practitioner becomes hard-pressed to resolve serious problems in his or her personal life or to handle equally grave professional problems which may primarily concern decisions of a technical nature, or the management and resolution of ethical and moral dilemmas, or the handling of psychosocial problems in a patient/family's life-and-illness situation.

Social workers, who are among those practitioners most vulnerable to such stress-producing factors, find it essential to be constantly alert to signs of disequilibrium in their usual balance of biopsychosocial integrity and to take full responsibility for restoring their equilibrium as rapidly as possible. Interprofessional consultation is a process that is very helpful in the restoration of a practitioner's inner balance.*

The individual family: an organic unit is intended to convey, first, the idea that the individual family member and the family unit to which he or she belongs are perpetually in a dynamic relationship and are perceived and understood as constituting a whole, and, second, the idea that the family, the basic social unit of our society, has characteristics and functions that are influenced from within by its individual members and from without by the institutions and systems organized and developed by the society in which the family exists. Interdependence is again a key: interdependence among family members, interdependence between each family member and the family unit, and interdependence between a family unit and society.

While this concept is understood in part through knowledge acquired by the social and behavioral sciences, a fuller significance lies within the context of social work practice. A good first statement is that stereotypes about the family are to be avoided: in our heterogeneous society many variations occur in accord with cultural and socioenvironmental forces and many changes take place during the life cycle of a family unit as its members live through developmental stages which call for modifications in behavior and personal relationships.[16]

Who constitutes a family varies so widely in this era that one can make few assumptions. The nuclear family of husband-father, wife-mother, and their children is still the expected structure, but there are large numbers of families composed of one parent with children. How these families function differs if the one parent is divorced, separated, widowed, or single; if the parent is a man or a woman; if the children are natural offspring or adopted; if the parent chose to be single or considers himself or herself to have been deserted by a legal or nonlegal partner.

---

* See the case history of Mrs. Riviera in Chapter 3, pp. 63–65.

There are other variations which the social worker has to understand and sometimes work with. There is the family of peers which some adolescents and young adults establish for communal living apart from their natural families, though not always alienated from them. Some minor children have lived all or most of their lives with substitute families or in institutions, and they have to be understood against their exceptional backgrounds. Adults, and in particular the very old, may have few or no connections left with persons related by blood or marriage but may have established their own families with self-selected "significant others." These people take the place of family members who are deceased or too distant geographically to be accessible or who are personally incompatible. It is of major importance to ascertain who stands for "family" in the eyes of the client or patient and what the relationships promise in the way of caring and helping.

It is important also to know and assess the memories a patient, who is the lone survivor of his or her kinship groups, has of his or her deceased relatives. Some patients find those memories strongly sustaining; for other patients the memories reactivate mourning and an acute sense of loss. A working principle for social workers is that the life experience flows from one developmental stage to another so that there is influence from the past in every present phase of an individual's life cycle.

Much has been said recently about the separation of the nuclear family in urban areas from its extended kinship groups, both horizontal and vertical. The social worker takes pains to obtain the facts about persons who appear at first to be isolated. At times there is a kinship group that can be counted on, or an individual member of a kinship group stands out as a natural resource in times of trouble. These connections are veritable life savers, especially for young families and the aging.

Customary patterns of individual/family behavior and relationships are susceptible to change when stress-producing factors are in operation. Will the change be in the direction of strengthening mutually supportive behavior or weakening it? How will the wage earner's loss of job affect him or her and the structure and functioning of the family unit? Specific questions such as these can be multiplied ad infinitum. All of them testify to the understanding that change in one element of the individual/family will produce change in other elements and in the family unit. This understanding obliges the social worker to weigh the probable consequences of his or her professional interventions which are intended to promote the greatest good for each family member and for the family as a whole, but whose ripple effects might be stressful for the family group or some of its individual members.

The interactions between individual/family and society's established institutions and systems are of great importance. Certain of the latter, such as systems of education, income maintenance, health care, and criminal justice, which set mandatory standards for the safety, protection, and health of children, have diminished what once were the near-absolute rights of parents over their children. How adequately does a given family act in accordance with mandated standards? If it does not, why? What will be the consequences? If a family does not so act (in regard, say, to children's immunization or attendance in school), can they be helped to do so? By what means? And with what consequences?

Some social resources are so hedged by restrictive regulations and are so scarce that they are available to relatively few eligible persons. For instance, what happens to a given family and to the working mother who heads it when there is no day-care center available at a price she can pay? What are the consequences when a center is available?

The foregoing comments and questions show something of the impact of institutions and systems on individual/families. There is less to be said for the influence wielded by the consumer of services upon institutions and systems, but the public is becoming educated about its rights to service and to protest and demand; voluntary organizations of consumers are showing both social and political strength; and the participation of consumer groups in establishing and improving community resources has, for some programs, become a legal requirement. In time, interdependence of individual/family and society should connote a more balanced state of interaction than now exists.

In the field of health care one may translate individual/family into patient/family and consider the relevance of the concept to situations of life-and-illness. The professional social worker has to determine what the significant stress-producing factors are and how they affect the patient, the other family members, and the family unit. He or she must determine what the nurturing and sustaining strengths of the family members and of the family group are and how they can be maintained, restored, or enhanced; and what their deficiencies are and how they can be minimized, neutralized, or compensated for. The social worker's understanding of patient/family includes an important principle: at any given time the patient may be the central figure, but his or her survival, recovery, and rehabilitation cannot be achieved at the expense of the others in the family, nor can their interests be protected at the expense of the patient's welfare. The more delicate the balance between the patient's needs and gratifications and those of other family members, the more effort is needed to maintain, improve, or restore the equilibrium of family members and of the family as a group.

The role of giver of health care carries within it the seeds of both hazard and support. The giver, too, is the product of experience within a family or surrogate family and is potentially able to perceive, understand, and respond helpfully to the varied ways in which patients and other family members feel and behave. In actuality, the giver's own experience with his or her family of origin or nuclear family may make it difficult for him or her to understand what is going on in a family different from his or hers in socioeconomic status, in ethnic and cultural customs and habits, in religious beliefs, or in political conviction, to indicate some of the variables in day-by-day living. Problems in perceiving and understanding differences may spring from problems of differing values and evaluation; a giver-of-service may look upon differences as wrong or inadequate unless he or she exercises self-scrutiny and self-discipline.

Evidences of the relevance of the concept to physicians and surgeons lies in the precept that they not take responsibility for the diagnosis and treatment of major illness in their own families. Adherence to this precept relieves the practitioner of a too heavy responsibility by recognizing that his or her judgment may be clouded and skills impaired by the emotional stress resulting from the patient's condition and his or her fear and desire for the patient's safety.

The potential for growth and adaptation [17, 18, 19] refers to the latent capacity of an individual to develop biologically and psychologically, to make social adaptations to the conditions under which he lives, and to create change in his situation when that is desirable. The sequence of biological and psychological

stages of growth makes possible the individual's increasingly mature psychosocial adaptations. Throughout the life cycle the individual is expected to meet the
demands of changing and multiple social roles and relationships and the
demands of his or her social milieu.

It has long been accepted by social workers that nature and nurture are
components in life which play upon each other in a circular process. At the same
time, there is a continuous debate in the scientific community about how to
differentiate those traits and characteristics that derive from the intrinsic nature
of the individual and those that reflect the influence of a nourishing or depriving
environment. While the geneticists and other scientists pursue their studies of
man's biopsychological nature, there is every reason to continue efforts to
improve the external forces, conditions, and institutions which are believed to
be significant factors in sustaining, nourishing, or impairing the individual's
natural ability to grow and adapt.

It is a major professional concern of the social worker that the external
conditions, that is, the environments in which people live, afford opportunities
that facilitate growth and adaptation and keep to a minimum the deprivations
which tend to block or retard people's progress toward self-realization.

Environment, then, as the social worker sees it, includes people who are
"others" to an individual, physical surroundings, socioeconomic conditions, and
institutions and systems under governmental and voluntary auspices.

One important characteristic of the environment is its variability among
individuals, families, cultures, and subcultures. Environment at its best offers
opportunities that afford nurture, protection, and invigoration suited to the
individual's changing biological and psychological status and changing social
roles and relationships—physical protection from natural and man-made threats
to survival; intellectual stimulation and sustenance; a heritage of values, beliefs,
and models of behavior; incentives for developing social relationships; and
favorable stimulation for assuming responsibilities in and deriving satisfactions
from new social roles. Stimuli that create manageable conditions of tension or
stress spur the individual onward.

There will always be depriving aspects in an environment in that opportunities may be withheld or delayed, may be quantitatively or qualitatively
inadequate, or may be unavailable—sometimes by the design of others and
sometimes by uncontrolled or uncontrollable accident. The occurrence of
privation is not always hazardous: among the factors that will determine the
individual's response to privation and its meaning are what the privation is, at
what age it occurred, how long it occurred, how healthy the individual's growth
and adaptation were prior to the state of privation, and, most important, how
privation was and is balanced by available opportunities. Some privations may
cause regressive reactions or irreversibly impair advancement toward maturity.
Others may be so timed, spaced, and limited that the individual can successfully
handle them by mastery, healthy defensive action, compensatory gratifications,
and the like; these depriving situations are thus converted into opportunities for
self-development.

Privation results not only from the absence of opportunity but also from
actions, events, and conditions that directly impose injury. Inadequate or
insufficient diet, chemical poisons, physical abuse, and disease processes result
often in irreversible damage to the body. Distressing emotional effects and
changes in social behavior may often follow biological injury.

Conversely, the immediate impact of privation may be psychological and social, but biological consequences may follow. The prolonged institutionalization of infants and children is a case in point. Inherent in these situations is the presence of too many different caretakers and excessive and prolonged periods of anxiety induced by delays in being picked up, cared for, and caressed. Infants are known to die under such depriving psychosocial conditions, and young children fail to thrive when they do not have close, trusting, and uninterrupted human relationships. They must have adequate nurturing and stimulation.

There is no secret about the similarly harsh privations that befall adults in our pockets of poverty and that are suffered by our untreated addicts, the delinquents and criminals in our society who are punished but not rehabilitated, and the neglected and helpless aged.

RELEVANCE OF THE CONCEPT TO HEALTH CARE

A very considerable volume of social work practice which takes place in social agencies and in health and health-related facilities has been for decades and continues to be directed toward improving the status of social-health.*

Social workers in the field of health offer direct services to reduce or eliminate environmental conditions injurious to human growth and adaptation, to make available rehabilitative services which will help people adapt to their changed situations, and to enable persons to use their inner strengths and community resources to overcome obstacles to growth and adaptation.

Social workers also contribute to improving the environment of the general public and special populations by means of indirect and instrumental services such as influencing legislation, encouraging and collaborating in research, and participating in the formulation of policy. More specifically, these efforts are directed toward correcting conditions such as poverty, inadequate housing, inaccessibility and unavailability of health care, and deficiencies in educational programs for children and adults.

Stress in human beings has numerous meanings—some colloquial, some technical—which are connected with the arts, with the physical sciences, and with the physiology and psychology of human beings. Within the context of social work practice, "(1) stress is equated with the stressful event or situation; (2) it is used to refer to the state of the individual who responds to the stressful event . . . ; (3) more often, stress refers to the relation of the stressful stimulus, the individual's reaction to it, and the events to which it leads."[20]

The second meaning will be used here with the understanding that stress is a dynamic state of psychological tension which arises when human beings face a demand for psychosocial adaptation. (The issue of physiological stress and adaptation in the human body is outside the professional experience and competence of social workers.) There are constant sources of stress in everyday life, because problems have to be solved, decisions made, conflicts resolved, frustrations tolerated, and relationships dealt with. There are also the adaptive tasks required by developmental and maturational stages in the life cycle and those that accompany unusual changes in social role.

* Social-health refers to the state of being that results from the interactions among socioenvironmental, psychological, emotional, and biological components in the life of human beings. The aggregate of these interactions is manifested in the social functioning of individuals, families, small groups, and populations.

If stress is thus considered as a normal and natural component in human life, the term is value free, and thus neither "good" nor "bad"; it signals a change or the threat of change and the need to adapt to change. Stress acquires value— for example, is benign, stimulating, or destructive—according to the perception of the person who experiences it. The perception is formed by the interactions of the person's native endowment and capacity with his or her life experience immediately preceding and concurrent with the stressful event or events, with the demands and supports currently in his or her cultural and socioeconomic environment and with the gratifications and deprivations derived from his or her personal relations. When stress is perceived as benign, it may stimulate mastery, learning, and creativeness. When perceived as harmful, it may lead to maladaptive acts of capitulation and a collapse in social functioning. Stress, then, may serve as an integrative or disintegrating force. "No one can live without experiencing some degree of stress all the time. . . . Stress is not even necessarily bad for you; it is also the spice of life, for any emotion, any activity causes stress. But, of course, your system must be prepared to take it. The same stress which makes one person sick can be an invigorating experience for another." [21]

Sources of stress are many. Stressful events may be large-scale disasters or one individual's personal loss. A most potent source from either kind of event is disruption of an individual's social frame of reference, especially those changes that deprive a person of basic emotional and intellectual gratification or reduce his or her sense of self-worth.

Events that signify great or unexpected improvement or good fortune in a person's life also cause stress and demand adaptation in values, feelings, attitudes, and patterns of behavior.

Finally, human beings have an unequaled ability to relate to symbols, that is, to representations as opposed to realities; thus they remember past experience and can also imagine or anticipate future events. An event, a person, or a situation may serve as a strong reminder of past stress-producing experiences or as indicators of future happenings; these phenomena may be stressful just as if the representations were in reality the events they symbolize.

Stress is manageable when the tension takes on the feel of challenge or excitement or just enough anxiety to spur people on. Their emotional reactions are not upsetting, and they can draw rationally on previous experience, knowledge, and tested skills to solve a problem. Altogether, they retain their image of themselves, their belief in their ability, and their place in a give-and-take relationship with others. The total situation as they perceive it is without danger to their integrity, and they can maneuver and master within their usual patterns of adaptation.

Unmanageable stress refers to that state of inner tension that occurs "only if a person lacks the capacity to cope with or master the event" [22] that produces such severe stress. In effect, unmanageable stress is what many call a state of crisis. The manifestations are emotional reactions that are extreme and upsetting; impaired thinking and judgment or confusion in the realm of cognitive functions; behavior such as agitated movements, inability to concentrate or perform usual tasks; and, at times, an appearance of disintegration, or of "going to pieces." [23]

Variability in adaptive capacity is shown by people who face similar demands to adapt but who differ widely in their ability to reduce states of stress and make appropriate social adaptations to the stress-producing event. The interactions of such variables as personal endowment, life experiences, demands and supports, and gratifications and deprivations are major determinants of the human capacity to deal with stress and stressful events. In addition, there are features in the occurrence of stress that exert a powerful influence on a person's ability to cope. They may keep stress manageable or bring a person to the breaking point of his or her tolerance for stress, for every human being has a limit of endurance.

Not the occurrence of stress per se but its cumulative impact, its timing and spacing, and its relation to the conditions of everyday life determine its significance and tolerableness. The meaning of stress is subjectively determined; no matter what the observer thinks it *should* signify, he or she must be guided in understanding it by the effect on the person under stress. The mastery of stressful events and the successful resolution of states of crisis tend to promote growth even when the processes involved have their painful aspects. In contrast, stress that is not strong enough to stimulate retards striving and growth.[24]

THE CONCEPT OF STRESS IN HEALTH CARE

The concept of stress in health care will be considered in relation to patients/families and their significant others, to the givers of care and the institutions and systems in which they work, and to the public which is composed of past, current, and potential consumers.

The Patient/Family

The occurrence of disease, injury, and disability inevitably makes demands for psychosocial adaptation and the resolution of states of crisis. The conditions that produce stress "create psychological strain on the adaptive capacity of the ego; first, through the threats that the [conditions] offer to the security and integrity of the person; second, through the impact upon the body image; and, third, through pain."[25] These are useful generalizations which the professional social worker must translate into specifics. The social worker must estimate specific consequences of stress and weigh them against the patient/family's capacity to cope with or without extra psychological supports and concrete social services available in the community.

The many and varied potential sources of stress that concern the patient who is the central figure in the life-and-illness situation have direct impact also on the other family members and on the structure and functioning of the family unit. The others, too, have to learn to live with and accommodate to conditions such as changes in the patient's body and bodily functioning, to the patient's decreased or loss of earning capacity, and to the patient's impaired ability to share household responsibilities. In fact, structural changes in the family unit may be necessitated by the consequences of the patient's illness. The social worker may indeed have the entire patient/family as his or her client.

SIGNIFICANT OTHERS

Persons such as the patient's close friends, minister, and employer are also vulnerable to stress-producing elements in the patient/family's situation in accordance with their own distinctive social values and attitudes. Some can be depended on for support and encouragement; others may drop away and thus add to the patient's sense of loss, weakened psychosocial integrity, and decreased self-regard. For example, while reemployment of the patient in his or her former place of business may be entirely unfeasible, in one organization management will collaborate with the social worker's efforts to help the patient become self-maintaining once again, while in another organization management may refuse to be involved beyond the bare minimum required by law.

RESOLUTION OF STRESS

Social workers with responsibility for giving direct service, regardless of field or setting, identify and build on the inner strengths and capabilities of the people they are helping. It is a major strategy in the social worker's efforts to facilitate another's problem solving, mastery of stressful events, and resolution of inner tension. People cannot effectively use supports and concrete services from outside sources unless they have at least a modicum of inner strength that can be mobilized. Hope, in the sense of realistic desire accompanied by an expectation of fulfillment, has a powerful influence on a patient/family's ability to cope with stress-producing factors in disease and disability. Hope may be for far less than cure. One patient's hope may be to live long enough to put his or her affairs in order; another's, that his or her physician will keep him or her as free from pain as possible.

For many persons faith is a personal attribute that serves the same purpose as hope and in fact reinforces it. To have faith is to have confidence in the trustworthiness of someone, something, or some situation; it is to believe even when there is no certain proof. Whether faith is religious or philosophical, whether it is trust in an individual giver-of-service or in a single institution, faith is an internal source of strength for coping with stressful factors in illness or disability. Strength derives also from the memory of past experiences when stress-producing events were overcome or endured.

Generally speaking, an individual's system of defense mechanisms is the strongest bulwark against overwhelming anxiety which might be aroused by dangers breaking through from within the human psyche and from the world outside as well. Defense mechanisms are essential to the successful integration and optimum social functioning of each human being. Under great stress some of an individual's mechanisms may break down, loosing a flood of anxiety which impairs the ability to function; in other instances of unusual stress and strain, certain defenses may tighten and strengthen in ways that help the individual to survive biologically, psychologically, and socially, but which under unfortunate circumstances may threaten survival.

Social workers have a special concern for the way in which patients and their relatives may use the mechanism of denial—by means of which painful realities are actually repressed—or the psychological protection of denying, which is a conscious way of easing or making tolerable an otherwise highly stressful experience.* [26, 27] Professional personnel in the health field may be experienced and competent in recognizing a patient/family's unusually strong protections and defenses which might impair their ability to decide upon or follow through on medical recommendations.

However, from the standpoint of professional education and training it

---

* Technically speaking, mechanisms of defense are developed and used unconsciously. Consciously, people may deny in the sense of disregarding, pretending, or fabricating.

may be only the psychiatrist who can determine (1) whether the patient/family's behavior, feelings, and attitudes are governed more unconsciously than consciously; (2) whether it will be psychologically therapeutic to help an individual strengthen a defense mechanism; (3) whether it will be psychologically safe to help weaken a defense; or (4) whether the individual should be left free of the influence of another human being to change his or her opinion and actions. These questions illustrate well how professional obligation and competence may confront the adult patient/family's right to self-determination, based on the patient/family's capacity to accept and deal with all or some aspects of the real situation. A person has a right to know and a right and need to hope; sometimes one right seems to contradict the other, and the individual may choose to know just as little as possible in order to sustain maximum hope.

THE GIVERS OF CARE

Stress experienced by the givers of health care can be a crucial factor in relations among staff members in an institution, in judgments and decisions made by medical and medically related personnel for the care of sick people, and in the relationships developed and promoted among personnel, patients, their family members, and populations in the community. Givers-of-service working in their various capacities are human beings first, each one liable to the impact of stress created by life-tasks, professional functions, environmental conditions, personal relationships, his or her own bodily distress, and other events and conditions that require adaptation within and beyond the usual day-by-day demands.

The giver of health care, regardless of profession or vocation, retains the ethical obligation to give the best service he or she can regardless of stressful events the practitioner may be experiencing. This situation identifies a task that confronts every giver-of-service: how to resolve the conflict between gratifying his or her personal needs and gratifying the needs of those he or she is pledged to serve, without damage to himself or herself or to the others. The required suspension or suppression of the practitioner's own needs has to take place without stifling his or her capacity for empathy and compassion. Having to care for and give support to a patient one can no longer hope to cure or perhaps save and coping with reawakened personal conflicts and feeling aroused by events in the life of a patient are two of the professional demands for adaptation to which physicians, surgeons, and related professional colleagues may react with feelings of severe stress which somehow must be kept within manageable bounds.

Givers-of-service also come into direct working relationships with colleagues in their own and different professions or disciplines and with many persons whose services on a technical or vocational plane are vital to health care. In situations which call for collaboration, such as consultation, administration of a program, or planning a new service, stress-producing problems do arise. Diversity in, and misunderstanding of, goals, concerns, and motivation; unreal expectations of one's self and of the others; unaccepted differences in competence and status; vested interests that clash and surface as biases or prejudices—these and other phenomena may retard achievement in collaborative performance.

Nonprofessional skilled and unskilled employees in the field of health care have stressful events to cope with too, such as unpleasant and frightening sights, sounds, and smells, the signs of pain and suffering, patient's complaints and demands, and tension in their relations with professional personnel. How they adapt to these conditions is a strong determinant of the quality of patient care.

There has been for decades a corps of dedicated volunteer workers in medical facilities who are also givers-of-service and whose vulnerability to stress-producing events must not be overlooked.

The Public

Consumerism has spread a wide umbrella, and health care is not the least of its concerns. The movement is supported by many volunteer organizations of individual consumers, some with powerful leadership, as well as by legislation which mandates advisory or decision-making committees on which the consumer-public is represented. When people who represent consumers meet with members of several professions and health-related disciplines and perhaps, of various vocations, it takes time, effort, and strong motivations to work out a modus operandi. Consumers and givers-of-service have to establish their respective boundaries in the decision-making process; they differ widely in knowledge and in skills, values, and attitudes and consequently will differ in the responsibility and authority they can assume. A complicating problem is the tendency of consumers of medical care to have higher expectations of physicians, medical science, and medical and medically related knowledge and practice than can currently be realized. There is also always the possibility that professional practitioners in health care underestimate the information and comprehension possessed by some lay consumers. Differences in socioeconomic class and in modes of living require mutual understanding of aspects of life such as education, professionalism, financial status, family roles and relationships, religion and morality, politics and government, and health and disease.

Accommodation to such differences does not imply achieving complete agreement; ours is a heterogeneous society, and its diversity demands recognition as a useful, even essential, component in a democratic society striving for social justice. Accommodation to keep tensions at a manageable level and stimulate problem solving may take such forms as reduction of bias by correcting misinformation and misunderstanding; learning that "different" is not synonymous with "bad"; and developing new roles and relationships with people of diverse backgrounds and new ways of thinking, feeling, and behaving to effect change in health care systems.

COMMUNICATION

Communication is a continuous form of interaction essential to the survival and development of human beings. It can be defined as "a process by which meanings are exchanged between individuals through a common system of symbols," [28] but symbols must be understood broadly to include a wide variety of signals. Less of a definition, but more descriptive and vivid, is the following statement: "No communication is, after all, nothing, emptiness, not having lived. . . . Communicating is struggling against mental decline and oblivion. It is the awareness of being an entity, an 'I,' an 'Ego.' . . ." [29] The implication is that communication is a two-way process: unless a message that is sent out or expressed is received, perceived, and responded to by a recipient, there is no communication.

Communication may be successful in that all the parties concerned have mutually conveyed and responded to their respective messages with mutual satisfaction. On the other hand, communication may be a partial or total failure because the sender's message is an incomplete or inadequate expression of his or her meaning, or because the recipient of the message has what Meerloo calls a "faulty antenna" and therefore responds to a message that was never sent, though it may have been the one the recipient heard.

Vehicles for communication are many and varied; they fall into categories that all human beings use as conveyors of messages and that persons engaged in giving human services must understand and interpret in order to carry out their responsibilities.

Verbal language—the use of words in speech and hearing, and in writing and reading—is the vehicle that seems to be the distinguishing mode of communication among humans. (The more one hears about the great apes learning to communicate, the more cautious one becomes in pronouncements of our uniqueness.)

A few important nonverbal vehicles common to human beings are the voluntary and involuntary signals of the human body, art forms, modes of self-expression such as choice of clothing and home furnishings and the quality of personal grooming, individual style in the performance of daily tasks, and the vehicle of silence. At the most specific level, communication takes place nonverbally through such phenomena as states of muscular tension, tone of voice, blushing, coughing, kempt or unkempt appearance, and the comfortable or the screaming silence.

Characteristics of communication, as defined above, range from its imperfect nature, its varied aims and intents, and its multiple levels and vehicles of expression to its possible ambiguities and inconsistencies. If these characteristics sound more negative than positive, that judgment derives more from the complexity of human beings and their behavior than from an innate deviousness.

The social worker who has not learned to check his or her intuitive understanding of another's messages against some corrective observations is lost. People who use the same verbal language may misread one another out of hostility. People who have no verbal language in common may understand one another's body language well. It is also necessary to recognize that messages can be sent by one party with such different intents as to clarify or to obscure, to present truth or to deceive, and to wield power or to be entrapped by it.

The inner consistency or inconsistency of the messages conveyed is a most important measuring stick of the meaning of messages and goes far in determining how to respond. Is the voice harsh while the hands tremble? Do the lips smile while the eyes glower? Or does the warm tone give credence to the words of compassion?

Facilitators and deterrents which commonly occur in the process of communicating need to be identified. Reasonably successful communication occurs when there is desire for mutual exchange and understanding, some concern or interest in common, shared values or beliefs, and some way of signaling that can be read accurately enough by the principals involved, especially when these facilitating conditions are strengthened by some capacity to be empathic and intuitive. These broad terms allow for the use of nonverbal tools for communicating feelings, attitudes, and moods when mutually understood verbal tools are lacking or call for reinforcement.

Because communication is essential to the life of human beings but is often imperfect or difficult to achieve, the more usual barriers to successful communication will be identified. In our heterogeneous society, not all people possess the same formal verbal language, regional speech patterns vary, street languages develop, and the vernacular of adolescents may be unintelligible to the contemporary adults.

Communication can be made difficult when cultural differences—for example, in family relationships or moral and religious beliefs—induce fear or dislike rather than a human desire to remove barriers.

Socioeconomic factors that deprive people of access to information, such as lack of educational opportunities and poverty, are impediments to communication. So too are sensory and other bodily deficiencies; technical inventions and special educational methods may exist to compensate for deficits but in our flawed system of social justice are often not available to those who need them.

Although there are people who purposefully create barriers to communication, many are frustrated by their inability. They may become angry and retaliative or, in defeat, withdraw from the struggle.

Communication in health care is a basic process exercised by the human chain charged with responsibilities for the delivery of health care.[30] The interdependence of consumers and givers of health care services leads to a constant flow of interacting behaviors, one of which, as might be expected, is communication. Givers-of-service, including professionals from many fields as well as technicians and paraprofessionals, may be concerned with planning, organizing, and administering programs of health care at various governmental and institutional levels and for many different populations at risk. Work of this nature now more and more requires that all principals have a voice in determinng what services are provided; where, when, how, for whom, and by whom they are provided; and how they will be paid for. The increasing numbers of collaborators, the conflicts of vested interests, and the range of sociocultural backgrounds of the participants make the process of communicating more arduous. The more heterogeneous the group, the harder it is for the individuals to identify common concerns and aims, to listen to and to hear one another, to strip away the stereotyped images and expectations, and to assume the role of colleague when one has been either leader or led.

There is a parallel demand for communication among givers-of-service and individual patients and their family members better suited to the changes in our social and professional environments. As health care has become more and more a public concern and more and more is considered a right, as the scope of services expands, and as scientific research and its findings appear daily in the mass media, people respond to the messages they hear. They expect more, question more, and want to know and understand more. Developments in knowledge and skill have, among other things, resulted in more specialties and specialists who then have to communicate constantly in order to keep reasonably current in one another's specialties and, at another level of work, in order to collaborate in the care of patients they have in common.

At this latter level, communicating by way of verbal and nonverbal symbols is an intrinsic part of the working relationship between patient/family and givers-of-service. The variables that influence how the messages go back and forth resemble those described for human beings in general, but they have special import when one party's status of social-health is at stake and the other party has an obligation to be caring and helpful. Not only do many patients nationwide talk and understand a foreign language more readily than they do English, but among the givers-of-service too are many who are not fluent in English. For some people the absence of easy verbal communication is not an unsuperable problem. For many patients the "feel" of the provider's interest, concern, gentleness, unhurried attention, and competence will compensate to a degree for verbal difficulties. But errors in diagnosis or in carrying out medical recommendations may occur when facts cannot be transmitted as accurately as feelings can by nonverbal signals. The risks and the advantages in the use of interpreters are matters for careful consideration.*

It is implicit in the role of giver-of-service that he or she bears the burden of promoting and facilitating communication with the patient/family. This affirmation does not cancel the obligation the patient/family has to carry a portion of the responsibility if they are seeking or using health care services. However, the patient and his or her relatives have the options other human beings have to withhold information (e.g., when they are afraid to learn what the symptoms mean) or to act against medical recommendations (e.g., to signal preference for a satisfying but shortened lifespan over a longer but unfulfilling existence).

Messages conveyed by givers-of-service to patients/families will be most meaningful when the messages are timed to be helpful to the persons who have to cope with stressful aspects of their life-and-illness situations, when they are responsive to the emotional reactions and attitudes of patients and their relatives, when they are couched in language suitable to the patients/families' conditions of life—in other words, when the messages have some immediately useful implications.

At the level of practical activity, social workers have learned that stereotyped ideas or biases they may have about people from cultures other than their own may result in failed communication with patients/families: a so-called uncooperative, noncompliant patient may be resisting a medical procedure or recommendation that is totally at variance with his or her customary way of life.

A giver-of-service must always be alert to the intent of the patient/family's messages. Are they signaling "don't tell me" or "don't ask me" or transmitting some other revealing instruction? Do the givers-of-service adequately assess how a patient reacts to their use of technical termimology among themselves as though there were a detached organ in the bed rather than a human organism? This kind of situation, for which the giver-of-service is solely responsible, may result in dangerously imperfect communication between the consumer and the giver of health care services.

In the current era of many specialties and subspecialties and of growing concern for a humanistic perspective on health care, there is a commensurate demand for inter- and intraprofessional collaboration in direct service.[31] It is a demand that must be met in part by ever-improving communication. This in turn calls for identification of compatible goals with and for a given patient/family, small group, or population; mutual respect for one another's expertness; and some values and attitudes in common which will inform their respective points of view about people, health and disease, and the delivery of services.

---

* For discussion of this problem, see p. 56–57.

In sum, communiction is a process indispensable to human life in general and to the health and social welfare of human beings in particular. It is the medium by which needs and wants are made known and help, caring, and curing are proffered.

REFERENCES

1. "[Social Work] values are—or should be—beyond intuition and amenable to socialization processes of social work education and supervision." Charles S. Levy, "The Value Base of Social Work," *Journal of Education for Social Work*, vol. 9, no.1 (winter 1973).
2. *Code of Ethics*, National Association of Social Workers Policy Statements 1 (Washington, D. C., as amended, 1967).
3. Alan Keith-Lucas, "Ethics in Social Work," in *Encyclopedia of Social Work*, 17th ed. (Washington, D.C.: National Association of Social Workers, 1977), pp. 350-356.
4. Charles Frankel, "Social Values and Professional Values," *Journal of Education for Social Work*, vol. 5, no.1 (spring 1969).
5. Lela B. Costin et al., "Barriers to Social Justice," in *Social Work Practice and Social Justice*, ed. Bernard Ross and Charles Shireman (Washington, D.C.: National Association of Social Workers, 1973), p. 1.
6. *A Patient's Bill of Rights* (Chicago: American Hospital Association, 1972).
7. Ruth I. Knee, "Health Care: Patients' Rights," in *Encyclopedia of Social Work*, op. cit., pp. 541-544.
8. Herbert H. Aptekar, "American Social Values and Their Influences on Social Welfare Programs and Professional Social Work," *Journal of Social Work Process*, vol. 16 (1967), p. 20.
9. Bess Dana, "Health, Social Work and Social Justice," in Ross and Shireman, op. cit., p. 111.
10. Ibid., p. 120.
11. Bernard Ross, "Professional Dilemmas," in Ross and Shireman, op. cit., p. 148.
12. Victor R. Fuchs, *Who Shall Live? Health Economics and Social Choice* (New York: Basic Books, 1974).
13. Marvin B. Sussman and Lee Burchinal, "Kin Family Network: Unheralded Structure in Current Conceptualizations of Family Functioning," in *Middle Age and Aging: A Reader in Social Psychology*, ed. Bernice L. Neugarten (Chicago: University of Chicago Press, 1968), p. 247.
14. *Standard College Dictionary* (New York: Funk and Wagnalls, 1968).
15. Samuel W. Bloom, *The Doctor and His Patient* (New York: Russell Sage Foundation, 1963), p. 70.
16. Marvin B. Sussman, "Family," in *Encyclopedia of Social Work*, op. cit., pp. 357-368.
17. Harriet M. Bartlett, *The Common Base of Social Work Practice* (New York: National Association of Social Workers, 1970).
18. Werner M. Boehm, *Objectives of the Social Work Curriculum of the Future*, vol. I, and *The Social Casework Method in Social Work Education*, vol. X (New York: Social Work Curriculum Study, Council on Social Work Education, 1959).
19. Ruth M. Butler, *Social Functioning Framework: An Approach to the Human Behavior and Social Environment Sequence*, (New York: Council on Social Work Education, 1970).
20. Lydia Rapoport, "The State of Crisis: Some Theoretical Considerations," in *Crisis Intervention: Selected Readings*, ed. Howard J. Parad (New York: Family Service Association of America, 1965), p. 23.

21. Hans Selye, *The Stress of Life* (New York: McGraw-Hill, 1956), p. vii.
22. Lydia Rapoport, "Crisis-Oriented Short-Term Casework," *Social Service Review*, vol. 41 (March 1967).
23. Ibid.
24. "Certainly one does not need to demonstrate that unstressful, aseptic conditions in the physical or mental dimensions of living can be catastrophic to the organism." Eli M. Bowe, "The Modification, Mediation and Utilization of Stress During the School Years," *American Journal of Orthopsychiatry*, vol. 34 (July 1964).
25. Charlotte G. Babcock, "Inner Stress in Illness and Disability," in *Ego-Oriented Casework: Problems and Perspectives*, ed. Howard J. Parad and Roger R. Miller (New York: Family Service Association of America, 1963).
26. David M. Kaplan and Edward A. Mason, "Maternal Reactions to Premature Birth Viewed as an Acute Emotional Disorder," in op. cit.
27. Joel Vernick, "The Use of the Life Space Interview on a Medical Ward," in Parad, op.cit.
28. *Webster's Seventh New Collegiate Dictionary*, 1963.
29. Joost A. M. Meerloo, *Conversation and Communication: A Psychological Inquiry into Language and Human Relations*, (New York: International Universities Press, 1952).
30 Barbara S. Hulka et al., "Communication, Compliance, and Concordance Between Physicians and Patients with Prescribed Medications," *American Journal of Public Health*, vol. 66, no. 9 (September 1976), pp. 847-853.
31. Martin Nacman, "A Systems Approach to the Provision of Social Work Services in Health Settings," Part I, *Social Work in Health Care*, vol. 1, no. 1, (fall 1975), pp. 47-53.

Chapter 2
The Practice of Hospital-Based Social Work:

MAJOR FUNCTIONS IN DIRECT SERVICE

A description of the major functions in direct service will be better understood against the background of several key assumptions. They provide a perspective for viewing the field of health care as a whole.

- Provision of adequate health care requires multiprofessional and multidisciplinary personnel, programs, and services which recognize and meet the biopsychosocial needs of individuals, small kinship and nonkinship groups, and populations to further their attainment of maximum social health.
- The programs and services exist within an extended framework of interdependent, multiple systems of care and services which contribute to the well-being of society.
- A working relationship among personnel and between personnel and the consumer-public serves as a dynamic medium for achieving objectives of health care in behalf of individuals, small groups, and populations.
- A goal held in common by professional givers of health care is to enable consumers to obtain maximum benefits from programs and services related to social-health.
- Two tasks shared by givers and consumers of health care are (1) the continual assessment of existing policies, programs, and services at all levels of planning and delivering care and (2) the projection of alterations and innovations that will result in more adequate provision of care.

Within the structure of a health facility, a department of social services has to fulfill its own professional mission and simultaneously be an integral part of the institution.[1] One expects that the full scope of work in a hospital's department of social services includes a range of responsibilities and functions and requires social workers with different kinds and degrees of competence on its social work staff. The size and organization of a department of social services and the areas of competence required of staff members will vary with the purpose, functions, and programs of the facility in which the department exists. In addition to giving direct service, a department may be accountable for administrative responsibilities, participation in research efforts, and contributions to the professional and vocational education of hospital personnel and students at various levels and in various kinds of educational programs. Thus a department of social services has obligations and objectives that influence the deployment of staff, the nature of assignments to staff, the methods employed to achieve its aims, and the department's internal structure and organization. However, certain functions are held in common by social workers who give direct services. These functions elucidate the most distinctive aspect of the social workers' professional practice; in addition, experience in these functions is a source of knowledge for the learning and teaching of students for the health-related professions.

The general purpose of direct social work services is to assist people, singly and in groups, to eliminate, reduce, master, compensate for, or defend against stress-producing factors in life-and-illness situations through the constructive use of internal and external strengths and resources, in order that they may achieve maximum status of social-health.

To fulfill this purpose social workers exercise specific functions, each of which requires a series of planned actions, directed toward goals that are expected to benefit those served and are compatible with the goals of members of other professions serving the same persons. The social worker may exercise more than one function simultaneously with the same person or persons. Or selected functions may be exercised in sequence because one function helps to prepare a patient/family or group to benefit from the second. While the major functions described below form a fundamental core of social work practice in hospitals, they are frequently carried out by a social worker *after* collaborative planning with members of other professions, or are carried out *collaboratively and in concert* with members of other professions.

Actions of these kinds afford some assurance of a cohesive, integrated plan of care which, it is hoped, will result in maximum benefits to consumers and givers-of-services.[2]

DETERMINATION OF THE POINT OF ENTRY

In 1905, when social workers officially entered the health care field, and for several decades to follow, they intervened in a patient/family's situation only upon the request of a physician. This pattern of case finding is no longer considered acceptable, and gradual change is taking place consistent with new ideas about professional authority, responsibility, and accountability that are affecting in particular physicians, nurses, and social workers in the health care field.

More acceptable patterns of case finding for social work services are being built on a wider recognition of professionalism in social work, on a more widespread expectation of collaborative, interprofessional, and interdisciplinary actions, and on more efficient deployment of hospital-based social work staff members. New patterns are needed to facilitate the access of social workers and patients/families to one another as well as to contribute from the social worker's educated perception of social need to collaborative assessment of life-and-illness situations and to effectively coordinate therapeutic and rehabilitative interventions.[3]

In the current period of transition from the original rigid caste-based system of physicians referring patients to social workers, there is a discernible movement forward. Where once the social workers could not initiate contact with a private patient, many hospitals have now opened the door. The step recognizes that the poor are not the only victims of anxiety and fear, strained pocketbooks, misinformation, and stressful family relations. But the most important recognition is that members of more than one profession have to work together with and in behalf of the same person—that the social worker's commitment to collaborative effort is just that and not a mask for a competitive power struggle.*

Where joint efforts are successfully taking place to identify what is needed, when it is needed and who is best qualified to provide the needed help, some interesting things happen which benefit not only an individual patient/family but whole patient populations in the institution. One valuable consequence is that often physicians tend to ask social workers to inquire into apparently problematic situations and recommend solutions; this kind of request is a far cry from an earlier practice that physicians had—and many still have—to "tell" the social worker what the problem is and how to solve it, or to be totally unaware that a social problem exists. There have been and continue to be endless complaints from social workers that they are called in at the last possible moment to make plans for a patient's discharge when there is no time to work out emotional entanglements or practical procedures in the scarce economy of resources. Leaving the hospital is amputated, so to speak, from the mainstream of the patient/family's way of life.

Another encouraging result of collaborative effort is seen in the establishment of intramural policy for the contact of social workers with members of specified patient groups. For example, physicians, nurses, and social workers may agree that social workers have an early exploratory function in regard to such high-risk hospital populations as hospitalized persons over 65 who live alone, unmarried teen-aged pregnant girls, and patients scheduled for laryngectomies or open-heart surgery.

The social worker's first exploratory contact need not be a face-to-face interview—logistics frequently do not permit that in any case—but may be in the form of a screening device such as a questionnaire designed to identify the patients/families who are potentially at high psychosocial risk.

An inescapable conclusion is that determination of the point of a social worker's entry into a life-and-illness situation is currently in need of solid, well-constructed research. How well does a hospital's deployment of social workers meet the needs of patients/families? Are the criteria for the social worker's entry different for patients in ambulatory care and hospitalized patients? What of the assumption that the earlier the contact, the more helpful the social worker is? How are governmental policies and regulations influencing the social worker's point of entry?

---

* This policy is not in force in every hospital. The social worker's contact with private patients is sometimes restricted to those referred by the private physician, by members of the patient's family, or by the patient himself or herself.

EXPLORATION AND ASSESSMENT
OF THE LIFE-SITUATION OF PATIENT/FAMILY

In the several fields in which social workers are employed, exploring and assessing psychosocial situations is a common and basic function.[4] Professional judgment determines how extensive and intensive the exploration must be and what the focus will be to guide the selection of data. The social worker in the health care field will explore and assess the circumstances and forces in the patient/family's life situation which are influencing or will influence the course and outcome of the patient's illness—the elements or characteristics of the illness which are having or will have impact on the life-situation. This kind of circular relation is an expected phenomenon dependent on the constant interaction of the biological, psychological, and socioenvironmental aspects of human life.[5]

The social worker's processes of exploration and assessment are based on the belief that problems are solved by people's exercise of their strengths and resources. Thus while psychosocial problem areas related to illness and disability must be uncovered, the social worker searches for capabilities, helpful motivations, and constructive attitudes possessed by patients and those close to them, and for socioenvironmental conditions and resources that can stimulate and enhance the patient/family's capacity to cope successfully with stress-producing events and circumstances of illness and disability. Personal and familial deficits and deficiencies and foreseeable demands for adaptation to significant changes which will threaten the social functioning of the patient/family must be assessed against the strengths and resources that are or can be made available when people struggle with illness, disability, and their consequences. Although it is the social worker's obligation to give focus and direction to an exploration which he or she undertakes, the competent interviewer does not exercise rigid control; he or she knows that what appears to be a wandering stream of thought may be closely connected with a major relevant theme—or it may be a significant evasion or a protection against a painful revelation.

While exploration and assessment of psychosocial situations is a major function of the social worker, the multi- and interprofessional implications deserve emphasis.[6] What the social worker observes and weighs has practical significance for his or her colleagues in other professions and vocations. And what others observe has relevance for the social worker's understanding of an individual illness situation. Thus the exploration can be multiprofessional or even interprofessional in the making and can form a base for interprofessional collaborative assessment, planning, and interventive action.*

Lest this function be mistakenly considered a one-time action, the likely need for reexploration and reassessment must be emphasized. The need is created for various reasons. The scope of a first exploration may be severely limited when the medicosocial situation is critical and immediate crisis intervention by the social worker is of the essence. Another reason may be important changes in the patient/family's external socioenvironmental conditions, calling for reappraisal of resources. And there are always the expected and unexpected developments in the illness or disability itself which require a fresh examination

---

* In this context, multiprofessional includes not only professional staff but also technicians and members of supporting staff such as orderlies, receptionists, and secretaries.

of the patient/family's current life-situation. The implied consequence of reexploration and reassessment is, of course, replanning of services.

The social worker's sources of information may, in principle, extend beyond the patient/family and hospital personnel. Some of the most useful sources may exist in the patient/family's natural social milieu, and these same persons may become valued participants in supportive, therapeutic, and rehabilitative activities. Teachers, employers, clergymen, or perhaps a landlord or staff members in community social agencies, may fall into the group of concerned, significant others.

Committed as the social worker is to the value-concepts of privacy and confidentiality, he or she is obligated to obtain the patient/family's informed consent before approaching their significant others. But the same values extend to those significant others. They must understand why they are being approached and consent to the social worker's use of the data they will provide.

This issue of ethical conduct is even more complex and difficult to resolve within the hospital setting. What do the rights of privacy and confidentiality mean in an institution where many members of multiprofessional, multidisciplinary, and multivocational staff have access to and a need to use information in patients' charts, records, and laboratory reports? In a given facility what are the policies that govern the use of available data? Who formulated the policies, and how are the actual practices monitored and evaluated? What happens when a staff member receives information from a patient/family that he or she is asked not to divulge to other family members or to other staff members who serve that patient/family?

Values and ethics are so incorporated into professional performance that they usually receive special attention only when they are breached. Because the process of exploration and the subsequent use of the data obtained afford such obvious opportunities to violate people's rights to privacy and confidentiality, knowledge of the hazards and risks is integral to an understanding of the function itself.

ANTICIPATORY AND PREPARATORY ACTIVITY*

Social work practice in hospital-based direct service reveals a large volume of work with patients/families that looks ahead and helps to prepare them to handle expected and probable stress-producing events and conditions of the future. Anticipatory and preparatory work aims to lessen feelings of shock, to cushion a blow, to enable people to plan ahead, and to make people readier to carry a burden or make a difficult decision. A secondary gain is to increase the patient/family's confidence in the social worker as one who knows, understands, and has the strength to face with them the unpleasant and the frightening.

Physicians carry the *initial* responsibility for informing patients/families about stress-producing elements, for example, in diagnostic procedures, in the patient's disease or disability, or in the therapeutic interventions that are available. There has to be a clear distinction between the primary, legal, and professional authority of the medical/surgical staff to anticipate and prepare,

---

* Any consideration of this function must take into account the patient's rights to know, to consent, and to reject, as established legally, ethically, and morally in our current society.

and the professional expertness of the social work staff to follow through on the psychological, emotional, and social consequence of such information which may threaten the equilibrium and functioning of the family and its individual members.

If social workers arrange to be present when the physician explains future conditions to a patient/family, they hear firsthand what the patient/family has been told and are in a good position later to correct misunderstandings and distortions, to understand the patient/family's emotional responses, to explore relevant factors in the patient/family's social situations, to eliminate or reduce obstacles to the patient/family's clear thinking and decision making, and to determine whether the patient/family needs more time with the physician to reply to questions that social workers are not competent to answer. Social workers would like physicians and surgeons to share with them more of the anticipatory and preparatory work that patients/families need. It would be a logical collaborative process resulting in the patient/family's greater confidence in the physician and in greater strength to tolerate and deal with what lies ahead.

Social workers who come in contact with private patients note frequently that they are not as well prepared for future events in their medical care as are patients who have had concurrent, coordinated services from medical and social work personnel on the hospital's staff. As a matter of fact, children are often better prepared than adults—a phenomenon that reflects a peculiar lack of empathy on the part of physicians and other health care personnel, as though they have forgotten or never realized how uninformed, apprehensive, and just plain frightened adults can be. Infrequently as yet, a private physician will arrange for a preadmission contact between a patient and a social worker in anticipation of a stressful event, for example, hospitalization or surgery. Much more frequently, private physicians refer their already hospitalized patients to a social worker on the staff for anticipatory and preparatory services, especially to plan for discharge.

There is an interesting variation on this function. It is not always exercised between social worker and patient/family. It sometimes provides an essential service to significant others, for example, a teacher or an employer; and there are the not infrequent occasions when the function is called into play by a member of a collaborating group who needs to turn to his or her interprofessional or intraprofessional colleagues for help in preparing himself or herself for oncoming events or conditions that are hard to face alone. The function may be called into play numerous times on behalf of an individual patient/family from the diagnostic period through the process of rehabilitation. The social worker's general knowledge, his or her accumulated experience, and his or her sensitivity to signs of anxiety and fear—sometimes masked by anger, irritability, excessive demands, and so on—lead him or her to recognize the need for anticipatory and preparatory work.

As usual, stereotyped conclusions do no good. There will always be people who clamp down hard on their feelings and seem to want nothing so much as *not* to know, *not* to foresee, and *not* to prepare. However, insofar as there are moral and legal reasons for someone in the patient/family group to be prepared for one or more aspects of the medical situation, important questions must be answered. Some of these are the following: What are the potential social and psychological costs to the patient/family if their protective mechanisms should be broken down? What is immediately essential for the reluctant persons to know? What can be currently left unspoken in order to conserve the patient/ family's inner strengths? What weight must be given to the influences of limited time, of medical and surgical procedures, of administrative and legislative regulations, and of how a social worker's colleagues in other professions perceive his or her role? What impact do and should these parameters have on the social worker's judgment?

If these questions lead to still other questions about desirable alterations in professional attitudes and behaviors and long-established, institutionalized perceptions and expectations among health and health-related personnel, that is a satisfactory first result. Then one hopes for disciplined inquiry and eventual change.

INVOLVING THE PATIENT/FAMILY AS PARTICIPANTS

The social worker's efforts to involve the patient/family as participants in processes related to medical care are prominent throughout the course of an illness or disability. This function reflects with unusual clarity the significance of "family" as a value and as an element in the social worker's knowledge base. The patient's participation helps to preserve his or her integrity as a human being, to maintain his or her self-regard, and to foster his or her functioning at his or her maximum level. The immediate purpose of participation shifts, for example, with changed environmental circumstances, newly determined medical needs, and successive stages in the course of the illness. In addition, patient/family participation is a process which lends itself not only to management of a current illness-situation but also to measures to prevent recurrence of illness and for the promotion and maintenance of good health. One now sees proposals and plans for programs of health education which will increase everyone's obligation to learn, to teach, and to practice sound ways of living and optimal use of resources related to health and medical care. For example, there is the development of advisory and liaison committees whose members are residents of the community served by a health care facility and whose influence reaches back into the community as well as into the institution. There are also established outreach clinics affiliated with hospitals and independent neighborhood centers which are oriented toward preventive medicine and employ educational methods in their contacts with the public.

Currently the involvement of patient/family as participants refers most often to the roles they play during periods of medical intervention. Full consideration reveals that participation is not of one kind or degree. It can be voluntary or involuntary, active or passive. Examples of the critical events that commonly require some form of participation are the decision to seek or apply for health care; making the necessary contact; giving medicosocial history, describing symptoms, and so on; making decisions, for example, to undergo diagnostic and therapeutic procedures; planning for living after ambulatory or in-hospital care is terminated; and carrying out agreed-upon plans. A large number of interdependent factors determine who in the patient/family become participants, the responsibilities they do or do not undertake, and the consequences of their actions and inactions. Among these factors are the patient's age, sex, and major role in the family; the relationships among family members; the goals of the family unit; the major characteristics and impacts of the patient's illness and its treatment; the patient/family's current sociocultural situation; and the probable outcome of the patient's treatment.

Then there are the variables in the commitments of personnel. The helpers and healers may have among themselves a range of attitudes, expectations, and behaviors which affect participation by patients, their relatives, and their significant others. To illustrate, a physician who has little faith in the elderly person's capacity for self-determination will expect passive participation in the form of unquestioning acquiescence in his or her recommendations. A nurse who believes in the human capacity for growth and adaptation and the importance of self-reliance will work patiently to enable a man fearful of "needles" to administer his own insulin. He would earlier have renounced his participation gladly in exchange for his wife's assuming the responsibility. A social worker who realizes that the most devoted relatives have breaking points under excessive pressure believes that the form of participation may be secondary to the supportive effects of participation per se. Thus, when a married daughter tells the social worker she could not bear the sight of her father's blood flowing in the hemodialyzer, the physician agrees with the social worker to shift the plan from treatment at home to treatment at the hospital. The daughter's participation will be in part to provide transportation for her father, that is, to give him access to treatment instead of exposing herself to excessive emotional pain. The first plan risked disruption of a cohesive family unit; the substitute plan, which was equally suitable medically, held little threat to the climate of love and mutual support that characterized this family group.

Since the influence of individual variables changes with different stages of life-and-illness, the pattern of participation within the family, as well as its purpose and significance, will vary over time. Ideally, changes in the pattern will be steadily in the direction of maintaining or improving the patient/family's quality of social functioning. However, life deviates from the ideal, and the social worker may intervene as an enabling external force to shore up or restore or provide a substitute for the kind of participation that once was possible. One becomes alert to people's eroded capacity to participate and searches for the reasons. Among them are the cumulative effects of such factors as physical, emotional, and financial drain and strain; deterioration in the patient's condition which necessitates that he or she—if able—and his or her relatives find a new pattern of participation and a new equilibrium in the family group; changes in recommended medical treatment of the patient which would violate cultural habits and religious beliefs and sanctions; and decision making regarding matters that threaten to disturb family relationships, bring dissenting viewpoints into the open, or otherwise create stress-producing situations.

Flexibility and rigidity as personal traits that govern whether and how a person changes his or her responses as conditions require are attributes important to assess and reassess. Considering the flow of events and conditions that can occur in the course of an illness, there are always changes in who participates with whom, for what purpose, and in what form. The capacity to assume and to relinquish authority and responsibility in a life-and-illness situation—for oneself or for another—is frequently central to participating successfully in activities in health care.

From the standpoint of a humanistic conception of health care, perhaps the most adequate explanation for this devotion to patient/family participation is found by returning to the social worker's values; the principles of maximum self-realization and feasible self-determination are lived out in helping people do with, rather than to or for, one another.

HELPING PATIENTS/FAMILIES COPE WITH REALITIES

The ability to separate the real from the unreal and to cope with stressful realities is an instrument for solving problems of living. Simultaneously, there is a human need for psychological protection and defense against realities that are painful and potentially disintegrative forces. Within ethnic and professional subcultures a variety of mechanisms exist for explaining, protecting against, and coping with the different conceptions of the real and the unreal.

Reality, defined as "that which exists as contrasted with what is fictitious or merely conceived of"[7] sounds absolute but is in practice an elusive concept; someone's reality may be another's fiction. In the field of health care the distinction between the patient/family's perceptions of reality and unreality is of major importance to professional personnel, whether the perceptions concern mind or body or the environment in which people live.

What patients/families believe about the origin, consequences, and treatment of diseases and disabilities has an immediate connection with their fears, anxieties, expectations, and hopes. Beliefs rooted in legends and myths may be sustaining and strengthening or may have the opposite effect of weakening the capacity to hope and to cope. Givers-of-service, therefore, frequently have to decide to leave people's irrational beliefs intact when they will not interfere with and may actually enhance the patient/family's use of scientific, medical facts and their positive response to professional opinion and recommendation. Fortunately, belief in the irrational often lives comfortably side by side with rational, logical understanding.

However, when legends, fantasies, and superstitions will impede the patient/family's realization of optimal social functioning, givers-of-service may then intervene if the "real" information they are offering can be made more satisfying and useful than the "unreal" information it is replacing. Although the influence of the irrational may be found in any patient population, it is apt to reach excessive strength in pediatric patients whose sense of reality is normally immature. At the other end of the life cycle, elderly patients also are highly vulnerable to fantasy and to confused or distorted ideas about their illnesses even when their psychological and intellectual functioning is relatively unimpaired. Many members of ethnic groups harbor as part of their philosophical outlook on life or their religious beliefs ideas about illness and medical care which to anyone steeped in the scientific base for medical practice appear unreal and irrational. For example, many patients/families practice spirtualism without serious threat to recovery or survival while concurrently following a physician's advice. Insofar as the patient/family's belief in the benign aspects of their cultural heritage gives them comfort, a sense of security, and hope, that belief can reinforce the efficacy of the physician's treatment. The power of prayer in the more traditional religions is also a reality to those who hold the belief, and is as a rule a beneficent one.

The lack of scientific information suffered by large numbers of patients and their relatives gives rise to all sorts of fantasies about illness and interventive measures and generates emotions ranging from the depths of discouragement to the heights of unfounded optimism. Ignorance of the structure and functioning of the human body is one important source of fantasies, especially those related to genitalia, sexual behavior, and procreation. People do not give up their fantasies easily, and corrective information may be thoroughly incorporated only after a long period of testing it out.

The symbolic meaning of certain foods in a given subculture, an habitual diet which is greatly relished, an accustomed way of cooking—factors such as these may have tremendous influence on following or not following a physician's instruction about diet. The realities of nutritional values, calories, and vitamins simply do not compete with years of pleasure derived from the patient/family's accustomed way of eating. Nor do they provide financial resources needed to meet recommended dietary changes.

There is an interesting phenomenon that might be called "idiosyncratic superstitions" which are real to a patient/family but unreal, false, and irrational to medical and health-related professionals: A woman is sure she will die when she reaches the age at which her mother died. A patient is convinced she will not survive surgery because two relatives died a few months after their respective operations.

Before leaving these matters of fantasy and legend, there should be mention of fantasies engendered in patient/families by the behavior of professional practitioners. One of the most stress-producing behaviors is the practitioners' tendency to talk among themselves at the patient's bedside or in an examining room while the patient is lying on the table, using their professional language or resorting to initials (e.g., "b.t." for brain tumor or "d.r." for detached retina). This linguistic behavior is intended to keep patients calm, unsuspecting, and unafraid but instead it often induces distressing emotional reactions in the patient/family, arousing fears and anxieties about the unknown, increasing the patient's feeling that he or she has lost control over his or her life and is being ignored as a person. Patients who are sufficiently sophisticated and self-assured can express reasonable anger and request that the physicians explain their conversation.

In the traditional hospital setting the physician plays a major and primary role in clarifying biological and medical realities about which patients/families are confused, misinformed, or ignorant. Nurses with specialized competence may share the physician's responsibility in this respect. Social workers, who may reinforce the information their colleagues have imparted to a patient/family and translate it into terms more easily understood, are concerned in general with reducing the patients/families' burden of stress and helping them to *keep related* to the realities of their situations. People try to slough off stressful conditions, forget them, deny them, or distort them into something more palatable. These defensive reactions may occur even when the professionals involved try to time and to partialize their responses to conform to the patient/family's capacity to tolerate and adapt to stress-producing phenomena. [8, 9]

The social worker can help patients/families and their significant others channel energy toward realistic expectations and goals. Patients themselves, as well as their relatives—or their significant others, such as teachers or employers—may expect too much or too little progress, at a tempo too fast or too slow, in the direction of restored or improved social functioning. People are often unprepared for problematic aspects of getting well; patients can find it hard to give up some kinds of dependency which were essential to their care in earlier stages of illness or disability. Or relatives may prolong protective care beyond the period of need or push the patient too hard and too fast to attain self-reliance. People need guide lines which, when necessary, will be corrective of unrealistic hopes and desires, fears and forebodings. Patients/families' expectations may be both general (e.g., the patient will be cured, will improve, will grow worse, will die) and specific (e.g., the patient will discard crutches in a month, will return to work in three weeks, will soon be bedridden, will not live to his next birthday).

Social workers need to be alert to what patients/families believe or want to hear in contrast to what some family member—perhaps the patient, perhaps not—has to know or acknowledge. Many realities that are hard to face and deal with are not inherent in the patient's illness but are related to it, exerting an important influence on some aspect of living. Some of these are the loss of income, the necessity for vocational retraining, the unsuitability of accustomed living quarters, the enforced relinquishing of prized personal possessions for which there will be no space in new quarters, and many other unpleasant realities which one hopes no one will have to struggle with alone.

Although time is never unlimited and frequently is far too short for fully incorporating and adapting to difficult situations, the social worker will recognize the limits people have for the endurance of stress and frustration and use all available resources to relieve them.

Encouraging the expression of feelings is helpful, as is the important technique of "holding the future before the patient/family." Since the future is not always bright, the intention is to help the patient/family maintain hope for living well whatever future there is for the patient. The challenge occurs particularly in those situations that have a guarded outlook. In this context, hope for living well may be quite restricted; yet because it serves a real purpose in the eyes of those who hold that hope, it will sustain and encourage them to live as fully as they can. Some patients/families derive their hope and strength from the physician's assurance that the patient will be kept as free from pain as possible; others will derive theirs from the knowledge that some form of third-party financing will be available for the remainder of the patient's life; still others will be strengthened by the realization that the patient can be transferred from home care to hospital care and back again as needed; and many patients who know or suspect their lives are ending believe that their remaining time will be well lived if they complete "unfinished business" which will fulfill their responsibilities to themselves and to others. The hope that they can accomplish the necessary tasks sustains their efforts whether they are directed toward the tangibles of money and property or to the impalpable legacies of personal relationships.

The passage of "time by the clock" has been mentioned frequently as a reality that has significance to both givers-of-service and patients/families. Other aspects of the reality of time need to be identified because of their importance in situations of illness and their relevance to the social worker's practice. There is no one concept or definition of time. Some ideas about time are clearly ethnic in origin; some are idiosyncratic, consistent with an individual's personality; and some are associated in our culture with phases of the life cycle.

Persons reared in a leisurely society, unused to planning ahead, may have a hard time with the firmly fixed appointments that prevail in our society. Children develop a sense of time as they mature, but when very young, "tomorrow" is as much as many can understand. Preparing a child for a visit to the doctor or similar event takes his concept of time into careful consideration. Adolescents tend often to disregard the conventional concept of time and timing in favor of their immediately felt needs and desires. Their reality, then, is what they want when they want it.

As one grows older a year is no longer an eternity, but day-by-day time may hang heavy if one is isolated or feels no longer needed by or useful to others. The social worker takes responsibility for converting this distressing meaning of time—real, not fancied—into a more pleasurable reality whenever the aptitudes and needs of the distressed person can be matched by an available resource.

ASSISTING PATIENTS/FAMILIES
TO USE RESOURCES AND STRENGTHS

Strengths and resources in this context are defined in the broadest possible sense in order to do full justice to this aspect of the social worker's practice. Resources include aids and supports available under formal, voluntary, and governmental auspices within and outside the boundaries of health facilities. These aids and supports are of three kinds: (1) They may be primarily tangible and concrete, such as money, prostheses, and recordings for the blind. (2) They may be psychological in nature, providing supportive attitudes or opportunities for emotional catharsis, advice, and counseling, and the like. These aids and supports are made available through a purposeful working relationship between those who are helping and those who are helped. Giving this kind of assistance is one of the social worker's major efforts, but at their best and most effective, these efforts will be made with interprofessional collaboration and the patient/family's participation. (3) They may be services produced by the labor of persons with recognized competence to perform them, for example, homemaking and housekeeping services, vocational retraining, or transportation for the physically handicapped.

Communities differ widely in the adequacy of resources that exist under organized auspices, voluntary or governmental. Whether a resource is *available* to a given patient/family depends not only on the supply but on the eligibility requirements, such as the amount of income an applicant can have, the length of time the resource can be provided, the illness from which the applicant is suffering, the geographical location of his or her residence, and the patient's age. Social workers are well informed about these conditions and how needed benefits can be obtained.

Of great importance are the resources that exist within the patient/family's natural milieu. They too may be tangible (money, living space), psychological (sympathy, compassion, communication about intimate concerns and personal experiences), and in the form of services (marketing, cleaning, giving medication, baby-sitting). The natural milieu of some patients/families may appear to be rich in resources, while that of others may appear impoverished. Whether existing resources will actually be delivered depends heavily on the character of the personal, psychological, and emotional relationships among people in the patient/family's natural environment. Thus a milieu potentially rich in resources may in actuality offer less adequate aid and support than a milieu that appears much poorer.

Voluntary organizations have been formed of persons whose common bond is the task of adapting to the consequences of a specified disease or disability. Essentially, these are organizations formed for self-help and mutual help.[10] Probably the best known of these are Alcoholics Anonymous and its related organizations, Al-a-non, for the spouses of alcoholics, and Al-a-teen, for their children. Others are Reach to Recovery, for women who have had mastectomies; Parents Without Partners, for those who do not have, or do not live with, spouses and whose members help one another to resolve problems of relationships and issues regarding the rearing of children; Parents Anonymous in New York City, whose members work with one another to prevent abusive and neglectful acts toward children; and National Tay-Sachs and Allied Diseases Association in New York City, which refers parents of children who have those diseases to self-help groups in their respective communities. In many localities there are chapters of national organizations. There are also numerous informal groups or clubs, for example, for parents of mentally retarded children, for parents of hemophiliacs, and for patients who have colostomies or laryngectomies. The leadership for these organizations usually comes from their lay members, although professionals are called upon as informants, consultants, researchers, and fund raisers.

Patients sometimes ask for immediate access to such organizations. Others do not feel ready but expect to use a resource later. There are those who want "nothing to do with groups" but do want a one-to-one contact with a knowledgeable and sympathetic layperson. And then there are the patients/families who need and ask for help from professionals. Patients/families who know of self-help groups frequently make their own contacts. Social workers consider these groups important resources to which they refer patients/families when their readiness for specific kinds of help is established and their consent has been obtained. Timing such referrals when patients/families can make the best use of available services is of the utmost importance.

There are representatives of some of these organizations who have relatively free access to hospitalized patients. At times these concerned individuals offer their services to patients without consulting any of the givers-of-service, who could suggest the most effective timing and approach and the problem areas for which a patient/family has the greatest need for help. These experiences are hazardous when they turn patients/families against a potentially valuable source of strength. The errors are often retrievable, but time better spent is lost while the patient/family recover from the first unfortunate, premature contact.

Strengths are a form of nonmaterial resource that originates within the person. They are basic elements in the human capacity to help and to be helped. It is axiomatic in social work practice, as mentioned earlier, that the processes of helping and being helped to cope with problems of daily living—with demands for adjustment and adaptation to changed conditions—are built on people's inner strengths.

It is expected that professional social workers are aware of their own characteristics and traits that have the greatest potential for affecting and influencing the people they serve or work with, that they correct or control personal qualities that might have damaging effects on clients or colleagues, and that they make disciplined use of those qualities that have potentially helpful impacts upon persons within the circle of their professional relationships.

The complement to required self-awareness is the social worker's obligation to identify and encourage maximum use of others' strengths that will facilitate their efforts to cope. These others are first of all patients and their relatives, but often the social worker's efforts are extended to the patient's significant others and to the social worker's colleagues in the health care setting. In regard to both helper and helped, the building blocks of inner strength are forged early in life.* At the same time, throughout the life cycle strengths and deficiencies are subject to change and are dynamically responsive to the course of an individual's life-experience. The social worker learns of a patient/family's strengths and deficiencies in large measure by talking over earlier critical problems and how the patient/family met them and by observing and discussing the current life-and-illness situation and the ways being used to cope with it.

Strengths and deficiencies can change in degree and significance from time to time. What is a strength under certain conditions becomes an impediment under others; for example, a patient's insistence on independence may be so excessive that he or she refuses to allow the appropriate dependence required for healing during illness. Keeping in mind that the significance of such personal qualities can shift, a social worker identifies certain ones as potential strengths in patients and their relatives and in himself or herself and his or her colleagues. Among the strengths are assured self-regard and an enlightened self-interest, but also included is the capacity to have concern for and trust in others, tolerance for frustration and uncertainty, the ability to renounce immediate pleasure for greater future gratification, flexibility, resilience, the desire to overcome obstacles, and the ability to give to and accept from others in a person-to-person relationship.

Social workers have responsibilities beyond knowing what aids and supports exist. They must either have or know how to obtain information about where and under what conditions a resource is available. They have to keep abreast of changes in such things as procedures and eligibility requirements which are made by the providers of the various aids and supports, and note the impacts of such changes upon patients/families and upon the quality of care. Whenever there are alternative resources and a real choice exists, the persons involved have a right to consider relative advantages and disadvantages.

The social worker must have a professional opinion about the nature of a patient/family's psychosocial needs, may have to reconcile dissenting opinions about those needs, and has to distinguish what is desired from what is needed and what is available. Having encouraged the best match possible between need and resource, the social worker may have to shift from helping to select resources to helping a patient/family derive the greatest benefit from the aids and supports that are available. For example, people who feel guilty, ashamed, or angry because an illness or disability has placed them among the medically indigent who must apply for Medicaid consume so much energy in emotional reaction to their need for financial aid that there is little energy left to use in behalf of restoring their social functioning. The social worker will encourage such persons to convert a fight against financial dependence into a fight to attain their maximum status of social-health. Buried somewhere there is usually a more rational attitude which a patient/family can be helped to use to rechannel their energy productively. The three kinds of resources that have been identi-

---

* For a fuller discussion, see the section on the potential for growth and adaptation, pp. 13–17.

fied—tangible, concrete aids and supports; services; and psychological aids and supports resulting from the influence of one person upon another and from qualities and attributes that have been incorporated into an individual's personality—are not completely disparate. Tangible aids and supports will have psychological effects which may be fulfilling and pleasant, unpleasant, or both simultaneously. Receiving services means not only that needed tasks are being done; the giver-of-service has some kind of relationship with the recipient of service, so that the human aspect may in itself become a resource and fill a psychosocial need when the relationship is mutually satisfying, or, under less fortunate circumstances, may interfere with the expected course of recovery from the illness.

The use of one kind of resource does not preclude the use of another kind concurrently or in sequence. One problem in a life-and-illness situation often generates others; and different aspects of these problems require more than one resource to meet the patient/family's needs. Need for a service or for a tangible aid can be met only by a service or tangible aid, although because of shortage and lacks, compromises are made and resources are used that only minimally meet a patient/family's needs. On the other hand—and this is important—not all problems that are manifested psychologically require psychological treatment. A tangible aid, a service, or both in combination may eliminate the basis for psychological symptoms of distress. Stated in reverse: when a substantiated need for a service or tangible aid remains unfilled, a reaction of frustration will occur, perhaps in the form of emotions such as anger, anxiety, a depressed mood, or apathetic resignation, or in active combativeness and insistent, demanding behavior.

Should such behavioral and emotional reactions threaten to interfere with optimal effects of medical care, the social worker will assist patients/families to bear with their frustration more benignly, although the lack of a resource is a reality that may produce a high degree of stress.

Many laypersons and social workers' professional colleagues in a hospital setting may rely on the wealth of information social workers have about resources. The nature and extent of the requests for their assistance may be marred, however, by a misunderstanding of the process involved. A common mistake is to think of locating and obtaining resources for patients/families as a mechanical cut-and-dried activity. The probability that emotions will be aroused when decisions and choices have to be made, that dissension and conflict are not unknown when patients/families participate in such determinations and are forced to make compromises, that almost always there is a waiting period before a needed aid or service can be made available—these are among the stress-producing probabilities that are not adequately understood or anticipated. In consequence, requests may be made of the social worker too late for him or her to make an adequate exploration and effective supportive efforts.*

Since many requests for resources are made immediately prior to a patient's discharge from the hospital, the strict regulations governing bed utilization add to the pressure of time and timing which is inherent in searching for the resource best suited to the needs of a given patient-family.

Another error is made when a colleague's request is couched in terms that predetermine both the psychosocial problem and its solution. This kind of

---

* See the section on determination of the point of entry, p. 27.

request creates a rigid framework from which the patient/family and the referring person may not wish to depart and within which the social worker cannot function. Like other professionals, social workers must be free to exercise their central competencies as a public trust, within the value system of their profession, and with due regard for the rights and obligations of fellow professionals.[11, 12, 13]

IMPROVING AND EXPANDING RESOURCES AND SYSTEMS OF CARE

The social worker who gives direct service to patients/families is inevitably drawn into aspects of indirect service such as assessment of existing resources and of the systems of care within which the resources are provided. The assessment is based variously on day-by-day experiences which social workers share informally among themselves as contributions to practice wisdom, on small, structured inquiries which cover selected patient populations in an individual facility, on formal surveys of populations in a community, and so on.

The seasoned worker who assesses resources also casts a critical eye on the related systems of care. These are often referred to in our society as nonsystems because, for example, they are seldom governed or guided by a consistent and logical public policy; the services they provide are fragmented and discontinuous; and their programs are uncoordinated at the operational level.

Flawed resources and systems of care are the concern of social workers— a concern that derives naturally from their basic concepts of values and knowledge.[14, 15] In consequence, it has long been a function of social workers to engage in efforts both to improve the quality, effectiveness, volume, and delivery of existing resources and to develop new resources that are needed but not yet provided. Substantial improvement in resources is often dependent upon prior improvement in a system or systems of care. This is the situation, it would seem, that currently exists in regard to both income maintenance and health care. Our piecemeal approach to improving these two patchwork systems continues to be as frustrating to personnel in the systems as it is depriving to the consumers of services and care.

Fundamental reforms in unsatisfactory systems—or total replacements— are long-term objectives which require the collaborative efforts of individuals and organizations representing different disciplines, professions, and lay groups. Also required are sophisticated methods that will be effective in persuading persons in dissenting or adversary positions to compatible points of view. Even when the financial costs are not a factor—and this is unusual—psychological, political, and legal factors may constitute barriers to change that must be reckoned with.

At this stage of the profession's development there are relatively few social workers who have become expert lobbyists registered at the various levels of government. The majority of social workers, each of whom has the usual obligation of a professional to improve the general welfare, do so through their professional and civic organizations, by exercising the voting franchise, and by using the established channels of communication in individual institutions and in our various systems of health and health-related care. These established channels, usually parallel to the hierarchical structure of the institution or system, are used as conduits through which pass the data that substantiate or refute the need for change in the human services related to health care.

It is the social workers at the operative levle of direct service to patients/ families who amass volumes of raw information that is basic—the bedrock of change and reform in programs and services. These data by themselves are seldom effective in producing change. The psychosocial data gathered by social workers have to be related appropriately to such components as financial costs, medical implications, available manpower, and the philosophic bases of professional education and practice before they can be put to optimal use.

Intraprofessional and interprofessional consideration as well as interdisciplinary examination are frequently in order for both short- and long-term change. Institutional and systemic change always meets with some inertia; is always accomplished over a period of time; and requires well-directed effort, competent use of the most appropriate methods, and collaboration with those personnel best qualified.

Short-term changes should not be downgraded because they happen to affect a relatively small population. Formation of a group of asthmatic women for health education, originally suggested by social workers who were concerned over the number of clinic patients who failed to keep regular appointments and turned up frequently for emergency service, is as valid and valuable for that population as are long-term efforts, for example, to shift the base for medical insurance from solo practice, fee-for-service to prepaid group medical practice for consumers nationwide.

To achieve change in health and health-related institutions and systems of care is the primary function of a few social workers with the required knowledge, values, skills, and authority, and it is a peripheral function for those whose expertness lies elsewhere. It cannot be ignored by any social worker whose perspective on life is broadgauged and whose conception of professional responsibility and accountability goes beyond the narrower here-and-now of today's assignment.

REFERENCES

1. Beatrice Phillips, "Social Workers in Health Services," *Encyclopedia of Social Work*, 16th ed. (New York: National Association of Social Workers, 1971)pp. 565–574.
2. Helen Rehr, ed., *Medicine and Social Work: An Exploration in Interprofessionalism* (New York: Prodist, 1974).
3. Bess Dana, "Health, Social Work and Social Justice," in *Social Work Practice and Social Justice*, ed. Bernard Ross and Charles Shireman (Washington, D.C.: 1973), National Association of Social Workers, pp. 111–128.
4. Max Siporin, "Situational Assessment and Intervention," *Social Casework*, vol. 53, no. 2 (February 1972), pp. 91-109.
5. Bertha L. Doremus, "The Four Rs: Social Diagnosis in Health Care," *Health and Social Work*, vol. 1, no. 4 (November 1976), pp. 120-139.
6. Arnold J. Rosin, "The Doctor-Relative Relationship: An Exercise in Interview Techniques in the 'Relatives' Clinic,' " *Social Work in Health Care*, vol. 1, no. 4 (summer 1976), pp. 499-505.
7. *Standard College Dictionary* (New York: Funk and Wagnalls, 1968).
8. Lillian Pike Cain and Nancy Staver, "Helping Children Adapt to Parental Illness," *Social Casework*, vol. 57, no. 9 (November 1976), p. 575.

9. Pauline Cohen, Israel N. Dizenhuz, and Caroline Winget, "Family Adaptation to Terminal Illness and Death of a Parent," *Social Casework,* vol. 58, no. 4 (April 1977), pp. 223-228.
10. Alfred H. Katz, "Self-Help Groups," "in *Encyclopedia of Social Work,* 17th ed. (Washington, D.C.: National Association of Social Workers, 1977), pp. 12541261.
11. Katherine M. Olsen and Marvin E. Olsen, "Role Expectations and Perceptions for Social Workers in Medical Settings," *Social Work,* vol. 12, no. 3 (July 1967), pp. 70-78.
12. Barbara Gordon Berkman and Helen Rehr, "Unanticipated Consequences of the Case Finding System in Hospital Social Service," Social Work, vol. 15, no. 2 (April 1970), pp. 63-67.
13. Barbara Gordon and Helen Rehr, "Selectivity Biases in Delivery of Hospital Social Services," *Social Service Review,* vol. 43, no. 1 (March 1969), pp. 35-41.
14. Darwin Palmiere, "Health Services: Health and Hospital Planning," in *Encyclopedia of Social Work,* 17th ed., op. cit., pp. 595-602.
15. Robert D. Finney, Rita P. Pessin, and Larry P. Matheis, "Prospects for Social Workers in Health Planning," *Health and Social Work,* vol. 1, no. 3 (August 1976), pp. 7-26.

PART *TWO*
PEOPLE AND PLACES

INTRODUCTION

The purpose of the following five chapters is to place in a useful, structured context the social worker's clinical data from which was derived the conceptual background presented in the preceding two chapters. In this sense, useful means viable, that is, living material which is capable of contributing to education for the health professions and, in the long run, to professional practice in the health care field.

The practice of hospital-based social work brings alive the impacts of illness and disability on people—not just on patients, their relatives, and their significant others, but also on the givers of human services; it describes the interactions of illness and disability, psychological and socioeconomic factors, and personal endowment; and it clarifies the special impact of the hospital as an institution, in itself a system of many parts which are in interaction with the community and with the individuals and the groups concerned with giving and receiving health care. The interplay of human elements and the structural organizational elements in health care is observable, and its consequences help to determine the psychosocial meanings of illness and disability.

The central concern of the hospital-based social worker is the welfare of human beings under stress of illness. This concern and the social worker's responsive professional exercise of it occur within a framework compatible with the mission, values, knowledge, and special skills of the social work profession. Traditionally, medical services in the hospital are made available in relation first to a disease entity and/or method of medical intervention and then within overall categories of age ranges designated as pediatric, adolescent, adult, and geriatric. Consideration by medical personnel of psychosocial factors connected with physical illness or disability depends largely upon their philosophy, their education and training, and their sensitivity to the human condition.

In contrast, the social worker's perspective is first related to personal and social needs assessed within a developmental frame of reference that includes chronological age; its associated and *expected* social roles, tasks, conflicts, and problems; and the *achieved* level of social functioning or status of social health. The patient's somatic condition is viewed as a stress-producing experience whose impact is determined by interrelated factors such as a person's age; his or her position in or significance to the family group; characteristics of the illness and its treatment; the socioeconomic situation; cultural influences; and available resources and strengths. As regards these resources and strengths, the hospital-based social worker emerges as an enabling, strengthening, and facilitating human resource for those who must cope with the problematic aspects of disease, disability, and dysfunction.

The coping has to do with the adaptations demanded by the impacts of illness and disability which are the immediate sources of stress under consideration. The impacts affect a wide range of social tasks and behaviors—impacts that apply with different force and effect, depending largely on people's natural roles and functions.

Considering social work's concern with the confrontation between people and the stress-producing events and conditions of illness, it is illuminating to observe how social workers fit the biomedical facts of a disease entity or of a disability into their own frame of reference. Their informal classifications do not constitute a scientific classification of disease entities (though social workers are well grounded in the medical facts) but represent in useful forms the social workers' understanding of the psychosocial significance of specific diseases and deficiencies. Their particular system of classification makes understandable their identification of the kinds of adaptation demanded by the varied impacts of illness and disability. As might be expected of social workers in hospitals providing secondary and tertiary care, most of their experience tends to be with patients suffering from acute episodes in long-term or chronic illnesses.

First, the social workers' psychosocial groupings or classifications put heavy emphasis on those diseases known as hereditary or familial. Illnesses of this kind not only reflect on the patient's heritage and disturb his or her image of it and of himself or herself but also threaten the health of his or her progeny—a double source of psychosocial stress that is frequently accompanied by such feelings as anger, frustration, guilt, and sorrow. Translated into personal-social problems, hereditary and familial illness demands solving such dilemmas as whether to marry or not; whether to have children or not; to whom to tell and from whom to conceal the nature of one's illness, chromosomal trait, and so on. Always there is a special concern for the welfare of those children already born into the patient's family: How can their health be safeguarded? Will they or will they not be victims of the disease? What should they be told?

Adult patients who have an inherited or probably inherited disease can often recall an older relative with the same disease—for example, diabetes—and memories of the changes that took place in that person and in the life of that person may become highly stressful. Those memories raise all the questions about the patient's own future that usually have no definite answers: Will he or she have to have an amputation? Will he or she lose his or her eyesight? Will he or she die an early death?

A second group of illnesses arouses a strong, unpleasant sense of personal difference from others. Some differences are directly and immediately observable by others, as when there is a physical anomaly such as a cleft lip; some are inferred from behavioral evidence, such as a diabetic patient's need to eat with strict regularity. There is wide diversity in human response to one's own difference and to differences one perceives in others. When the differences derive from a physical deficit or anomaly, the primary sense of inferiority may be tempered by, for example, the patient's mastery of a handicapping condition; by acceptance of a therapeutic agent, medical intervention, prosthesis, and the like as compensatory, enabling elements; or by enjoyment and utilization of secondary gains in the form of special privileges and attention which may be gratifying to the patient but sometimes impair his or her motivation and ability to cope. In brief, it is dangerous to assume that one knows the exact meaning of a stressful experience to an individual unless there has been communication which reveals what particularizes the experience for him or her.

Progressive diseases form a third group which social workers identify as peculiarly stressful. Progressive diseases, however else they differ, have in common the certainty of a worsening condition which demands, over time, continuous readjustment to a decreasing status of social-health and social functioning. A progressive disease like uveitis, which affects a sensory organ but leaves the rest of the body and intellectual capacity intact, must be differentiated in its demands for adaptation from a progressive disease like Huntington's chorea, which eventually affects the entire body and mental faculties as well. Also, since some progressive diseases are fatal and others are not, there is in the former instance the heavy burden of stress that for many people accompanies the expectation of the death and loss of a loved family member or friend. When the threat of another's death confronts one with the thought—so often pushed away—that death is also one's own and everyone's destiny, feelings of stress may mount to a crisis of panic, despair, and retreat.

It may be the patient's relatives who feel the greater stress when the disease is progressive, especially if there is a steady loss of the patient's capacity for self-awareness and for assuming life-tasks and roles natural to his or her age, sex, and status. One has in mind not only adult relatives who are active in the situation but young and growing children who must adapt not only to a changing parent who is ill but also to a well parent struggling with his or her own readjustment and often to their own new and different responsibilities and relationships as children in the family unit.

Children of a patient with a progressive, and in particular a fatal, disease need special attention. They are seldom adequately prepared for the course of a parent's disease or for his or her death. By all accounts the well parent is the best person to prepare them, and he or she usually can, given support and help to face and assimilate some of his or her own anticipatory sorrow.

The characteristic of chronicity is the major stress-producing attribute of a fourth group of illnesses.[1] An increasing number of patients—now nearing a majority—who receive care from acute general hospitals are patients with chronic diseases. They come for medical care when an acute episode of their chronic illness occurs, when interventive measures can be applied to stabilize or arrest the disease, when a rehabilitative program is in order, and/or when they are participants in a medical program of research.

Advances in medical knowledge and skill keep some contagious and infectious diseases under control, have eliminated others, and are leading into an era of considerable concentration in medical care and in medical research on chronic diseases, congenital defects, and genetic disorders. Improvements in the availability and accessibility of medical care, increases in the provision of health-related resources such as services for family planning, and regulatory controls over consumer goods and pollutants in the environment—these and other developments contribute to the general welfare but create some inevitable problems, too. People are surviving diseases, anomalies, and deficiencies that would once have brought early death; many of them survive, however, with chronic conditions that impair their social functioning, that sometimes require special treatment—medical and social—throughout the life span, and that often make unusual demands for adaptation on the part of the patient/family and their significant others. It is doubtful, of course, whether we ever make what we call progress without paying for it in problematic consequences. In this and similar situations the payment is the stress-producing element, chronicity.

A fifth grouping is characterized by the attitudes and feelings of repugnance or aversion that they call forth in our general society or in a subculture of it. Fear, shame, loathing, disapproval, and guilt are among the most potent reactions to conditions that vary widely in their medical and social implications. Thus for some people hepatitis is associated always with drug abuse, a disorder of the liver with alcoholism, and venereal disease with forbidden sexual behavior. When there is the possiibility of contagion, for example, the patient may look upon himself as a danger to others and an undesirable to be avoided; those close to the patient may be torn between concern for him or her, fear of the risk to themselves, and shame or anger if they believe the patient's conduct is responsible for the infection.

When reactions of aversion reach a high pitch, they may evoke the use of various protective and defensive actions and devices which reduce feelings of stress but which at times may take the form of disregarding medical advice.* Identifying such acts of noncompliance is an exercise without value unless it leads to a more fundamental understanding of the behavior: Is the patient reacting to a changed self-image? Is the patient frustrated by restrictions on his or her freedom of choice? Is the patient trying to disregard the implications of his or her disease for the health of his or her spouse and children?

These five groupings and their associated characteristics are cited to illustrate a useful perspective on illness and disability. It is hoped that the data will not be used to stereotype patients/families but to guide exploration and assessment of an individual patient/family's situation and of situations faced by specific patient populations. Generalized knowledge derived from professional practice in any field of human service has to be transmuted into terms that are suitable to specific individuals, families, other small groups, and populations of various sizes.

An examination of the impacts of illness and disability on people brings into focus the importance of place and space—more generally referred to as the environment. Specifically, the impacts of the hospital as a system emerge and call for understanding. Among the sources of these impacts are the structure and organization of the institution and of its many subunits; the qualifications of staff and the way in which they are deployed; whether medical care is disease and organ oriented or people oriented; and the degree to which authority, responsibility, status, and power are shared among a multiprofessional, multidisciplinary staff. Some of the ways in which people and institutions interact will be manifest in the chapters that follow.

*See the section on resolution of stress, pp. 18–20.

To assist the reader's appraisal of the data in Part Two of this text, a listing of common demands for adaptation that spring from the stressful events and conditions of illness and disability is presented below. The demands are described in general terms which allow for a wide range of specific experiences. No order of priority is intended; the demands apply with different force and effect to patients who are in different stages of the life cycle. In a given situation some demands for adaptation have greatest significance for the patient, some for the other family members and persons in close relationship, and some for the givers-of-service:

- adaptation to change or threatened change in self-image and self-regard and in the regard of others for oneself
- adaptation to change or threatened change in the status of one's authority, responsibility, and freedom of choice
- adaptation to change or threatened change in one's socioenvironmental pressures and supports
- adaptation to change or threatened change in one's ability to carry out an accustomed pattern of daily living
- adaptation to loss or the threat of loss of persons, possessions, bodily integrity, psychological capacities, control over one's environment, and so on
- adaptation to separation or the threat of separation from sources of personal security
- adaptation to uncertainty
- adaptation to pain or the threat of pain

The organization of specific data in Chapters 3 through 7 starts with the focus on adult patients (aged 21 to 65), who constitute a numerical majority in the acute general hospitals in the urban area from which the data in this text derive. In addition, adults are in a central position in our society as the major generative group economically, culturally, and biologically speaking. The age range is so wide that it permits observations of many natural social roles and tasks and the effect of illness and disability upon them. Thus the adult patient may be seen as homemaker, earner, spouse, sexual partner, parent of young and of grown children, grandparent, grown offspring of elderly parents, and social companion. In any of these natural roles the adult patient is vulnerable; how the adult assumes and adapts to the role of patient is related to his or her natural roles at a given stage of life. Because of the many possible definitions of social role, it is advisable to state the meaning adopted for use in this text: "Individuals (1) in social locations (2) behave (3) with reference to expectations and . . . these mutual expectations (4) are affectively charged."[2]

In Part Two, Chapters 3 and 4 focus respectively on the adult patient's experiences during the processes (1) of diagnosis and assessment and (2) of treatment and rehabilitation in the hospital and its subunits. Chapter 5 has to do with the impacts of care in selected loci of the hospital on the persons involved.

Chapters 6, 7, and 8 are devoted to selected patient groups which merit attention for reasons such as their being at high medicosocial risk, unusual impacts resulting from the nature of their medical conditions and their treatment, and special characteristics of stages in the human life cycle.

Chapter 9 contains the author's assessment of current social work practice in the participating acute general hospitals; some speculative comments on future goals; and suggestions for further developments in professional education for social work.

REFERENCES
1. Elsbeth Kahn, "Disability and Physical Handicap: Services for the Chronically Ill," in *Encyclopedia of Social Work*, 17th ed. (Washington, D.C.: National Association of Social Workers, 1977), pp. 252-260.
2. Leila Calhoun Deasy, *Persons and Positions: Individuals and Their Social Locations* (Washington, D.C.: Catholic University Press, 1969), p. 227.

Chapter *3*
The Adult Patient

Before there is any certainty for patient/family or health personnel about the nature of the patient's illness and its implications, there is a diagnostic process and period to be lived through. Although some patients undergo most or all of their diagnostic procedures in the offices of physicians in private practice or in prepaid group practice, many experience the entire diagnostic process in the service units of a hospital, either in the units for ambulatory care or in hospital or a combination of both. The hospital-based diagnostic process considered here is experienced in large and complex institutions, staffed by hundreds of personnel and equipped with strange, frightening machines and instruments which cannot be disguised even when there is an attempt to soften the surroundings and make people comfortable. The sight of other patients in various stages of undress, in wheelchairs, or being moved on rolling stretchers through busy corridors does little to allay anxiety. To those who need privacy, a calm atmosphere, and quiet, the usual ambulatory care service can offer only a minimum. To those whose discomforts, apprehensions, and fantasies are all too personal and unique, quick, brusque questions, unexplained transfers from one staff member to another and from one room to another, long periods of waiting between one procedure and the next, repeated visits to the hospital at hours that do not conform to the patient's routines and responsibilities all tend to exacerbate the tensions the patient/family are already enduring and in general have a dehumanizing effect at precisely the time when the patient and his or her relatives most need to feel respected, cared for, and sympathized with. How to balance individual, personal needs and wants against the demands upon the institution for efficient service to masses of people is a troublesome issue. It is a recurrent issue whose resolution will stem not only from changes in the regulations and procedures of a single institution but also from a viable sociomedical policy—a policy that is still lacking at the governmental and administrative levels of this nation. It is necessary to keep in mind the current conflicts and contradictions between many of the institutionalized operations of a hospital as a system and the needs and desires of the human beings who enter its walls for medical care.

The diagnostic period and process may be short or prolonged, but in either case it is likely to be stressful. Concern about the implications of the diagnostic process for the patient and other family members has special significance. Although many patients/families have contact with social workers during the diagnostic period and are helped to deal with their fears and apprehensions, patients/families who do not have this opportunity early are often found at a much later stage of medical care to be still striving to cope with the unresolved tensions, strains, and personal problems of the earlier period. One may make the assumption that the process of medical diagnosis affords a major opportunity to assess persons and their life-situations and, at its best, entails individualized responsiveness to the patient/family. Formal history taking is essential to making these assessments, but the value of informal exchanges, both verbal and nonverbal, between givers and recipients of services should not be underestimated. Can hard-pressed personnel give the time it takes for these communications? Or better yet, can personnel afford not to take the time? There is also the matter of timing—of sensing that a patient/family is ready or not ready for the exchange that hospital personnel would like to have, then and there, if the patient/family were able to cope with it.

More and more hospitals are arranging for assessment by social workers of the high-risk factors in patients/families' situations, either just before or at the point of a patient's hospitalization. This arrangement, however, may pass over the diagnostic process except for those relatively few patients who are admitted for diagnostic procedures. And, of course, no one has yet devised a satisfactory plan for discovering and reaching all the patients in ambulatory care who are at high social risk during the diagnostic period.* Even in this early stage of medical care patients may begin to feel less in control of their lives and less self-reliant. In instances of anxious waiting for reports on tests and examinations, they live apprehensively in the limbo of uncertainty and are faced with unknowns; when they are hospitalized for diagnostic procedures, they are deprived of their familiar surroundings and the presence of the people who usually give them comfort and support. Wherever a patient's examinations and tests take place, he or she may be asked to give consent to unfamiliar procedures, some of which require bodily contact and may involve pain and risk. The patient is asked to share facts and experiences in his or her life that are often intensely personal and private.

Many events that produce anxiety during the diagnostic period are those for which the patient/family are unprepared. There is more than one side to the state of unpreparedness. It is possible that no one in a position to do so has given the patient/family an adequate explanation of what will take place or when, where, and by whom the procedures will be administered. In other instances attempts have been made to explain, but communication has been unsuccessful. Perhaps the patient and relatives have been too frightened and distracted to

---

* It is worthwhile to note that a number of social service departments are engaged in developing screening devices to identify patients/families at risk medically and socially. These devices will include criteria other than serious illness per se as indicators of an immediate need for comprehensive psychosocial assessment. There are intersting historical implications in the revival of concern for the social worker's early engagement with the patient/family that are related to a broadening sense of mission and reformulations of values and social policies.

hear; perhaps there is a language barrier; perhaps too many technical terms found their way into the physicians's or other staff member's interpretations; perhaps the physician tried to make known too many things at one time, and half of what was said has been forgotten, especially the half that the patient/family prefers not to hear. Unexpected occurrences cannot be anticipated, but their adverse effect on the patient, relatives, and friends should be observed and reduced to a minimum. For instance, a patient was taken for x-rays in the morning, as expected. What was not expected was that she did not return to her room for five hours. The patient was frustrated, furious, and "all stirred up"; she had not brought "so much as a magazine" with her to while away the waiting time. The friend who had arranged to visit her was frantic with worry, could get no information, and had to leave without seeing the patient. Much of the distress these two friends felt could have been alleviated. Someone could have told the patient that a breakdown in machinery caused a delay and that two of the x-ray plates had required retaking. A simple message to the friend who the patient knew was waiting would have been a worthwhile service.

This story is told to illustrate that the patient can get lost as a flesh-and-blood human being if hospital personnel are not at least as much patient oriented as disease and organ oriented. In effect, the plea is for as much personalized, humanizing behavior as possible on the part of personnel at all levels of responsibility. There cannot be complete administrative or professional control over stress-producing events; but it can be urged that maximum control be a matter of policy and good practice. For example, a physician's unexplained instructions to repeat a diagnostic procedure or add a new one may cause alarm, not only because the patient/family is medically unsophisticated, but much more because anything that is ordered by medical personnel takes on a special significance for all but the most passive persons. Instructions that are not unusual in the eyes of health personnel (who know that first findings may have to be checked or that records inexplicably get mislaid) may in the eyes of the patient point toward danger and disaster. Mysterious orders for "a repeat Pap test" may rouse fearsome fantasies in the patient when in truth there was a technical error which had no medical implications. The common denominator in all these situations is a deep, pervasive, and potentially frightening uncertainty.

For people without a continuing relationship with a primary physician—a description that fits far too many patients/families—it cannot be overemphasized that the inevitable stresses of becoming a patient and undergoing a diagnostic process in a service unit of a hospital can be raised to high magnitude by encountering a strange physician with each new episode of illness or in sequential clinic visits during an episode of illness. The continuity and familiarity that are maintained through other personnel, such as clinic and floor nurses, social workers, and clerical staff, are important and compensatory to a degree. Yet they cannot really make up for the constant rotation required by the educational programs of medical students, interns, and residents in teaching hospitals. Some organizational arrangements do provide continuity of medical care with the same physician throughout a period of rotation and sometimes over a prolonged period of time. For instance, in some hospitals comprehensive medical care clinics staffed by attending physicians only and specialty clinics with similar arrangements do offer patients medical care with the same physician over intervals of many years. Large numbers of patients, however, do not have the relative comfort of knowing their physician and of having physicians who are familiar with their patients, their patients' families, and their way of life. Lack of such security is a source of stress that can be expected to augment the effects of all the other stressful factors. The peculiar kind of uncertainty that accompanies these situations is easily understood: "Does this new doctor know what he or she should know about me?"

Another source of stress associated with the diagnostic process when the patient uses a hospital clinic lies in the risk that privacy and confidentiality of communications may be breached by such conditions as crowded space, inadequate provision of closed cubicles for examinations, and lack of a quiet place where conversation between patient/family and medical care personnel will not be overheard.

Women who require gynecological examinations are apt to experience considerable psychic stress and strain from a combination of factors—when the examining physician is a stranger, when the patients are not helped to relax, when the room seems crowded with observant residents, and when the door to the examining room is not kept closed. These are sources of stress that are not inherent in the diagnostic process or in hospital care; they are avoidable if the primacy of the patient's interests and well-being is accepted. However, there may also be sociocultural factors that increase the problem for some women but cannot be controlled by the institution or its personnel. For example, women whose cultural background strictly prohibits touching the genitalia may need repeated visits to the clinic before they can undergo an adequate examination, and then only if the physician is a woman.

What does happen to the many women with this kind of background whose values are not understood? What happens to any patient in any setting in which there is a discontinuous pattern of physician's care? There is a distinction to be made between the fragmented and intermittent *medical* care so prevalent in our society and the discontinuity of *physician's* care which may occur even when a patient's medical care is continuous. Even continuous medical care is impaired when no relationship between physician and patient can develop. Considering the range of stressful events that can be associated with the diagnostic process, it is timely to note the importance to the patient/family of knowing that there is one physician who has assumed primary responsibility. The need for such security is heightened by the nature of current sophisticated diagnostic processes which may involve many people—perhaps several physicians, a number of laboratory technicians, nurses, a social worker, and possibly others. In consequence, bewilderment, confusion, and anxiety are reactions common to both the socially sophisticated and socially unsophisticated. Neither financial affluence nor a college degree is insurance against impacts of illness; most patients, regardless of socioeconomic background, need access to a professional who can explain, listen, and reassure and who can coordinate prescribed medical care when it becomes a matter so complex as to be beyond the patient's ability to manage.

COMMUNICATING IN THE DIAGNOSTIC PROCESS

A constant flow of communication between patient/family and health care personnel at all levels is implied in becoming a patient and undergoing a diagnostic process.* Much of the exchange is anticipatory and preparatory in

---

* See the section on communication, p. 20.

nature as one procedure and its findings lead to the next step and finally to an integration of data for consideration of their full biopsychosocial meanings.

Communication has different functions during the diagnostic process. Successful communication makes it possible for the patient/family to undergo the necessary diagnostic procedures with the least psychosocial discomfort and for the physician to learn what procedures are required and how best to present and explain them to the patient/family. After an interval—perhaps only a matter of minutes but sometimes a matter of weeks—the time comes when the physician, as the authentic source, has to have a purposeful give-and-take with the patient/family about the findings. If there are significant positive findings, there has first to be communication about "what is wrong." This phrase is used instead of "what the diagnosis is" because it conveys flexibility in what the physician tells the patient/family—that is, flexibility that allows the physician at a given time to avoid or minimize significant sources of stress. Some people never hear and never want to hear the technical word for what is wrong with them. Others insist on knowing "everything," but only some really want to know much or are helped by learning everything. In fact, it would be dangerous to assume what a patient means by "everything." It is far better to encourage the patient to ask a series of questions until he or she feels satisfied—at least for the time being. There is sure to be another series of questions later. Some people are too frightened or too limited intellectually to hear what the physician is saying, forget most of it, and distort the rest. Some listen stoically and let themselves feel the shock and fear too late for the physician to handle in that session. Some look upon the medical profession with awe, say "hm, hm" as the physician talks, never ask a question, but immediately afterward turn to a relative—or the social worker—and ask, "what did the doctor say?"

On the other hand, with rare exeptions patients and relatives want to know *something* and from a medical standpoint *must* know something, however simple and incomplete, in order to participate in decisions about diagnostic procedure and recommended treatment, to say nothing of taking part in the therapeutic process itself.

Although the authority of medical knowledge rests with the physician, who has the prime responsibility for sharing diagnostic findings with the patient/family, social workers have an equally authentic role to play. That role may start with the social worker and the physician discussing and deciding together the approach that will be most fruitful and least distressing in a given patient/family situation. The more complicated the total life-situation and the more threatening the symptoms or characteristics of the diagnosed or suspected illness, the more desirable it is for the physician and social worker together to hold one or more interviews with the patient/family on what is wrong or, even earlier, on recommended diagnostic measures. There are many advantages to this collaborative effort. The patient/family perceives the positive working relationship between physcian and social worker to be reassuring and strengthening. The social worker hears firsthand exactly what the patient/family is told but may not hear or may distort; in continuing contacts with the patient and relatives the social worker is able to repeat, reinforce, and clarify information; encourage expression of feelings and fantasies that should be aired; help clarify the realities of the illness and its consequences; anticipate the need for specific resources to deal with those realities; and see to it that the patient/family has access to the physician for further discussion when that is necessary.

In order to decide what to tell and what to withhold, how much to say today, to which family member to say it, and which questions to answer fully and which in part, the physician will have to include in the diagnostic procedures, as has already been said, an assessment not only of a disease process but also of the people significantly involved and of their relationships and life-situation, on which the illness will surely have some impact. As has been seen, the physician may make his or her assessment in concert with others, one of whom may be a social worker whose knowledge of the patient/family can contribute to the physician's understanding.

On the whole, the emotional reactions of patients and their relatives tend to be similar. However, members of the family group will vary in the intensity of their feelings, in the degree to which they try to conceal their feelings or protect themselves from full awareness, and, of course, in the specific worries that they have. The phenomenon of similar reactions disappears when the adult patient's illness renders him or her incapable of recognizing that he or she is ill or making decisions in his or her own behalf. When the patient was formerly a self-maintaining member of the family, such a change in the balance of interdependence in family responsibilities and relationships is a source of considerable stress: there can be guilt—however irrational—for taking matters out of the patient's control, sadness and a sense of loss, anxiety lest one has made the wrong decision, and so on. A married patient's spouse and their children have to adapt not only to his or her changed responsibilities and ability to function in their family roles but to changes in their own authority, responsibility, and enforced need to make decisions and choices they would not have made alone before. It might be said that each of the patient's limitations due to illness is likely to make a counterdemand for the other family members to take on new or expanded tasks. As early as the diagnostic period patient/families may begin to face these demands for adaptation; they do not arise only during the phases of treatment and rehabilitation. Patients and their relatives need ample opportunity to express their reactions to these demands among one another and to medical care personnel. Often the expression of feelings and attitudes leaves people freer to make their own realistic adjustments and adaptations; some people need, in addition, direct help from professionals who know how to enable others to use their own strengths and to provide available resources most suitable to their needs and desires. Since a successful process of enabling others depends first of all on a successful process of communicating between and among human beings, it will be useful to describe conditions that are most likely to impair, weaken, or destroy that process. They can be classified into four kinds of stress-producing phenomena that can occur when patients/families and medical care personnel try to communicate.

STRESS-PRODUCING PHENOMENA IN COMMUNICATIONS

First, there is language unsuited to the intellectual and emotional capacities of the patient and his or her relatives. If the patient and physician do not have a common language, the use of an interpreter can pose serious problems when the latter is not thoroughly oriented to his or her function and responsibilities in the health care field. Using a family member or friend as an interpreter may be the most feasible arrangement, but it can also be the most dangerous. For example, in the emergency service of a hospital a woman who spoke only Spanish was being palpated. Her husband, who knew some English, was acting as interpreter. He was visibly agitated and worried, and something about his distress made a nearby nurse keep careful watch. Suddenly the nurse heard the patient say in Spanish "it hurts on the right side," but her husband translated it into "left side." At this point the nurse intervened and, as unobtrusively as possible, took over as chief interpreter. An emotionally involved person may be at the same time the most well-intentioned and the most unreliable informant and interpreter.[1]

At times the difficulty arises because the patient/family are emotionally ready for only simple and brief explanations in colloquial language, and the physician has trouble finding the right words. It is always desirable to find out what the well-read patient has in mind when he or she asks such questions as "Do I have coronary disease?" The information the patient has may be too generalized to be useful to him or her, or it may be applicable to the personal experience of a friend or friend of a friend, but not sufficiently pertinent to his or her own condition. In those instances the patient is likely to be enlightened and relieved by having his or her medical problem explained authentically in language that the patient can relate to his or her own symptoms and life situation. Another patient, however, who correctly suspects his or her diagnosis before consulting a physician may have read professional references that were well selected and that he or she understands and applies accurately. Still another may become similarly well informed after his or her physician has discussed diagnostic findings with him or her.

On another plane, there are the cultural differences in language and word usage that are associated with differences in age, educational experience, socioeconomic status, or other factors. These differences have somehow to be bridged, though not always by the physician's adopting the patient's way of self-expression; unless it is natural to the physician, it may sound contrived—even mocking and disrespectul—subverting a sincere intention to be understanding and helpful. It is more important that the physician grasp the meaning of the patient's language, both verbal and nonverbal; the physician's response can be in his or her own style.

How important easy communication is to patients and relatives is illustrated every day as they cluster among themselves or form a group around a staff member who shares their language or style of expression. As one social worker described it, "They make a kind of village green out of the clinic and the clerical staff can learn more than the professionals do about the patients. The receptionists are important members of the staff."

Second, there is *inadequate partialization* of information. The physician and other givers-of-service do not necessarily tell all or tell all at one time. Partialization in the process of communicating refers to breaking down the substance of what is to be transmitted over a period of time. It means (1) giving the patient/family as much information at a given point as they are ready to hear, assimilate, and use and (2) giving the patient/family enough information at a given point to handle their anxiety and to understand and make informed decisions about recommended next steps. The physician can usually rely on patient and relatives to indicate in words and manner what they understand or suspect, what they need to understand, and what they want to hear or want not to hear. It is not easy to read and respond to all those messages from the patient/family. One plea, protest, gesture, or question can contain several levels or layers of meaning.* In addition, the several members of a family do not necessarily have the same needs and wants, and the physician may have to anticipate, among other things, how his or her responses will affect the balance of relationships in the family group.

For example, by partializing their interventions and communications, a collaborating physician and social worker helped to keep a patient in command of herself and her family situation even as they prepared her over a period of time for eventual loss of vision. The patient's pride in supporting herself and her two adopted children was intense and needed to be left intact insofar as possible. As is so often the case, especially with progressive diseases, the first diagnostic period was followed at necessary intervals by numerous periods of reassessment. Careful partialization was an integral factor in patient-physician-social worker communication during each of the successive periods. The original messsage the physician conveyed was that the patient's right eye was infected and inflamed; the medicine he was prescribing would clear up the infection, and he expected that her vision would remain as it was for a time. Later he had to tell her the same thing about her left eye. Still later he said that if the current medication did not work, he would have to operate. And that led to the patient herself taking the painful step of asking whether that meant removal of her right eye. Parallel to the physician's partialization was the social worker's. She made consistent efforts to uphold the patient's ability to take appropriate action, step by step, and prepare the children for each new aspect of the situation. Resources for financial assistance and for retraining were made available when the patient could use them to greatest advantage. The children were gradually brought into active participation and came to understand how they, the physician, the social worker, and various staff members of the community's agency for the blind would share responsibility with the patient for care of the total family while sharing was necessary.

But sometimes the giver-of-service is blocked by his or her human emotions and all but fails to partialize. For example, at the time of the first overwhelming shock of learning that he or she has cancer a patient may say, "What can you do for me?"—meaning "right now." The physician who misunderstands the patient's request for (partial) information leaps silently to the knowledge that there is no assurance of cure. The physician stumbles in responding, "thinking five years ahead of the patient," so that the communication is faulty and unsatisfying when the patient's anxiety is high. Fortunately, the situation is usually recovered quickly because the physician naturally says something about immediate treatment. But the different levels at which patient and physician may be speaking and thinking can threaten the development of a good working relationship between them.

Third, there is the untruthful message sent by a giver-of-service and perceived by the patient/family as an untruth. Human beings, as we have seen, can function at more than one level at a time. So it is that personnel in health care—sometimes knowingly, sometimes unwittingly—speak words or make gestures that are not believed by the patient/family because the conveyer of the message is uncomfortable about what he or she is saying or doing. It is the incredibility that comes through and that is distressing to the patient/family,

---

* See the section on communication, p. 20.

even when the intention of the giver-of-service was to be compassionate and helpful.[2, 3]

It is important to distinguish between this form of perceived fabrication (which does not assure but rather undermines strength and confidence) and *partial* information which is truthful as far as it goes and can be made more complete in ongoing communication without retraction of what has gone before.

An "untruth" that responds to the patient/family's wish to hear something they know is untrue is still another matter. Often when this happens no one is deceived or betrayed; everyone knows the truth but conspires in a pretense shared silently with everyone else. It is their mutually accepted protection—perhaps only for a time, perhaps throughout a patient's illness. Truth, when linked with hope, is accepted and acted upon constructively by a large number of patient/families. The essential element of hope takes many forms but to be consistent with truth needs to be realistically presented by health care personnel. Whereas cure is an appropriate hope for some, for others assurance that pain will be kept at a minimum or that vocational retraining will be available or that there will be time for the terminally ill patient to plan for the family's future may be the impetus for looking forward and living as fully as possible in whatever time there is.

Fourth, there is the *disconnected message*—the message from health care personnel that is not made relevant to the patient/family's life-situation. Transmission of medical information, to be intellectually and emotionally incorporated and usable, needs to be specifically and openly connected with individual and family conditions for optimal effectiveness. Explanations about recommended diagnostic procedures and the findings that result should be not only medically but also socially oriented to the circumstances of the individual patient/family. Most medicosocial connections have both cognitive and emotional connotations, again illustrating the indivisibility of the biopsychosocial nature of human experience. Physicians and their colleagues are comfortably aware of some connections, may anxiously anticipate or exaggerate others, and perhaps try not to see those connections with execptionally painful implications. Following are a few of the most common and the simplest kinds of medicosocial connections which need to be brought into the open, either as being problematic or as strengths to be relied on and used.

Connections between medical conditions and financial circumstances are frequent and anxiety producing even during the diagnostic period. There are innumerable ways in which these connections manifest themselves. The laboratory tests and examinations are a strain on many people's incomes. The adult with a modest income and either no health insurance or insurance that covers only the costs incurred during hospitalization is among those in a tight financial squeeze from the beginning stages of illness and throughout its course. The patient may not be old enough for Medicare or poor enough for Medicaid or eligible for federal disability insurance unless completely disabled.* Yet at the beginning of the patient's illness, he or she already feels financial strain or anticipates it with anxiety. Even when the adult patient is eligible for public financial aid for medical care (Medicaid in New York State), such financial assiatance may not include the cost of transportation between home and medical

---

* In 1972 amendments to the federal law made some adults under 65 years of age, with specified diseases, eligible for Medicare.

facility. Furthermore, there are patients who do not know what benefits they are entitled to and may not even realize that they should ask about them. A frequently anticipated consequence that causes worry and dread concerns the possible loss of a job and therefore of income should the diagnostic period require too much time away from work.

Failure to keep clinic appointments is often due to such practical but emotionally laden problems rather than to lack of concern or denial of illness. Even if the United States establishes a funding mechanism and a system or network of systems that provides a continuum of medical care for everyone, there will be problematic connections between illness and finances at all stages of illness. For the most part these connections will exist as long as health-related programs and services are fragmented, discontinuous, uncoordinated, and, at times, not available or not accessible to those who need them. For example, inadequate and bad housing is so closely related to low economic status that one has to be alert to significant connections between it and events in the diagnostic and treatment periods. When bathroom, cooking, and sleeping quarters in an overcrowded tenement apartment afford no protection to the patient and other members of the family and when there are strict regulations for bed utilization but too few or no facilities in the community for less than hospital care and more than home care, then the patient/family are caught in an ugly situation which may be handled (not resolved) at the cost of family relationships and, no doubt, at considerable cost to the patient's health status.[4]

Other connections have to do less with finances and more with personal relationships and social tasks and values. For instance, the young mother who needs a series of diagnostic tests is fortunate if she can arrange with a family member or reliable neighbor to care for her children of preschool age or make lunch for the older ones who come home at noon. Many mothers in this position have no choice but to come to the clinic with their children. The play-waiting room available in a hospital to children of adult ambulatory patients without question meets an important need. But there are days when the children are better off at home, or they just seem too much for a woman who is "dragging herself around." Elderly or sick relatives in the home may need protection and care while the patient is at the clinic. The patient may need help to get to the clinic because of a physical disability coupled with a problem of transportation and the inconvenient time of his or her scheduled appointment.

There are inevitable problems created by medical needs, such as having to arrive at clinic at eight in the morning without breakfast and after an hour's subway and bus ride in order to have a barium enema. There is the conflict-of-interest situation as when a mother's obligations toward her children clash with her own need for medical care. And there is the problem of decision making which does not involve external circumstances or the welfare of other people but expresses an individual's internal conflict about his or her personal situation—say, a conflict between the desire to be well and the fear of surgery—which makes it difficult to accept fully his or her medical diagnosis or give consent to recommended intervention.

For example, a woman whose concern about the care of her husband, children, and household was vastly reduced when she was assured of a homemaker's services still could not decide about a recommended herniotomy. The surgeon, who described the operation as minor, could not understand the patient's continued indecision until the social worker uncovered the private drama.

A few years previously, when the patient was first hospitalized for a hernia repair, the physicians discovered that she was pregnant, and the surgery was not performed. She recalled her depression and despair; she had not planned the pregnancy, nor did she want a fourth child. She did have a tubal ligation after the child's birth and knew that this time she was not pregnant. Still, she had a persistent fear that the doctors would "go in and find something" and she might not live after the operation. Encouraged to talk more about her fear, the patient described the experiences of two close relatives. An uncle died because he neglected to have his hernia taken care of. An older brother did consent to surgery, but the surgeon discovered he had cancer, and after several more operations the brother died. "So,". said the patient, "I know I might die if I do have an operation, and I might die if I don't." Three staff members—the surgeon, a resident, and a social worker—worked with the patient to help her make a decision. They reviewed the predictable risks and benefits of the operation, made all possible distinctions between the patient's situation and that of her uncle and brother, and duly recognized her ability to make sound judgments in previous crises. In two months the patient said she was ready to enter the hospital. She made a quick recovery after surgery and resumed her family responsibilities with a sense of satisfaction.

On a broader scale there are cultural influences that bear on the meanings of the diagnostic process and should be instructive to givers-of-service obligated to establish successful communication with patients/families and their significant others. Cultural influences are realities to be understood and evaluated, not disregarded or overruled as evidence of irrationality and ignorance. To some people drawing blood for a laboratory test does literally mean taking away their strength. There can be true resistance to going through a diagnostic process if the patient believes that it is the will of God to test his or her faith through illness. Similarly, the patient who believes her sister-in-law has put a curse upon her will tend to disbelieve that laboratory tests and x-rays will help her. When near and distant family members pour into the hospital, it has to be learned whether the gathering is an expected sign of solidarity and mutual support or whether it is a panic reaction in the family circle or a warning signal of less than complete trust in the hospital.

It has to be understood whether moaning and groaning are the natural responses of a people who freely express their sorrow and fear, indications of severe pain, or idiosyncratic distress signals of an individual in crisis. It has to be understood, for example, whether a patient's silence reflects the reluctance of people in his or her ethnic group to discuss personal and private matters with anyone outside the family, whether the patient usually has difficulty in relating to others, or whether the patient is simply cautious about confiding in someone whom he or she has not yet learned to trust.

What may be legends, myths, or strange folkways to physicians and their colleagues can be integral parts of the patient/family's way of life. The patient/

family need not be restrained from acting upon their beliefs unless their actions endanger their own or others' safety. When the patient believes the diagnosis of benign tumor is the result of all the novenas that were said for him, there is no need to disturb his faith; to the contrary, the support he receives from prayer merits everyone's approval. One need not interfere with a patient's sprinkling a mixture of her excretions and nail parings on her neighbor's doorstep to make her stop seducing the patient's husband. But it calls for intervention if a psychotic patient hears voices that tell her to put poison in her neighbor's coffee.[5] "Magic (of which gambling is a functional equivalent), science, and religion are a 'three-cornered constellation.' They are distinct but interconnected modes of adjustment which enable men to meet uncertainty, attain rational mastery of their environment, and deal with problems of meaning, respectively.."[6]

Cultural and idiosyncratic factors affect personnel as well as the consumers of health care. All practitioners in the field of health should be aware of the effects that their own attitudes, behavior, feelings, and values have upon others and of the ways in which others affect them. The corollary principle is that practitioners in the field are responsible for controlling and regulating their own reactions and responses in order to avoid harmful effects and enhance beneficial effects on patients/families and colleagues alike.

The professional staff member has a double responsibility insofar as he has been socialized into the subculture of his profession. He needs to recognize what the subculture is and how it affects him and others. Such knowledge can be a powerful instrument in achieving good staff relationships which in a complex, highly structured institution are essential to establishing and maintaining good patient care. Also, one must question whether givers-of-service who are not sensitive to the significance of the cultures and subcultures that nurture them and their colleagues are capable of sensitivity to the culture of a patient/ family or patient population and are able to shape the communications within the framework of that culture. In any case, however, the greater the distance between the cultures of one party and another, the greater the difficulty in mutual understanding and acceptance of differences. In particular, different expectations regarding roles, responsibilities, and relationships within the family; differences in attitudes toward accepting help from community resources; and differences in responding to illness, discomfort, and pain are capable of calling forth responses from personnel that are stress producing to the patient/family.

Thus a physician who values reserve and constraint may look upon an expressive, demanding patient as a complainer and a bad patient. Personnel whose culture puts a high price on self-reliance may look with disfavor on a patient's receiving supportive services from the community for which he or she does not pay. Again, foreign-born personnel (who are currently in great numbers in hospitals in metropolitan areas) often cannot accept cultural differences in outlook on families and family responsibilities. Physicians brought up to believe in the dignity of old age and to behave with respect toward the head of the household can become so indignant over our ways of behaving that they try to impose their patterns upon the patients/families they are treating. It is incomprehensible to many physicians raised in an oriental culture that in our society many of the elderly live apart from younger members of their families. In the eyes of those physicians, children have abandoned their parents; it is hard for them to understand that physical separateness does not inevitably mean social and psychological separateness or to believe that, in many instances, the older person wishes to maintain his or her own home.

The great diversity of values, attitudes, and customs that characterizes this nation is mirrored in its regions, states, and other subunits and institutions. In the narrower focus of the hospital, as in the larger society, that diversity is a challenge, a basis for perpetual conflict, or a basis for richness in opportunity for communicating and problem solving during the diagnostic process and the processes that follow.

The events in the adult patient's experience during the diagnostic period which lead into the conditions that confront him or her during treatment and rehabilitation are exemplified in the following case histories by observing how two families, the patients' physicians, and a social worker participated in and coped with a stressful and critical diagnostic period which terminated in each patient's consenting to surgery. In each instance the adult patient's physician called on the social worker for assistance, but with a difference in perception and perspective that affected the social worker's activities and the patients/families' decision making. There are also other significant differences, such as differences in the quality and strength of family relationships, in the degree of medical-social risk that confronted these two patient/family groups, and in the degree to which the members were able and enabled to use the help of physicians and the social worker. Each of these medicosocial histories bridges the way to the processes of treatment and rehabilitation which will be discussed in the chapter that follows.

Mrs. Perez, the social worker, was asked by Dr. Roberts, the attending gynecologist, to talk with him and the chief resident, Dr. Powell, about Mrs. Riviera and her family. Dr. Roberts thought an assessment of the home situation was needed. In addition, he asked her to arrange interviews in which he, Dr. Powell, and Mrs. Perez could discuss first with the patient and then with the patient and her husband the findings and recommended surgery. The surgeons hoped that the patient would consent and her husband approve.

Mrs. Perez learned from the medical record that Mrs. Riviera was 36 years old, born in the Caribbean, and married to a man of 42 from the same island. They had a boy and a girl in their teens who visited the patient regularly, as did her husband.

Mrs. Riviera had been admitted to the hospital on an emergency basis two weeks before Mrs. Perez was called into the situation. The patient's presenting symptom was rectal and vaginal bleeding; the decision to admit her immediately was made because seven years ago she had had radiotherapy for cervical carcinoma. Although Mrs. Riviera said she had had no medical problems for the past seven years until the bleeding started three weeks before coming to the clinic, the gynecologists who examined her believed that recurrence of the carcinoma was a possibility.

Mrs. Perez met with the two surgeons who explained that following two weeks of diagnostic procedures, they and two consulting gynecologists had decided to recommend surgery that would be complex and lengthy. They could not predict the extent of the surgery or whether it would result in cure. If the patient and her husband refused surgery, it was estimated that Mrs. Riviera would have a life expectancy of about one year. If they consented, there was a chance, but no guarantee, of cure. The surgeons realized that many factors were involved in the patient's making a decision and wanted to be sure that both she and her husband understood clearly what the risks were. The surgeons were certain a complete hysterectomy would have to be performed; cystectomy and colostomy might also have to be performed.

The significance of this extensive surgery was so laden with emotion for Mrs. Perez and the surgeons were so attuned to the probable impact upon her that the three of them spent a long hour examining the recommended surgical plan and discussing the potential emotional and psychological consequences for the patient/family. Each of the professionals understood that Mrs. Perez had to have time to resolve her own emotional reactions before she could be of help to the Rivieras. The surgeons' feelings were by then unambiguous and free of ambivalence about their recommendation.

On the following day Mrs. Perez joined the gynecologists when they told Mrs. Riviera what they recommended and why, the risks, the hoped-for outcome, and the alternative outcome if she did not have surgery. In the social worker's words, "The impact of what the doctors said was so great that, even though she understood English, Mrs. Riviera asked me to tell her in Spanish." Mrs. Riviera's first response to Mrs. Perez's interpretation was silence and withdrawal; then, when urged to say whatever she wanted, she expressed her horror of becoming disabled, "a vegetable." The surgeons repeated their explanations, bit by bit, emphasizing the advantages of her age and general state of good health, the opinions of the two consulting gynecologists, and describing again her bodily functioning should her intestinal tract be involved. The surgeons left Mrs. Riviera's bedside, encouraging her to think things over, and promising further talks with them and Mrs. Perez.

Mrs. Perez stayed on, hoping that Mrs. Riviera might express herself more freely than in the surgeons' presence. At first Mrs. Riviera cried, then said, "I think I have cancer. With the operation or without it, people die from it anyway. If I am to die, let it be God's will. It is better to leave me the way I am than to be useless as a woman."

Mrs. Perez agreed that God's will is undeniable but reminded her that on earth we all had to make hard choices. Mrs. Perez expressed her and the surgeons' confidence in Mrs. Riviera's strength to make a decision. Spontaneously, the patient reviewed her illness. She repeated that she had been told seven years ago that she had cancer. She followed this remark immediately by saying that the vaginal bleeding which brought her to clinic two weeks ago started after she carried a heavy bundle of laundry. Mrs. Perez disregarded this transitory attempt to deny and spent the remainder of the hour engaging the patient in a discussion of how Mrs. Riviera would be thinking about her husband and children while she made up her mind about the operation.

Mr. and Mrs. Riviera were seen together on the following day when the two gynecologists and Mrs. Perez went over the ground again. The couple were encouraged to ask questions and to express their hopes and fears. They were reluctant to consent to surgery but were obviously asking for help in reaching a decision. In this joint interview Dr. Roberts prepared Mrs. Riviera for some further examinations and tests. There was no pressure in this or subsequent interviews for the patient to make a quick decision.

The surgeons and the social worker were constantly available during the next two weeks, largely because the patient found it hard to have more doctors and technicians "work" on her and because her tolerance for pain and discomfort was running out.

It was during this interval that Mr. and Mrs. Riviera began to talk to each other more openly about her illness and the future. They drew Mrs. Perez into their discussions, which contained both happy reminiscences of their family life and apprehension about Mrs. Riviera's predictably long hospitalization, whether or not she underwent surgery.

The financial situation was eased when the family was declared eligible for Medicaid and when, with the surgeon's help in completing the forms, Mrs. Riviera filed for and received sick benefits from her trade union.

Despite the children's ages, the parents wanted an adult woman to be "in charge" when their father was at work or visiting Mrs. Riviera as he now did daily. An aunt of the patient agreed to move into the home for two or three months and take over some of Mrs. Riviera's tasks during this period of uncertainty.

These two weeks of indecision were marked by the patient's moods, which varied from depression to her first show of violent anger in protest against "these tests." It was a time, too, when Mr. Riviera saw Mrs. Perez frequently. Shy and passive though he was, he spoke with emotion of his wife's condition but without acknowledging that she had cancer. The children now began to notice their mother's sadness and silences and spoke to Mr. Riviera of finding her in tears several times. He could not bring himself to tell them how serious their mother's condition was, nor did he and the patient want anyone else to tell them. The hospital staff honored this wish as a protective device for the parents which should not be disturbed at that time.

It was under these stressful circumstances—a month after diagnostic procedures were initiated and two weeks after the patient, her husband, two surgeons, and a social worker started working together supportively in a process of crucial decision making—that Mrs. Riviera, with her husband's approval, gave signed consent to the recommended surgery.

Mrs. Perez, the social worker,* received a call from Dr. Russ, surgical resident in the gynecology clinic, asking her to obtain homemaker service for Mrs. Fernandez, who was to be hospitalized in five days for a hysterectomy. Mr. Fernandez worked, and there were three sons and two daughters ranging from 9 to 17 years of age. Dr. Russ expected the patient to be in the hospital for about ten days.

The hospital records first described the family situation eight years

---

* The same social worker worked with both the Riviera and Fernandez families.

earlier. Mr. and Mrs. Fernandez, then 36 and 33 years old respectively, were born in Cuba but had been on the mainland since adolescence. They were bilingual, as were their children. The patient at that time was Carla, the third child, then five years old. She had a complicated cardiac lesion; surgery had been considered but was postponed indefinitely and never performed. The child was found to be disturbed, overactive, and difficult to control; although psychiatric treatment was recommended for her, the parents decided against it. Both Mr. and Mrs. Fernandez were said to be rigid and controlling; while both parents seemed frightened of illness, Mr. Fernandez's overt reaction was to become angry when the children were ill.

Approximately a year later Mrs. Fernandez came in with a menstrual problem, though she was more concerned about limiting the size of her family. She asked for tubal ligation, which Mr. Fernandez opposed for several months. He finally gave his signed consent, and the procedure was completed. There were no further entries until the current ones concerning Mrs. Fernandez's recommended hysterectomy.

Mrs. Fernandez had one more clinic appointment before being admitted to the hospital, and on that day Mrs. Perez talked with her at some length. She was tense, anxious about how the children would be cared for during her absence, and worried about the operation. She feared that she would hemorrhage if she had intercourse after the operation. She said her husband "wants things his way," but that she "makes the decisions." He was opposed to the operation, but she chose to go through with it; if it made her healthy, she could take proper care of the children. "He won't even discipline them; he's afraid they won't love him."

Mrs. Fernandez described the children so that the social worker could tell the homemaker about them. Pete, 17, was in high school and doing well. Frank, the 16-year-old, was in another high school and making poor grades. He tended to fool around and distract the other pupils as well. Mrs. Fernandez seemed overprotective as she spoke of Carla, now 13, but the child was doing well in seventh grade, she was less excitable, and her heart condition was said not to interfere with her school and play life. Fred, 12, and Rosa, 8, were said to be good, healthy, active children doing average work in school. Mrs. Perez noted that Mrs. Fernandez talked about each child with concern for his or her well-being but with little warmth in her voice or manner and no evidence that either parent was openly affectionate; distance and rigidity seemed descriptive of the home atmosphere, the social worker thought.

The family's physical environment seemed adequate as Mrs. Fernandez described it. They occupied a six-room apartment in a two-family house outside of Manhattan; the furnishings and equipment would make it possible for a homemaker to keep the rooms clean and orderly.

Mr. Fernandez earned a modest income at his regular job and augmented it by working overtime. All members of the family were eligible for Medicaid at the time of Mrs. Fernandez's admission to the hospital for the hysterectomy.*

---

* Eligibility requirements for Medicaid are liable to change, the tendency being to "cut," that is, to lower the amount of family income permitted for approval for Medicaid.

In the one interview Mrs. Perez had with the patient before her surgery the marital relationship emerged as the most conflicted and problematic facet of her life-situation and the most closely related to the operation. During the past two years sexual relations had been difficult, largely, Mrs. Fernandez believed, because of her gynecological complaints. She had been fearful of intercourse because of "bleeding several times a month." Mr. Fernandez became very angry with her, and they were not talking to each other at all; nor was he talking to the children. The only verbal communication among family members was among the patient and the children. Mr. Fernandez's opposition to the operation, the patient explained, was due to his belief that they would be unable to have sexual intercourse for many months. Both spouses had the idea that the operation would permanently deprive the patient of all desire for intercourse. Mrs. Perez gave the patient correct information, limiting herself to the distorted ideas specifically expressed by Mrs. Fernandez. The patient was pleased with Mrs. Perez's offer to talk with Mr. Fernandez about plans to care for the children as well as about the surgery.

Mr. Fernandez refused an interview with the social worker in person but talked with her, albeit angrily and fearfully, over the telephone. He said he would not consent to his wife's operation; she was old enough to decide for herself. He did not want her examined and operated on by so many male doctors. Nor would he come to talk with the surgeon, either, to get answers to his questions.

The five-days' interval between the social worker's entry into the family's situation and the patient's hospitalization was sufficient to obtain homemaker services, an achievement that allayed Mrs. Fernandez's anxiety about the care of her family. On the other hand, the patient had to take responsibility for consenting to surgery not only without the support of her husband but under the cloud of his disapproval and anger.

The experiences of these two families during the period of diagnosis and assessment can be examined in several dimensions. The interaction of biological, psychological, and socioenvironmental elements in each instance is vividly illustrated; among these the quality of familial relations and their significance in the medicosocial situation of each family are highly instructive. The painful impacts of the diagnostic process itself are open to analysis; they can be seen in the context of personal characteristics, family relations, the kinds of medicosocial risks, and the complex nature of deciding whether to consent to the recommended intervention. The different ways in which the physicians perceive the patient/family's life-and-illness situation and their determination of the social worker's point of entry lead logically to questioning what elements in the organization and structure of the hospital and in the deployment and functioning of hospital-based social workers account for the case-findings by physicians rather than by a social worker.

Not all patients/families have similarly stress-producing experiences in their first period of medical care. However there are sufficient numbers who do to suggest that they be afforded appropriate, adequate assistance in coping and that there be full recognition of the influence these experiences will have on the subsequent period of treatment and rehabilitation.

Throughout this chapter social workers, implicitly and explicitly, connected their exploratory and explanatory activities with the primary role of the physicians in the diagnostic process. The efforts of both groups serve to anticipate with patients/families what lies, or may lie, ahead and to help prepare them for informed decision making.

In all three of the detailed case examples* there are repeated references to patients having to decide whether to follow physicians' recommendations. The data in these brief medicosocial histories illustrate how the professional activities of social workers complement those of the physicians in enabling patients to make informed decisions, whether they concern diagnostic procedures or therapeutic interventions. The physician's and the hospital's legal obligation to obtain the patient's informed consent complements the social worker's value-beliefs, especially the worth of the individual and maximum feasible self-determination.[7]

Social workers have an ethical commitment to the client's right to informed consent in regard to the psychosocial components of diagnosis and treatment. For example, social workers and their clients agree explicitly to work together to solve specified problems and strive toward agreed-upon goals.

Perhaps the oldest and most frequent occasions for the social worker's seeking the client's informed consent concern the social worker's contacts with other people in the client's behalf. The social worker is obligated to obtain informed consent before giving to or eliciting from others information about the client that is intended to be of benefit to him or her.

Since so much of the social worker's activity is to make resources available to the client, the volume of contacts with those others and the range of resources tapped can be quite large. In hospital-based practice these may be the patient's key relatives and friends, employer, clergyman, physicians, and so on, whose sympathetic support, compassion, and ability to contribute some form of assistance will increase the well-being of the patient.

Added to the list of individuals are those community organizations and agencies whose services would benefit the patient and his or her relatives. The hospital-based social worker has to convey to the representatives of these agencies information that proves the patient/family's eligibility and clarifies as precisely as possible the kind of help needed, the length of time it will be needed, and so on. Similarly, the social worker in the hospital, in order to continue his or her role responsibly, may need to inquire how the client used and responded to the services provided the the client in the past or how he or she is benefiting from services currently provided.

In all of the foregoing circumstances informed consent is intended to safeguard the privacy and confidentiality that can be waived legally only by the mentally competent adult patient himself or herself. In operational terms, the client's informed consent** helps to protect him or her and the givers-of-service against the risks of hidden agenda and concealed or secret professional actions. Within this framework, the social worker, like the physician, has to consider the scope of information and understanding a given patient/family should have at a

---

* The patient in need of a herniotomy (pp. 61), Mrs. Riviera (pp. 63–65), and Mrs. Fernandez (pp. 65–67).

**Although informed consent is often given in an oral exchange, it is given to the social worker in writing and signed by the client whenever legally required.

given time; the merits of interprofessional collaboration versus parallel coordinated efforts; the best means of achieving successful communication with a given patient/family in the process of obtaining informed consent; and the distinctive responsibilities apportioned to physician and social worker respectively, in accordance with the legal and professional authority invested in members of each profession.

The hospital setting poses a special problem in respect to preserving the client-patient's privacy and confidentiality. There must be records, chart notations, consent forms, laboratory reports, and other documents which are guides to the patient's medical care and help to minimize the risks incurred by him or her and by the multiprofessional, multidisciplinary staff members who provide services. Secretaries and typists, nurses, social workers, and numbers of technicians have access to patients' records in the course of carrying out their officially assigned tasks. How confidential is confidential? Do all patients/families realize how accessible their records are and have to be to numerous persons within the hospital walls without the patient's explicit, formal consent?

Social workers constantly have to formulate concisely and accurately for the medical chart what could be lengthy narratives about a patient/family's psychosocial situation and the social worker's projected plans and ongoing activities. A major problem for the social worker in writing these notations is to make them useful to himself or herself and others without revealing details that should be kept out of the chart, with its many prospective readers, but that may be conveyed, with informed consent and by other means, to givers-of-service who must have them in order to do their work competently.[8] Eternal vigilance rather than the perfect solution seems to be the answer to meeting our legal, moral, and ethical obligations.

REFERENCES

1. Hugh James Lurie and George Lawrence, "Communication Problems Between Rural Mexican-American Patients and Their Physicians: Description of a Solution," *American Journal of Orthopsychiatry*, vol. 42, no. 5 (October 1972).
2. L. Beaty Pemberton, "Should We Tell the Truth?" *Resident and Staff Physician*, vol. 18 (May 1972).
3. Alan Keith-Lucas, "Ethics in Social Work," in *Encyclopedia of Social Work*, 17th ed. (Washington, D.C.: National Association of Social Workers, 1977), pp. 350-356.
4. Nora Piore, "Health As a Social Problem," in *Encyclopedia of Social Work*, op. cit., pp. 525-540.
5. Lurie and Lawrence, op. cit.
6. Renee C. Fox, *Experiment Perilous: Physicians and Patients Facing the Unknown* (New York: Free Press, 1959), p. 232.
7. Ruth I. Knee, "Health Care: Patients' Rights," in *Encyclopedia of Social Work*, op.cit., pp. 541-544.
8. "No Secrets," *Observer Review*, (London) February 6, 1972.

Chapter 4
The Adult Patient:

THE PERIOD AND PROCESS
OF TREATMENT AND REHABILITATION

Whereas the period and processes of diagnosis and assessment can be bounded by becoming a patient, which is the beginning step, and making a decision about continuing into treatment, which is the final step, social work practice in the acute general hospital makes slight distinction between treatment and rehabilitation. In explanation it can be said that the dynamic psychosocial orientation of social workers and their perspective on social functioning account for their consideration of treatment and rehabilitation as a continuum. From a social work perspective, minimizing or preventing disability in social functioning has to start early in the process of medical care; and rehabilitation should be thought of in reference to all patients and not only in regard to those with marked physical impairment or exceedingly impoverished opportunity, or, as it once was, in reference mainly to vocational retraining. These ideas are compatible with current definitions and concepts expressed by experts in rehabilitation in the field of health care. For example, Spencer and Mitchell define disability as "a reduction in personal coping and adaptive function which causes significant limitations in overall performance in daily living." After defining handicaps as forms of impairment and the rehabilitative process as aiming to control or reverse handicapping conditions, the authors go on to say, "The process of limiting disability must begin in the acute disease hospital. . . . [1] And Phillips underscores this notion in a companion article when he says, "Ideally, rehabilitation is initiated *at an early stage of treatment* to avoid complications of further limitations that might later retard or prevent a return of function."[2] Naturally, the physicians cite examples of early control of disability for the purpose of preventing physical handicaps such as bedsores, contractures, and muscular weakness. But they refer also to early measures directed toward the social, emotional, and vocational aspects of daily living. It is here that one sees a firm congruence with the social worker's point of view about rehabilitation. However, all three processes—diagnostic, treatment, and rehabilitative—are related by the prior experiences of the individual patient/family, which influence their current ability to cope and their hopes, aspirations, and belief in a future.

The impacts of the treatment and rehabilitative processes derive from many events and conditions peculiar to these processes. However, there are others similar to, or repetitious of, earlier experiences in the diagnostic process. Difficulties in communication, uncertainty, hospital regulations which are stressful and distressing for the patient/family, the interactions between biomedical factors and socioenvironmental conditions—these and many others will appear and reappear as possible and probable sources of stress. The specifics of these events and conditions will differ, but they will fall within the categories of demands for adaptation previously described.* The issue of illness begins, for the patient, with the first symptom. For the physician it often begins much earlier. Once a patient seeks medical attention, the course of the illness becomes a major strand of experience. It intertwines with the course of treatment and rehabilitation and with all the psychosocial aspects of living connected with the situation of illness. These strands are difficult to disentangle; they have little meaning when they are arbitrarily separated because then they are out of the context of human living. Thus, in what follows an attempt is made to put emphasis first on one strand and then on another, while maintaining the dynamic relations among them.

STRESSFUL EVENTS AND CONDITIONS INHERENT IN ILLNESS

A wealth of material emerges from the social worker's keen perceptions of psychosocial and emotional distress in others and from their unflagging—sometimes even stubborn—efforts to alleviate it. Their perspective requires that they note how significant phenomena that occur in the course of an illness impinge on patients/families and health care personnel and make heavy demands for adaptation. Most frequently the social workers identify uncertainty, pain, the occurrence and recurrence of acute episodes in a chronic condition, and the recurrence of symptoms after periods of remission; changes in bodily strength, functioning, and appearance; changes in intellectual and emotional capacity; and changes in the ability to perform the tasks of daily living. Some changes herald worsening conditions; many changes are for the better. Some are more predictable or gradual than others and do not result in the crisis and shock that sudden or unexpected change produces.

Uncertainty— one of the distressing anxiety-producing attributes of the diagnostic process—is also a pervasive, inherent element in the processes of treatment and rehabilitation. It is so pervasive and so impelling in its demand for adaptation that a highly concentrated and lengthy discussion of it would not be as useful as keeping it in context, that is, discussing it wherever it appears as a significant aspect of the treatment of disease, deficits, and disability. Uncertainty is openly expressed by many patients in such questions as the following: What will happen to me? Will I have to live with this disease? Can I be cured? Will it come back? Will it get worse? Will I die of it?

Many laypersons do not realize that the practice of medicine is not an exact science, that the etiology of many diseases is unknown, that the outcome of most forms of therapy can be estimated over a range of probabilities but not

* See Introduction to Part II, pp. 45–50.

precisely predicted, and that, among many other uncertainties, medical research, whether basic or applied, at times leads to further uncertainties rather than to indisputable truth.

The patient/family is therefore likely to undergo disappointment and continued uncertainty when the physician cannot guarantee "cure" or satisfactorily explain how the patient got sick in the first place. Along the same lines, contradictory opinions and recommendations from two or more physicians add to the anxiety that uncertainty creates, although it must be noted on the positive side that diverse opinions offer the patient the choice to which he or she is entitled. But making the choice is not a responsibility every patient wants to take, and he or she may suffer from another level of uncertainty after deciding on one rather than another.

Physical pain— frequently the precipitating factor in an individual's search for medical care, and likely to occur also when certain diagnostic procedures are made — is an inescapable element in the course of many diseases and in the use of some interventive measures. Adult patients sometimes suffer more fear of anticipated pain than they suffer distress over the actual experience. Relatives also suffer from the patient's anticipated and actual pain. Health care personnel need to be sensitive to this elemental fear — a fear that they often share, especially when they know they can do little, or not enough, to eliminate it.

Just as patients/families have their distinctive ways of reacting to pain or the threat of pain, so do hospital staff members respond variously to the reactions of patients/families.

Patients/families reflect their cultural traditions and heritage in the way they bear or do not bear pain. Some people are frightened by any kind of pain and seek relief freely—they want to know the source of their pain and what can be done about it. Some people who have learned to deal stoically with severe socioeconomic deprivations react to pain in the same way.

Patients brought up in awe of medical authority may not tell their physicians of their pain but want a nurse or social worker to act as an intermediary in the quest for relief.

Some cultures encourage free expression of emotion and others encourage restraint and concealment of emotion. Reactions to pain usually follow a person's general cultural pattern; for example, he or she openly complains and moans or endures silently.

However diverse people's reactions are to their own or other's pain, all observers agree on the subjective character of pain and of tolerance for it. The social worker's recognition of pain as a highly individualized and personal experience within the structure of a cultural pattern is reflected in his or her careful listening to complaints of pain and in being alert to the absence of complaint when complaint is expected:

> *Pain and illness are stress situations to which individuals respond*
> *as people, as humans equipped with intricate biophysical, bio-*
> *chemical, physiological, and psychological mechanisms which*
> *enable them to adapt to stress, whatever its origin. However, stress*
> *is also a cultural experience in perception as well as in interpreta-*
> *tion and, as such, is responded to by behavior and attitudes*
> *learned within the culture in which the individual is brought up.*

> To ask whether the man's biopsychophysical endowment or his
> cultural background is more important in allowing him to survive
> under stress is pointless and futile. The most we can hope to
> achieve is to assess the functions of different components in the
> biocultural process of man's struggle for survival.[3]

Even when pain can be alleviated or eliminated the actual experience of
pain is always a lonely one, seldom describable, and not measurable by anyone
other than the patient. Current experiments may discover a way to measure it.

The situation that creates patients/families' most stressful dilemmas,
frustration, discouragement, and perhaps despondency or uncontrollable anger
occurs when pain becomes intractable and serves no purpose. This is the
situation that givers-of-service and patients' relatives and close friends abhor
and, in time, may find unendurable. Sympathy and empathy may persist, but
they may be overwhelming to powerless onlookers. When the capacity to help
the sufferer is played out, that is, when no further techniques or drugs for the
relief of pain are available, then the time may come when the giver-of-service is
tempted to turn his or her back on the unendurable. It is then when the patient
most needs human contact and emotional support. The giver-of-service who has
not developed the attribute of detached concern is liable to become a needy
person who can no longer satisfy the needs of another.

The human voice and the human touch in themselves do not relieve
physical pain or eradicate its source. But they are indispensable conveyers of
comfort, support, and strength.

Recurrent episodes of illness are common among patients with chronic
diseases. These episodes bring many patients to the clinics of acute, general
hospitals and precipitate the hospitalization of many others.

A composite picture of the asthmatic patient will be used as an illustration.
It will show emotional reactions of patients/families to recurring attacks, the
effects of such episodes on the patient's daily functioning and on the lives of
others in his or her natural milieu, and the significance of methods of delivering
medical care. The data that follow are not comprehensive, nor do they describe
a random sampling of asthmatic patients. The description is suggestive of the
kinds of data that should be known about other patient populations whose
clinical symptoms recur at unpredictable intervals.

A large majority of the patients described below were women between 20
and 40 years of age, most of them wives and mothers, but emotionally immature,
dependent, and prone to manipulating others to meet their own needs. During
this period of diagnosis they were impatient and made several false starts before
they realized that tests had to be completed before treatment began. Once in
treatment they continued to show the same difficulty in returning to clinic for
medication or keeping appointments with the social worker. Not all these
difficulties are to be attributed to personality traits. Other obstacles will be noted
later.

The asthmatic patient cannot be sure when an attack will occur or how
severe it will be; this is the condition of uncertainty he or she must live with. For
many patients the most fearsome uncertainty of all is whether the next attack
will be fatal. When an attack occurs, the patient's normal functioning is
impaired. As one social worker put it, "When a woman has an attack and is
gasping for breath, she runs for her medication. She can't do her household

chores, care for the children, or cook at these times." If the patient goes into a panic or becomes too impatient, he or she may forget the physician's intstructions and swallow one medicine after the other, not waiting the required interval for results. Many of the asthmatic patients come to the emergency service when the medicines they have been given to use at home do not relieve them or when their acute attack occurs on a day when the clinic is closed. Also, since the worst and most frightening attacks occur during the night, most of these patients have to use the emergency service because they have no physician with primary responsibility on whom they can call.

Patients who turn up again and again in the emergency service rather than at the clinic in which they are or should be registered are obviously in need of special help. Some may fail repeatedly to take their medication in the prescribed way; some have practical problems, such as not being able to have their children cared for on clinic days; some need much help to conquer a tendency to seek medical care only in a crisis; and so on. In any case, as one social worker put it, "It is insufficient to leave the asthmatic patient in a corner of the emergency service with his IV bottle. He needs a chance to talk out his emotional reactions and his worries about the practical aspects of daily life." A working man may fear that his job is jeopardized—this is his third day out in three weeks. A housewife may have an immediate concern because her children expect to be called for at school and will want their lunch.

The use of emergency service in the absence of continual ambulatory medical care results inevitably in fragmented, discontinuous medical and physician care.*

The recurrent attacks of the adult asthmatic patient exact a toll from others in the patient's life-situation. Children of an asthmatic parent suffer repeatedly from fear of the patient's death. Also, they at times suffer neglect or are overburdened with family responsibilities. In many instances, an older child has to stay home from school with younger siblings while the mother is at clinic, or when she is suffering from an attack at home. Extra household responsibilities may fall on children whose mother cannot do the dusting and cleaning without suffering an asthmatic attack. Relations between spouses are not immune. The more immature and manipulative asthmatic women, especially those who cannot express their anger directly, frequently vent it by refusing intercourse on the grounds of their illness. At that point of conflict the husband may threaten to leave her. She counters with "How can you leave me when I am sick?" The husband starts feeling guilty, then furious, and a real fight is on.

Work roles suffer too. The asthmatic woman is often unable to work outside the home as other women do to add to the family income. Some do manage to earn during the warm months of the year, but they are unable to work from November to May in New York City. The asthmatic man has to stop working when he has an attack. If he is well integrated he may rest a day and then return to work. Less well integrated patients may panic and give up

* Changes in procedures can improve the quality of medical care. There is a notation in the *Mount Sinai Medical Center News* (May-June 1971) that "Each night a card file from medical clinics with patients' names, diagnosis, and current treatment noted, is delivered to the Emergency Room so that, should a regular clinic patient come in, doctors can check on his current medical problems and medication."

A similar procedure was established at Beth Israel Hospital (New York City) a year or so earlier when the comprehensive care clinics began to function.

working. The other side of the coin is that employers may refuse to keep on persons with records of irregular attendance. .

The phenomenon of recurrring episodes in a chronic disease can have an important impact on physicians in regard to the patient's work role. In compliance with policies and regulations governing eligibility for financial assistance and other benefits, physicians are asked to attest in writing to the patient's ability or inabilitity to work and the conditions under which he or she will or will not be able to work. This requirement poses many problems for the physician because there are so many uncontrolled and uncontrollable variables that determine the patient's work role. The physician needs all the data and expert opinions available from other medical specialists, nurses, social workers, and other personnel who know the patient to supplement his or her medical findings. In most instances of this kind, collaboration among givers-of-service is the key to their decision making as professionals obligated to consider the patient/-family as a totality. This means assessing such relevant factors as the patient's family relationships, the strength and weaknesses of the family unit, the patient's response to challenge and frustration, and the patient/family's hopes and expectations.

On the socioenvironmental front, an inadequate income puts the asthmatic patient at a special disadvantage. His or her vulnerability to dust, poor ventilation, climbing stairs, extreme cold, and vermin, for instance, makes decent housing and living arrangements of great importance in reducing the frequency and intensity of attacks. But low income is one of the strongest obstacles to obtaining adequate living quarters. In our urban areas asthmatic patients are not always given priority—as are cardiac patients—for public housing. If the use of public transportation is out of the question because of the crowding, dust, and dirt; if a taxi is the only means of reaching the Emergency Service quickly; if the asthmatic patient needs a telephone for emergencies but hasn't the money for it—then what?

These are the conditions that forcibly bring home the fragmented, incomplete, uncoordinated programs and resources in what should be closely related systems of human services. Were these patients to have ready access to a physician and a larger supply of medication at home to relieve their most acute and severe attacks, what difference would there be in their social functioning? Would the accessibility and availability in themselves serve as measures of control over anxiety and recurrent attacks? And—one of the most general fundamental questions of all—what can adequate income do and what can it not do to provide the physical and human environment that will encourage the patient/family's maximum social functioning?

In the light of existing medical and socioenvironmental conditions as described above, the pressures of unmet and inadequately met needs, added to the pressures created by the characteristics of the disease itself, make ready access of these patients/families to social workers, social services, and social resources imperative. The social workers can often fill some gaps, remove some barriers, reduce some anxieties, relieve some emotional tensions among family members—all of which will improve people's ability to cope, and increase their chances of benefiting from medical care and of restoration to optimum social functioning.

These questions relate to social and health policies regardless of the illness or disability under consideration. It will take many kinds of experimentation and controlled research to find the best answers to which services to deliver, how to deliver them, how to pay for them, and how to assure the high quality of service that is demanded by a sense of social justice.

Modes of intervention used by physicians for therapeutic purposes differ in the impacts they have on patients/families, for example, in the attitudes and feelings they arouse, the risks they pose or that people think they pose, the disruption they cause in people's lives, the immediate and long-term consequences that are expected, and the predictability of outcomes. Under the large headings of medical, that is, conservative treatment, and surgery, both major and minor, there are many specific measures among which choices have to be made by patients/families and their physicians. As medical knowledge and technology expand, the number of available specialties, subspecialties, and techniques increase, but at any given time their effectiveness and safety may be under official scrutiny. Some measures will be frankly experimental and restricted to use in controlled research programs which are required to operate under specific guide lines in order to protect human subjects from undue risk and danger.

The discussion of drug therapy and major surgery that follows is suggestive in specific terms of what givers-of-service should know about specific interventive measures, what patients/families should understand before consenting to or rejecting recommended interventions, and the importance of observing and reporting the signs and signals of stressful impacts.

Data such as these bear a direct relationship to the physician's obtaining and the mentally competent adult patient's giving informed, signed consent to specifically recommended medical and surgical interventions. By law, by institutional policy, and by the ethical principles and evolving ethical practices that guide the practitioner, there are a mere handlful of exceptions to the adult patient's rights to know, to give consent, and to refuse it.* But compatible with these rights is the practitioner's obligation to understand the patient's ways of reacting to stressful events, tolerance for stress, and capacity to adapt—and to use this understanding when he or she enters into the process of seeking informed consent. On such knowledge of the patient's person and temperament and on the course of the two-way communication that must take place depend the practitioner's manner, timing, and dosage when he or she makes disclosures that in themselves are mandatory. There is no longer much that is discretionary for the practitioner who is recommending a certain procedure; yet the tone of voice, the words used, the time allowed for the patient's assimilation of information, the give-and-take the practitioner encourages, and the site where the conversations take place are not to be minimized as factors that influence the patient's all-important decision.

While acquiring bits and pieces of information about the use of drugs, laypersons often attach their own meanings which were learned through personal, familial, and ethnic experiences. Thus "medicine," considered by one cultural group as "good," is believed to be more efficacious if it is a liquid rather than a pill. On the other hand, if medicine is referred to as a drug, it is perceived as "bad" by residents of a neighborhood familiar with drug pushers; furthermore, these residents may believe that any drug that has to be injected, for example, insulin, marks the person as a drug addict.

* For fuller discussion of the concept of informed consent, see pp. 68–69.

Medical terms that have rather recently become known to the general public are subject to misunderstanding, or at best to partial understanding, either of which may be accompanied by some strong feeling of dread and anxiety on the one hand or undue expectation of miracle working on the other. An example is chemotherapy, which connotes to many people the use of dangerous drugs administered only to patients who are at very high risk in the terminal stage of illness. Some people think that radiation therapy is a form of chemotherapy which always has the same grim connotations of pain, hopelessness, and imminent death. In general, people know what is meant by side effects of chemotherapy and radiation therapy, and, it is not surprising, dread them; but they seldom realize that current medical science does not permit a precise prediction of the side effects an individual patient will experience.

The layperson's limited understanding and medicine's own limitations account in part for the patient/family's frequent conclusion that the newer therapies are experimental even when they have legal and professional approval. The specter of uncertainty cannot be eliminated from the practice of professions committed to continuous progress and development in the field of health.

This sample of patients/families' misunderstandings and fallacious assumptions is a reminder of the importance of clear and accurate communication between patients/families and givers-of-service. Givers-of-service know from experience that there is at least one assumption they should not make, that is, that there is a positive, perfect correlation between the educational and economic status of a patient/family and their understanding and use of information given by medical and medical-related personnel. Neither material wealth nor educational opportunities nor intellectual prowess can guarantee victory over emotions, fantasies, and myths which may impede and impair rational thought processes.

The very power of irrational thought and feeling adds to the problem of enabling patients/families to deal with potential adverse consequences of various modes of treatment—not only the consequences unusual or bizarre enough to frighten patients and their relatives, but also mild consequences which can make people apprehensive because they do not know the source or importance of what is happening. Some cruelly disturbing experiences result from a patient's lack of preparation for significant side effects. Take the instance of a male patient in his eighties. During a course of drug therapy he confided to the social worker assigned to his clinic that he had been greatly distressed and ashamed for several weeks because he was having erections. He thought something terrible, "something mental," was happening to him until he read in the New York *Times*, with enormous relief, that the drug he was taking often caused that uncontrollable reaction.

Because it is known that frequently patients, and relatives too, at first neither hear nor understand explanations, instructions, and recommendations, the major responsibility for initiating and developing a process of successful communication rests with medical care personnel, primarily with the physician. While social workers can help by clarifying the patient/family's understanding of medical and surgical information and can do much to help patients/families deal with their emotional and attitudinal reactions, they have neither the professional competence nor the professional and legal authority to be the primary conveyers of that information. It is essential for the physician to take a substantial part in maintaining the patient/family's anxieties and emotions at manageable proportions.

Since patients undergoing chemotherapy are frequently ambulatory, they may be at special risk if they fail to understand or to follow medical instructions, fail to report significant reactions or report them inaccurately, take an unprescribed drug that is contraindicated medically, and so on. In some instances the ambulatory patient's relatives or close friends exert a helpful control and are reliable informants. In other instances there are no available relatives or friends, or they cannot be depended on to do the needed monitoring and reporting.

In a hospital with the traditional structure of clinics for ambulatory patients there is special need for procedures and collaborative efforts among givers-of-service to protect patients from the errors inherent in multiclinic, uncoordinated care. In regard to chemotherapy, the potential dangers are of such nature as prescribing drugs that do not "mix," or of prescribing a drug for one pathological condition that is contraindicated for another condition.

Again, because the patient is ambulatory, he or she may be employed or enrolled in a vocational retraining program or be active with some peer groups or otherwise in contact with significant others. Among them there may be some people who should be reliably informed about medication that might affect the patient's emotions, intellectual processes, or overt behavior. For example, a man in a chemically induced euphoria may be certain he is cured of his illness, able to return to his previous occupation, and ready to drop out of his retraining program.

Surgery is almost automatically connected with the hospital-based practice of medicine and so will serve well as a second illustration of the impacts and meanings of interventive measures. Both social workers and the physicians and surgeons with whom they work use harsh words to describe what surgery means to most patients: an insult to the body, a violation of the body, an assault upon the body, and sometimes "a small death" when the idea of surgery is pervaded by anxiety about anesthesia. Seldom do patients and their relatives look upon surgery as a method of treatment; too often they perceive it as a last resort. "Insult," "violation," and "assault" connote not only the physical onslaught but also the emotional onslaught that accompanies the experience of surgery and some of its consequences. One cannot overemphasize the importance of preparing patients and their relatives for what is going to happen on at least two levels: the technical procedures that will be employed to effect hoped-for, specified results and the emotional and psychological reactions that can be expected prior and subsequent to surgery. Patients/families need simple explanations about the anesthetic, the expected length of time the patient will be in the operating and recovery rooms, when and how the relatives will hear from the surgeon, and so on. A certain amount of worry and anxiety is alleviated when patients/families are given time to ask questions and be informed about procedural matters. Beyond this is the compelling need for patients and their relatives to have adequate opportunity and time to air, discuss, and reduce the anxieties aroused by their anticipation of the operation itself and of the consequences of surgery. As one social worker phrased it, "The time of the surgery itself is a time for emotional containment, not for spilling over." Thus, the emphasis is on time for spilling over *before* surgery takes place.

One of the most stress-producing requirements for the adult patient is that he or she must give consent, that is, take responsibility for surgery to be performed. It is a particular hardship when the patient knows that the treatment will result in bodily disfigurement or impairment in functioning. The natural response to being required to make this kind of decision is anger, regardless of the probable benefits. An occasional patient will react strongly to a surgical procedure that most patients recover from without a sense of bodily loss. For example, one patient had a prolonged period of psychological recovery following removal of a gallstone. For almost a year he kept the gallstone on display in his livingroom to show "what they took from me." One can only guess at the hidden significance of the surgical assualt to this particular man. To most patients a gallstone is a foreign body that should be removed.

The patient's early expression of anger is usually healthy and lessens the chance of prolonged mourning and depression following the surgery. However, not all patients and relatives can talk out their anger and anticipated sense of loss; social workers respect such silence but often verbalize something to the effect of "it must have been a very hard decision to make." At the least the patient/family will hear the message of sympathy; more than that, the ability of the giver-of-service to voice emotion may encourage the patient and his or her relatives to begin a healing process of more open communication among themselves and with concerned personnel.

Many patients are admitted to the hospital one day before surgery is scheduled, and a large number of them will have had no contact with a social worker either in an ambulatory care clinic or a physician's office. Thus, when a social worker finds, or is referred to, a patient in need of help before surgery is performed, the situation often presents an urgent need for rapid, concise exploration and assessment and for first aid in the psychosocial sense. In other words, the situation is apt to call for some form of crisis intervention. In order to avoid crises as much as possible, social workers in a number of hospitals are experimenting with screening instruments such as questionnaires to reach patients at high psychosocial risk in a matter of days or a week or two before they are admitted to the hospital. Although in these instances much of the surgery may be elective, it cannot be assumed that there is no need for social work services. Indeed, there may be many indicators—the size of the family, the ages of the family members, financial status, and the nature and characteristics of the illness, among other factors—that point to the need for a social worker's early intervention. Not least among the reasons for intervening before surgery is to insure, as far as possible, the patient/family's understanding of, and readiness for, the scheduled operation. Even after what appears to have been an adequate disclosure of facts and an adequate exchange between surgeon and patient, a severe emotional reaction will wipe out all rational response. For example, a social worker cited a woman patient who had had breast surgery, telling her in a rush of tears and fury, "They told me nothing, nothing. I woke up and found this." The facts were different, as the social worker knew, but at this point her concern was to help the patient express her anger, fears, and repulsion, which were reactions directed more to what had been done to her than to the persons who had done it. No anticipated event is a fully realized reality until it happens, and from this point of view no preparation will be foolproof.

Yet there must be preparation, not only for the surgical intervention per se but for the appearance and use of appliances or equipment—intravenous tubes and bottles, a urinary bag, catheters, and so on—along with clear explanations of why they will be used and how the patient will benefit. Learning the realities from authentic sources will help to counteract erroneous information gleaned from friends and copatients, as well as to correct a given patient's or relative's fantasies and speculations. Part of the patient/family's preparation may have to include the timing and sequence of the use of certain appliances, as, for example, when the patient is faced with a laryngectomy. Knowing that he or she can expect eventually to eat normally, that suctioning will not be necessary forever, that he or she can learn new ways of breathing that will make verbal communication possible—this knowledge makes the period of recovery more endurable and by extending hope starts the rehabilitative process even before treatment starts.* It is necessary to qualify the foregoing recommendations with a reminder that false assurance is no help, nor is it usually believed. Disclosure of both short- and long-term effects of surgery is important, as the foregoing comments on laryngectomy make clear.

The short-run consequences of a hysterectomy—limitations on heavy lifting, the length of the convalescent period, the need for homemaker or housekeeper service, and so on—are all conditions that the patient, her spouse, and other relatives need to understand and be helped to plan for. The nature of the permanent change in the patient's procreative functioning and the fact that her sexual functioning—desire and responsiveness—need not change are, of course, the long-term consequences women and men worry about the most and understand the least. Particularly at stake in most marriages is the mutual adaptation that the partners have to make in regard to their sexual relationship. It never suffices for the surgeon to *tell* the couple that they can have a normal sex life, nor is it enough to answer all their questions, necessary as these communications are. The couple must, in the end, have time to experience the truth of the surgeon's assurances, and that experience may occur only after a stressful period during which inhibiting fears and anxieties are gradually overcome. Self-fulfillment can be deeply violated for the woman who under-goes a hysterectomy during her childbearing years and for the male partner who desires fatherhood. It may be easier for both to adapt to the woman's sterility if they already have living children. However, the process of accepting this critical form of loss can be made more difficult by commitment to cultural values that measure manhood and womanhood by the ability to procreate.

A different kind of stress and adaptation occurs when the nature of the surgery reactivates childhood conflicts and problems. Alteration in the function-ing of the intestinal tract is a case in point. When still a small child, the adult patient learned to control the elimination of bodily wastes, learned to value self-control, and learned that others valued and loved him or her for exercising this control. When through surgery or disease he or she loses this control, the patient goes through a bad period of self-devaluation and of expecting others to be repelled because of his or her strange, artificial, and imperfect means of control and self-care.

Surgery undertaken to perform amputations on adults creates one of the most stressful changes in bodily structure, appearance, and functioning and in turn usually has great influence on the social functioning of the patients and those significantly related to them. Previous patterns of adjustment can be

* In some hospitals each patient who is to undergo a laryngectomy meets both the speech therapist and the social worker before the surgery takes place. This practice illustrates not only preparation for treatment but the psychological start, in the form of hope, of social rehabilitation as well.

assessed for their clues to inner strengths and external resources and to lacks in personal equipment and outside supports. The important components in the patient/family's ability to cope may shift in amount and direction as life-situations shift and change. Thus, medical care personnel need to consider the components as they currently exist even while they attempt to revive all the strengths that are in abeyance. Special care is urged in evaluating the influence of a patient's expectation of self. This is a major motivating force, but, if he or she holds too tightly to this expectation, the patient will find it difficult to make compromises. The patient may expect too much or too little of himself or herself, and friends and relatives may also err in either direction in their expectations of the patient. Eventually there has to be a compatible meeting of these expectations and the limitations imposed by the amputation and its psychosocial consequences.

Previous attitudes are crucial factors in a patient's outlook and striving to cope. One patient in her late fifties told her social worker that she had always "despised anyone in a wheelchair." Now she expected that others would have the same attitude toward her. The social worker understood that the patient was unable to say, and might never say, the deeper truth—that she was directing her profound feelings of disgust toward herself. The scope of this patient's task was enormous; it encompassed relearning how to regard herself and others in a much more drastic turnabout than many other patients are faced with. Her long-time derogatory attitudes could be expected also to slow her relearning to walk with a prosthesis and perform her usual chores of self-care and home responsibilities. Her known strengths and the healthier aspects of her self-expectation would have to be exploited from the beginning of her ordeal: every rehabilitative activity that could be built into the recovery process would be essential to her restoration to a satisfying balance of interdependence.

The patient's anger, depression, and mourning felt for the actual loss of a leg may be delayed if the surgeon puts on a cast with a "foot" attached. The real shock then comes several weeks later when the cast is removed and the patient sees the stump for the first time. In their anger, some patients make complaints they had never voiced before, such as a diabetic patient contending that the clinic's improper treatment of an infection had made the amputation necessary. It is essential for the patient to express anger, fears, apprehensions, and worries. All doors should be open—all cues should be used, as one social worker put it— to encourage the patient to communicate with medical care personnel throughout the entire period of treatment and rehabilitative care. The force of the patient's anger and its persistence, if too great and too long, may stand in the way of eventual acceptance of and adaptation to his or her loss and impaired functioning. Special measures may have to be taken, sometimes with the help of a psychiatrist, to reduce the anger and make easier the patient's acceptance and adaptation. One pauses here to speculate on the numbers of patients with such adverse reactions who become litigants in malpractice suits, no matter how fully informed they were before giving signed consent.

Observers have noticed that the amputee in hospital who is bent on survival, recovering, and relearning may be less upset at that time than his or her relatives. In such instances, the relatives may not be concentrating on the present, as the patient is, but thinking fearfully about his or her and their future. For example: How much care will the patient need when he or she leaves the hospital? Will he or she ever be able to go back to work? How much will he or she be able to earn? Will the wife be able to continue to work, or will she have to stay home and care for the patient? The specific questions differ from family to family, but these questions, with their accompanying emotions and attitudes, need to be openly discussed, as do the patient's questions.

While patients are still in the hospital, one can note how different they are in striving or not striving to cope with their problems in physical and social functioning. Some of these differences result from cultural attitudes toward illness, for example, that dependence on others for physical care is acceptable in illness. This idea may become a trap unless the patient/family are also motivated toward a better balance of interdependence in the future. In some hospitals all amputees are located within a circumscribed area. The arrangement helps personnel to stimulate the patients early to do what they can for themselves— each patient within his or her own medically imposed limits—and makes it easier for the patients to help one another by demonstrating their newly learned skills and by giving one another social support. In other hospitals, where amputees are located throughout the building, it works well to introduce them to one another for mutual help. Some patients initiate requests to talk to people who have successfully resumed their lives after amputation. For example, one woman who was walking well and taking care of her household came to the hospital regularly once a week and was very helpful to the patients who had asked for someone to talk to. The physical arrangement in the hospital may make little difference for the patient in the end. So much of the impetus for coping and recovery is an inner motivation that the patients often learn by themselves how to get from bed to chair and back, how to dress themselves, and so on. This observation is not meant to invite withdrawal of care, attention, encouragement, and direct teaching of patients. It is rather an appreciation of people's spontaneous striving to cope because they do have inner strengths and they do use them. But like most human beings, they benefit also from others' recognition, respect, and reassurance. It has been observed that when hospital personnel foster patients' dependency after it is no longer needed for therapeutic reasons, it is usually for the convenience of the staff rather than for the well-being of the patients.

Patients with amputations have many ups and downs; feelings of depression are common and natural. Any permanent, serious condition that will handicap a patient or is liable to recur or to increase in severity calls forth a series of adjustive emotional and attitudinal processes. They include denial, rejection, anger, and depression before the final stages are reached of acceptance and incorporation into one's changed self-image. It can be said that while the patient is still in the hospital, the presence and ministrations of medical care personnel often prevent the depression from being severely immobilizing. Some of the greatest hurdles and hazards occur after discharge from the hospital. To quote a social worker highly experienced in programs for home health care, "It is when he [the patient] gets home and realizes more fully how he has to live with himself that he faces his greatest mental health hazard. He needs continuity of attention and caring." The process of resuming maximum social functioning at this stage is made more difficult by the patient's still awkward use of his or her prosthesis. (Many patients, in fact, have to return to clinic for further training.) The patients, like the social workers, believe that they experience the greatest impact of loss of limb upon their discharge home.

One patient described the experience with moving clarity: "The first month was full of problem solving; the second month I coasted; the third month my limitations hit hard."

It is at this point, too, that the matter of vocational rehabilitation may have to be faced squarely, and along with this many patients/families have also to face a period of unemployment, an appreciable decrease in income during the period of retraining, and often a lessened earning capacity when reemployment is achieved. There are instances of the reverse, that is, an increased earning capacity following retraining, when the upward mobility makes its own demands related to the possession and management of more income rather than less.

At the other extreme are the patients who are unlikely to return to work at all. Age, cultural and educational background, and even difficulties in transportation may be deterrents. For example, a male garment worker nearing 60 years of age, with an amputation above the knee, will not be able to return to the standing job at which he worked for thirty years. The Department of Vocational Rehabilitation will make decisions about his capacity for retraining—whether he can shift from hand to machine work, how long a working day he can tolerate, whether his educational background and language skills are commensurate with the demands of retraining, and whether he will be able to use public transportation from his home in an outlying district to the garment center in Manhattan for regular employment.

Toleration for a full day's work and for the rigors of urban public transportation is important because the amputee—especially the older person—finds it harder to do things than before. The end of the day may leave him or her exhausted even if reasonably good psychological adjustment has been made to bodily changes and a decreased ability to function in day-by-day living.

Uncertainties and problems like these take their toll from the patient's relatives, too. They may not realize it, but the social worker is forearmed by the knowledge that the most devoted family members can reach a limit. Physical fatigue, frustrations, and impatience with a long period of the patient's physical dependence do finally set in. And when the patient senses such feelings, he or she may in turn vent anger upon his or her relatives or retreat into depression. For everyone, then, a firm hold is essential on the realities of what to expect, what one can and should do, and who can be called on for help when these feelings develop and result in conflict. When patients are in home care programs, they and their relatives can call on a social worker at these critical points for help in restoring family equilibrium. Patients discharged home but not in home care programs seldom have easy and continuous access to the social worker they knew in the hospital. Hospital-based social workers are still largely hospital-bound in their giving of service, with notable exceptions for specific programs that reach out into the community.

The process of the amputee's social rehabilitation illustrates well the relation between this process and the patient/family's socioeconomic condition. One needs to know, for example, whether an apartment house is furnished with an elevator; whether the apartment is too crowded or too small for the use of a wheelchair; whether the doors are too narrow for a wheelchair; whether the height of the patient's bed will permit his or her movement to a chair and back again; whether bathing, toilet, and cooking facilities are functional for the patient's continued progress in self-care and social rehabilitation. The big question comes when living space should be altered or refurnished to suit the patient's condition or when a move to more suitable quarters is desirable. The patients cover a wide range, from those receiving public assistance, to the "medically indigent," to the "working poor," to the many people whose incomes are moderate but utterly inadequate for remodeling living space or paying higher rent in a better building. Money for these purposes is in scarce supply and usually available on a highly selective basis. Even within the program there are distinctions; the Veterans Administration can provide money for housing alterations, for example, only if the veteran's disability is service connected. The situation of the amputee and his or her family members offers an opportunity to bring the housing situation into focus but only as illustrative of how an unmet social need interacts with fragmented systems of medical care. Uncoordinated systems of services are at times not much better than no services at all.[4,5]

Technologies have been developed that permit replacement of parts of the human body with either human transplants or man-made substitutes. Scientists have successfully invented machines that monitor, control, or regulate a human biological system or take the place of an impaired human organ. These and similar devices have become fairly familiar instruments within the past decade or so, although not always completely trusted or universally approved by the consumers, providers, and givers of health care services. The formidable appearance of many of the machines; the patient/family's knowledge of risks involved and of uncertain outcomes; the peculiar sensations, real and imagined, of foreign bodies implanted in the body, and sometimes in control of a vital organ or system of the patient's body—these are among the factors that arouse fear and anxiety, which are reactions that givers-of-service can help the patient understand and tolerate but that the patient has to learn to cope with in his or her day-by-day encounters with life and illness.

Bodily change, often resulting in changed bodily and social functioning, is a well-known characteristic of many disease processes and physical deficiencies. The idea of oneself as a person is closely connected with the way one perceives and thinks of one's body and the way in which other people perceive and react to it.[6] Bodily changes in the course of illness and treatment can be in the nature of impairment or improvement; adaptation is necessary in either case, causing some anxiety and requiring some learning and relearning and some modifications in attitudes, feelings, and behavior. Bodily changes as a major stressful event include bodily impairment caused directly by a disease process; bodily change occasioned by interventions such as surgery or chemotherapy, which may occasion simultaneously both impairment, and improvement, loss and gain; bodily changes requiring the use of appliances and prostheses which may at the same time augment and ease adaptation to differences in appearance and functioning; and bodily changes that occur normally in the cycle of human growth and development.

The most frequent and significant types of bodily change—those that seem to have major social and emotional consequences—are in the patient's altered appearance, in the different way his or her body functions, in the control the patient has over his or her body, in sensory acuity, in the ability to move, and in bodily energy or strength. These changes seldom occur singly; the multiplicity of adaptations that are required of so many patients/families is an element to be heavily weighed in projecting therapeutic and rehabilitative measures. Everyone has limits of patience, resilience, and adaptiveness, to name but a few helpful attributes needed to cope successfully with unwanted, and at times even with desired, change.

The consequences of these changes are manifested in psychosocial changes, such as the ability to carry out one's usual tasks at home or to continue as an earner, the emotional response to family members and significant others, and any aspect of daily living that is vulnerable to the stressful conditions of illness and disability.

It is common among givers-of-service in various professions to say that some of these changes in social functioning induce "reversal of roles" but does this phrase describe accurately what takes place? Tasks and the balance of interdependence among family members do shift, but is there really a reversal of roles between spouses or between children and parents, to mention the most common so-called reversals? Don't the marital partners continue to be men and women, husbands and wives, fathers and mothers—albeit struggling to adapt to new responsibilities and the loss of old ones, and to new personal needs? What are the effects of the struggle to adapt? Do the children continue to regard themselves as children even when assuming unaccustomed and perhaps undesirably heavy responsibilities? Under what circumstances do a husband and wife actually incorporate and function in a reversed social role? Is it likely that in some unions each maintains his or her previous self-image and regards the enforced shift in tasks and functions as alien, and perhaps violations of self? Is the sense of violation a function of deep-seated values which prescribe what men and women should do and proscribe those tasks that negate manhood or womanhood, fatherhood, or motherhood?

These questions lead naturally to queries regarding measures that can be taken when the shifts in tasks and interdependence result in strain and crisis which threaten the integrity of relationships and of the family group. Assessment of each family's life-and-illness situation becomes a crucial process if one needs to answer such questions as the following: Are there serious threats to the mental health and social functioning of family members and the integrity of the family group? Are there community services available to families that are vulnerable to social disintegration resulting from psychological pressures? Can neighbors or relatives in the extended family or members of a church group, for example, be enlisted in a rearrangement of tasks that would have healthier psychosocial connotations for all the family members? What inner, psychological strengths can medical care personnel help the patient/family use to the fullest in order to adapt to unmodifiable conditions in the life-and-illness situation? When a patient's disability is severe and permanent, can the shifts in tasks and interdependence be so managed that they will not impede the process of the patient/family's restoration to their maximum social functioning?

A decrease in or loss of sexual potency, the possibility of such an occurrence, or a fear that it will develop constitute perhaps the most stressful, critical, and belittling changes in bodily functioning that the adult patient can experience. It strikes to such an extent at the central core of an adult's self-image and at cultural values concerning intimacy and privacy that patients, their closest relatives, and even givers-of-service tend to avoid communication about sexual problems. This flight resembles the tendency in our society to flee from contemplation of dying and death.

Insofar as some givers-of-service in the field of health care are struggling to cope emotionally with fundamental matters of life, illness, and death, those patients who are in grave need of psychosocial support at times of crisis will not obtain it or will do with far less adequate help than they should have.

It would be grossly inaccurate to imply that all bodily changes bring negative consequences in daily living. Many are enabling and enhancing changes in the long run. but adaptation to beneficent change has its own potential for producing stress and even distress. Inertia, insecurity regarding the future, fear of failing in a new situation, reluctance to give up familiar gratifications for those unknown—these are some of the attitudes and feelings that may slow down the process of social rehabilitation. Not only the patient but the total family unit and all its members may be vulnerable when a man who has been unemployable for two years becomes fit for retraining and returning to work, when a solicitously cared-for wife and mother is enabled to resume her tasks and fulfill her obligations, or when a walker or a cane or a wheelchair partially restores a patient's control of his or her movements. These and many other conditions of an improved status of social-health hold the possibility of some degree of conflict—not always conscious—and some problematic elements in the process of adapting to the "good." Perhaps the common denominator is the apprehension experienced by many patients and shared by many of their closest relatives and friends when the dependence on others which is so desirable for therapeutic purposes is expected to give way to a more normal, balanced state of interdependence.

BEHAVIORAL CHANGE AND SOCIAL FUNCTIONING

In each of the previous sections in this chapter on treatment and rehabilitation the phenomenon of behavioral change has been cited. Its links to the course of an illness, to the psychosocial impacts of a mode of intervention, or to the biological consequences of a therapeutic agent are clearly discernible. Even so, there is justification for elaborating on and reemphasizing the significance of behavioral change in its own context.

First there is the decided shift in the balance of the patient's interdependence which manifests itself as regression in both psychological and social functioning. Regression takes place in most patients as a response to what they perceive as highly stressful events and conditions—a severe injury, serious illness, surgery, periods of grave uncertainty, and the like. The operative point here is how the patient/family perceives the situation rather than how it is perceived technically by givers-of-service. In this context regression is a partial retreat to an earlier, less mature level of psychosocial functioning in which the gratifications derived from being taken care of physically and being cared for emotionally by others greatly exceed the gratifications resulting from self-reliance and giving of one's self to others. Ordinarily the patient's regressive behavior is temporary, serving as a useful mechanism for survival and for early progression toward physical and social recovery. In truth, the temporary regression is best perceived as an acceptable, even desirable, yielding to the patient's increased need for dependency on others which results from being ill or disabled. "In our society, a sick person is considered to have some degree of impairment or disturbance in his ability to carry out his normal tasks and responsibilities. . . . He is not simply 'allowed' to withdraw if he wishes. To some extent he is encouraged—and even required—to do so."[7] Although much of the regression is manifested in physical dependence, regression in social functioning is also usual and equally justified therapeutically. However, the mentally competent adult patient cannot, even temporarily, renounce responsibility for making informed decisions about his or her medical care.

The qualification of regression as partial is important, even while one recognizes that dependence is total at times, for example, when the patient is under an anesthetic or in a coma. Mrs. Riviera's behavior in the intensive care unit is a good case in point.* Although she was physically in need of many appliances, life-supporting equipment, and constant nursing care, she was nevertheless able to respond to medical care personnel, to talk with the social worker daily, to visit with her husband, to understand and react emotionally to what the surgeons had done and were doing, and to make some momentous decisions. The patient with specific areas of incapacity—temporary or permanent—is not necessarily an incompetent, totally dependent person. As one social worker put it, "Even a patient with some memory loss can participate in decision making—about his living arrangements, for instance."

It has already been noted that adult patients differ in the intensity of their motivation to work their way out of regression toward restoration of less dependence or greater independence in social functioning. Some need more stimulation and support from without than others to take the necessary steps to reattain an optimum balance of interdependence. In this process one notes the influence of medical care personnel, whatever their function, and of close family members during both the period of desirable therapeutic regression and the subsequent period of active progress toward more self-reliant psychosocial functioning.

People's expectations of themselves and of one another have particular significance for their behavior in situations of illness. There are all kinds of matching and mismatching of expectations held by the patient, relatives, and medical care personnel. If all three parties expect and approve the patient's regression while it is therapeutically desirable, there is no problem. A few common examples of problematic situations are the following: when the patient's justifiable need for unusual care, protection, and dependence is not or cannot be met by his or her relatives; when the patient wishes to continue his or her regressive behavior when it is not medically necessary and his or her relatives either fall in with the patient's wishes or become impatient and angry over the prolonged dependence; and when the patient does not allow himself or herself the kind and degree of regression that is therapeutically desirable, perhaps only because he or she is ill-informed but perhaps because he or she fears being controlled by others or fears that once in a regressive state, he or she will not want to resume an expected state of self-reliance. The patient usually does not express in so many words the fear of wanting to remain in a regressive state. It is a speculative interpretation observers make when the patient's resistance to regressing takes on the flavor of protesting too much.

To understand such problematic situations and to be of help in resolving them, the givers-of-service need to assess the patient's family situation and become aware of the family's own part, if any, in creating a problem. Leaving aside relatives' lack of knowledge as a factor in these problems, the nature of the relationship among family members, their solidarity in times of trouble, and their mutual sympathy and compassion for one another are among the significant attributes that need to be evaluated.

Physicians, nurses, social workers, and others who give direct health care services at times discard their professional attitudes and conduct and revert to

* See p. 63.

lay reactions. For example, on an unusually busy hospital floor the patient who is enjoying and prolonging his or her regressive state may make things so much easier for some harried staff members because of his or her passivity that they indulge the patient rather than stimulate him or her to greater activity. But the same patient may arouse irritation in other staff members if they perceive him or her as not trying to be self-reliant when there are less able patients who need their care. The patients who do not like to be helped and resent having things done for them are similarly subject to the ways others see them. They may be perceived by some as upstanding individuals, using their strengths effectively under siege, while others may view them as recalcitrant and noncompliant.

To note these and similar differences in interpretation is not a condemnation but a recognition that professional attitudes and conduct are achieved and maintained—with lapses—at a personal cost through a never-ending process of professional development. Although the statement quoted below is directed to physicians, it describes well the central obligations of all professional practitioners in the health care field:

> In the "emotional aspects" of his relationship with the patient, the physician is expected to maintain a dynamic balance between attitudes of "detachment" and "concern." He is expected to be sufficiently detached or objective toward the patient to exercise sound medical judgment and maintain his equanimity. He is also expected to be sufficiently concerned about the welfare of the patient to give him compassionate care.[8]

A breakdown in detached concern occurs, as a rule, because the practitioner has removed the patient/family from center stage. Someone else is occupying that place—perhaps the practitioner himself or herself. With the help of hard-won self-awareness and a deliberate effort to understand the patient's signals, the practitioner can restore his or her detached concern; the loss is temporary and retrievable.

Behavioral changes in the patient other than regression may be symptoms of or reactions to a particular disease process or consequences of interventive measures, as mentioned in previous sections. Then there are the behavioral changes occasioned by changes in the patient's human and material environment. The patient may lose or gain when these changes occur, but in either case they can have a direct effect on the patient's response to treatment and rehabilitation.

The patient's behavior may become bizarre, irrational, and inappropriate; his or her thought processes may become illogical and manifest themselves in confused, garbled, and unintelligible speech; moods and emotions may become excessively labile and appear unrelated to the realities of the patient/family's day-by-day life. To illustrate: in progressive diseases symptoms usually become more severe, requiring the patient/family's readaptation to new and different phenomena; an exact picture of the patient's future behavior is seldom predictable except in the broadest terms which offer the patient/family rather meager preparation; and the chronicity of most diseases that result in these changes and the fact that treatment is often coterminous with life create an excessively heavy demand on human adaptability.

The value of preparing the patient/family for what is going to happen is indisputable. The problem is the unpredictability of the patient's specific behavioral changes. Here again the gaps in medical knowledge are hard for patients/families to accept, and the specific behavioral changes, unexpected as they are, may create hardship and crises. For example, a patient's wife and adolescent daughter knew that his brain tumor "would progressively worsen his condition." But they were shocked beyond belief when, one day, he made sexual advances to the daughter. Social workers, who are often the first of the practitioners to be accused by the patient's relatives of not preparing them properly, recommend strongly that the physician in charge go one step beyond the prediction of "worsening condition" to the more specific probability of strange behavior, uncharacteristic of the patient (as spouse and father, in this case). If the physician and family members pursue such a statement to the point of understanding that the behavior might, for example, be assaultive or sexual, so much the better; there is more time then for an early consideration of available measures to control the behavior, or the possibility of removing the patient from the home to a facility which can offer the care the patient will need.

Insofar as serious behavioral changes may be unavoidable consequences of medical care in research programs, the peculiarly stress-producing combination of hope, risk, challenge, fear, and uncertainty calls for discussion. These are stress-producing factors for patients/families and for research personnel alike. Everything already said about the processes of the physician's seeking and the patient's giving informed consent can be heightened exponentially for everyone involved in programs of biomedical research. Physician-participants in these programs confront unusual situations which make great demands on their ability to adapt to, or cope with, psychosocial stress. The problems are so fundamental as to influence the usual nature of the physician-patient relationship. They are frequently colleagues in the research effort, in somewhat the same sense that patients/families who come before medical students to discuss their life-and-illness situations are assuming a teacher's role. Sometimes a personal relationship develops between physician and patient which makes living and working within the research design practically infeasible.

One of the keenest observers in the field, speaking of physicians' stress when they are experimenters, noted especially "problems of uncertainty and therapeutic limitation, problems concerning the ethics of human experimentation, the selection of patients for research subjects, the conflicts between standards of rigorous investigation and those of good medical practice." [9]

Social workers are often on call by physicians in medical research programs to help patient-participants and their relatives when patients' home situations get out of hand, their anxiety becomes critical, their isolation begins to feel unbearable, their doubts mount concerning the research program and its value, they feel worse instead of better, and so on.

Social workers are, on the other hand, too infrequently members of the research staff or of the preliminary research planning group. They are nevertheless deeply concerned for the rights of human subjects in medical research programs. They put considerable weight not only on the patient/family's being well-informed about the aims, methods, and techniques of the research project; the risks; and the possible benefits but also on the safeguards for privacy and confidentiality. These rights in particular require informed consent, well in advance, to the plans for reporting data about the design, execution, and findings of the research program. Some patients feel rewarded and gratified by the prospect of appearing in print, but other patients shrink from the idea, despite promised anonymity.

The exceedingly high degree of uncertainty that pervades the atmosphere in which medical research takes place delves deeply into the participants' sources of inner strength. That much uncertainty can be a powerful influence on how patients perform their expected tasks, such as getting out of bed, self-grooming, eating prescribed diets, reporting accurately about symptoms and reactions to medication, and carrying on their family roles insofar as possible even while they are hospitalized.

The period of treatment and rehabilitation, which has been surveyed illustratively rather than comprehensively, discloses many stress-producing factors, events, and conditions that are commonly experienced by adult patients receiving hospital-based medical care. It is the impact of these elements that gives meaning to illness and disability. The people who are affected cover a wide range: not only the patient and his or her close relatives, but other persons in the patient's natural surroundings who have special significance and most particularly those who are involved directly as givers-of-service in numerous professions and technical and nontechnical occupations. The enormous burden that has to be borne by the givers-of-service becomes clear through descriptions of the psychological and emotional reactions they may have to their patients and their patients' experiences; through revealing the heavy responsibility of decision making inherent in established diagnostic, therapeutic, and rehabilitative processes and in research programs; and in fulfilling the legal and professional obligation to obtain informed consent—an obligation that contains within itself the total spectrum of professional values, attitudes, and conduct.

From the standpoint of the patient, whatever the meanings may be of elements such as pain, unpredictable remission and recurrence of symptoms, and biological and behavioral changes, the most pervasive, universal element, and one that often strains to the utmost an individual's power to endure, is uncertainty. It is no accident that this chapter starts and concludes with observations about that distressing, often undefinable, and unfocused feeling of doubt, not knowing, and fearful suspicion.

With more or less success patients/families, their significant others, and givers-of-service make their highly individualized adaptations to the stress-producing components of the period and process of treatment and rehabilitation.

REFERENCES

1. William A. Spencer and Maurice B. Mitchell, "Disability and Physical Handicap," *Encyclopedia of Social Work* 6th ed. National Association of Social Workers, (New York: National Association of Social Workers, 1971), pp. 204-218.
2. Harry T. Phillips, "Disability and Physical Handicap: Services for the Chronically Ill," in ibid., pp. 218-228.
3. Mark Zborowski, *People in Pain*, (San Francisco: Jossey-Bass, 1969), p. 250.
4. Janice Paneth, "Definition in an Inflationary Period: Some Current Social Health Need Provisions," *American Journal of Public Health* (January 1972). See also Eli Ginzberg and Charles Brecher, "New York's Future—A Manpower View," *City Almanac* (Center for New York City Affairs of the New School for Social Research), vol. 7, no. 3 (October, 1972), p. 12.
5. Bess S. Dana, "Health Care: Social Components," in *Encyclopedia of Social*

Work 17th ed. (Washington, D.C.: National Association of Social Workers, 1977), pp. 544-550.

6. Leonard Kriegel, "Uncle Tom and Tiny Tim: Some Reflections on the Cripple as Negro," *American Scholar*, vol. 38, no. 3 (summer 1969).

7. Renee C. Fox, *Experiment Perilous: Physicians and Patients Facing the Unknown* (New York: Free Press, 1959), p. 115.

8. Ibid., p. 86. See also the description of compassion in this text, p. 7.

9. Ibid., p. 58 ff.

Chapter 5
The Impacts of Medical Care
in Selected Loci of the Hospital

In this chapter hospital-based medical care and its impacts on patients/families, on their significant others, and on hospital personnel are viewed within the framework of the various sites in which the care is delivered, for example, in clinics for ambulatory care, in the emergency service, in the coronary unit, on the floors for hospitalized patients, and in the home-bound patient's natural environment. The same range of demands to adapt to situations of life-and-illness occurs within this framework as within the framework of specific illnesses and interventions. Certain demands to adapt occur more noticeably in one site than another, but there are no demands that are unique to one locus or to one group of patients/families or personnel. The diversity in demands for adaptation is more than equaled by the diversity in the impact of and response to the demands. For example, hospitalization means to many patients a stressful loss of freedom of choice and control over their environment as well as separation from their usual sources of personal security in the form of familiar people, possessions, and places. But it is equally clear that such generalizations are not universally applicable. The patient who feels resistive to the professional and administrative controls over moving about, eating, and sleeping may have as a companion in the next bed a patient who enjoys the same controls because they symbolize being cared for. Among the crucial demands for adaptation that face patients/families in all loci are changes in the balance of psychosocial interdependence which spring from changes in the patient's ability to function, such as changes in socioeconomic circumstances which, whether temporary or permanent, call for adaptation to phenomena such as a modified standard of living for the family or the supplementation of the patient/family's natural resources by community resources, or changes in personal relationships which may occur in response to frustration, anxiety, fatigue, and loss of mutual emotional gratification.

There is an important distinctive element in ambulatory care in the requirement that patients/families assume considerable responsibility for carrying out aspects of treatment as prescribed or recommended, often by a multiprofessional group of personnel. Carrying out treatment in the home may impose upon the patient and his relatives a considerable demand for compliance and good management of time, effort, and money. The clinics for comprehensive care frequently offer the much-needed service of patient education for which public health nurses have official responsibility. Although the benefits of patient education are frequently referred to, such programs are both scarce and fragmentary. They tend to be established for selected patient populations at high risk, for example, unmarried pregnant teen-aged girls.

The fundamental impact of any locus in the hospital is derived from the nature and potential outcome of the patient's disease or disability in conjunction with the diagnostic or treatment procedures required at a given time, together with the age and sex of the patient. The service units, many of them highly specialized, affect the patient and those close to him or her through the quality of the atmosphere—calm, tense, orderly, or confused; the special skills of the people who care for the patients; the responsiveness of professional and nonprofessional staff members to the needs of patients/families; and the known or fantasied functions of the technical equipment that is a fixture in the environment of the modern hospital.

Different service units require different adaptive behavior in respect to patient/family participation, professional collaboration, coordination of procedures, the quality and substance of communications among the parties concerned, and so on. The descriptive data that follow illustrate the need to understand experiences that patients have in common and those that are differentiated by the characteristics of the intramural settings in which they occur. The service units described in this chapter are selected but diverse enough to be suggestive of the kinds of circumstance that strongly influence an individual's or family's experience.

Through understanding the nature of the patient/family's experiences, it is possible to help them cope with the stress-producing aspects of the hospital setting and to encourage them to use their strengths and resources to benefit fully from the medical care they receive.

HOSPITALIZATION: GENERAL CONSIDERATIONS

The consumer of medical care in metropolitan areas is likely to have some understanding that the practice and technical equipment in teaching hospitals is sophisticated and advanced. To such persons, while the thought of hospitalization normally produces anxiety, it bears less often than previously the stigma of being the place of last resort. This statement is not necessarily true for patients, many of them with chronic and fatal diseases, who enter the hospital in the terminal phase of illness and know that their lives will end there.

With the prevalence of third-party payments—by voluntary insurance plans, public funding mechanisms, or both—the immediate costs of in-patient medical care cause less worry and strain for more patients/families than ever before, despite the incomplete coverage of our current systems of payment. At the same time the policies and practices that have been and will continue to be instituted to control the costs and assure the quality of medical care in the hospital have their effects on patients/families, medical practice, and adminstrative procedures.

In the following material three aspects of hospitalization are singled out because of their specific and immediate impacts: preparation for admittance to the hospital, the period of hospitalization, and care subsequent to discharge. *Preparation for hospitalization** is essential for every patient whether or not hospitalization is a new experience. To be effective, preparation has to be tailored to the patient—his or her intellectual ability to understand verbal explanations, emotional temperament, general apprehensiveness, and specific sources of anxieties and worries.

Patients admitted on an emergency basis, as in cases of trauma or acute symptoms threatening survival, will not have had time for preparation. But in general, patients other than these will, in principle at least, have had the opportunity of being prepared by private physicians or by a physician and other personnel in a hospital's service units.

A major element of preparation is assuring that the patient/family understand why the physician recommends hospitalization, what the other choices are, and what their consequences might be. In other words, the patient's decision to be hospitalized should rest on a process of full and honest communication between the patient or the patient's guardian or surrogate and the physician. It is expected that the greater the patient's participation during the period of preadmission, the better he or she is enabled to cope with subsequent stressful events and circumstances.

Preparation also includes considering predictable psychosocial problems and the resources to resolve them. The most common of these problems are related to financial status, the care of the household and family members during the patient's hospitalization as well as after his or her discharge. Adult and elderly patients often need to review their own resources—insurance coverage from various sources, for example—and how to apply for benefits to which they are entitled.

Patients whose hospitalization is planned in advance usually receive several forms to complete and return; nowadays one of these may request information intended to alert the social service department of the hospital to a patient/family's possible need for help from a social worker, that is, information that will indicate the kind or degree of psychosocial risk to which the patient/family is or will be exposed. In some instances preadmission contact with a social worker may serve to avoid or minimize problems; in other instances, contact at the point of admission or very soon thereafter is highly effective in reducing unavoidable stress and strain with which the patient/family will have to cope, and on occasion, in avoiding some stressful situations altogether. Thus the nature of a patient's scheduled surgery in combination with the number and ages of children in the family, the estimated length of hospitalization, and a lack of medical insurance may add up to probable need for financial or homemaker service or both during and following hospitalization and for help in coping with the probable outcome of the operation.

The patients of private physicians seldom have access to a social worker prior to hospitalization except through screening devices such as those described above. Patients who are referred for hospitalization by physicians in ambulatory care clinics are more likely to have had contact with a social worker who collaborates with the patient's physician in preparing him or her for becoming an in-patient. There are, however, many clinic patients who do not have contact

---

* See the section on preparatory and anticipatory work, p. 30.

with a social worker, and it remains an open question whether those about to enter the hospital have all the preparation they need. This issue requires further study, along with numerous other questions related to the larger problem of deploying social workers in health care facilities.*

Finally, the aspects of preparation for hospitalization are related to the characteristics of the service unit where the patient will be and to procedures he or she can expect. Selecting what the patient/family should know immediately before or at the point of hospitalization is important. There is a limit to what people can absorb and use well, so both dosage and timing are matters for consideration.

The period of hospitalization takes on a meaning that depends in part on how personnel respond to the attitudes and behavior of the in-patients and their visitors and on how staff members perceive their own functions and experiences as givers-of-service. Thus personnel become major contributors to the meaning of hospitalization for patients, relatives, and others in the patients' natural milieu.

Social workers, when they are observing and assessing the meaning of hospitalization to the patient/family, use a frame of reference related to significant psychosocial aspects of the experience: How alien is the setting to the patient/family and in what specific ways? How do the patient and his or her relatives express their reactions? What is the culture of the floor, the lounge, the patient's room? How do the patient and his or her relatives show their reactions to the culture of the service unit?

How does the patient perceive himself or herself in the hospital setting? How do the relatives perceive the patient? How do the members of the hospital staff perceive the patient/family? What is the nature of the interaction between staff members and the patient/family? What is the interaction between the patient and his/her fellow patients?

A hospital is usually perceived as a symbol of authority in that it is a place where other people are in control of what will happen to the patient. How comfortably the patient adapts to the hospital's status of institutionalized authority is influenced by the size, architecture, and interior design as well as by the behavior of personnel, all of which are elements in the general atmosphere of the hospital. Upon entering, the patient/family may sense a calm and supportive, orderly, uncrowded, and unrushed atmosphere, or one that seems excited, hurried, and agitating. The atmosphere in Emergency Service may be different from that in the regular admitting office of the same hospital, or it may be the same. There may be one kind of atmosphere on one day and another kind on another day.

The patient is frequently in great need, psychosocially speaking, at the point of admission: he or she is apt to feel alone, helpless, and frightened. When patients are scheduled for a critical diagnostic or treatment procedure, feelings of abandonment and powerlessness may peak when the hospital is emptied at night of visiting relatives.

On the way to his or her room and in the room itself, the patient (and usually a friend or relative who comes along) will encounter some of the strange and unfamiliar aspects of the setting: people in various uniforms, from a volunteer to someone in the crumpled-looking garb of the operating room and

* See also the section on determining the social worker's point of entry, p. 27.

machines and equipment about which he or she knows nothing and which may precipitate disturbing fantasies. Some stress-producing particulars are unaccustomed noises generating from people in distress or produced by machines; numbers of persons who come singly or in clusters to ask questions, examine, touch, poke, and talk to one another over the patient's head; smells that cannot be identified; the sharing of a room with other patients who may become friends and helpers or sources of irritation; and other patients' friends and relatives who may be kind and sympathetic or who may invade the little privacy that is available in a multibed room. For example, a 35-year-old woman and an 85-year-old woman were sharing a two-bed room, each of them suffering from a disease of the gastrointestinal tract. The younger woman found the experience fatiguing and upsetting on two counts—the older woman's frequent bowel movements and her staying awake all night and sleeping all day. The incompatibility of these two patients was extreme, to be sure, but serves to illustrate some of the stressful conditions that may accompany hospitalization. At the other end of the curve are roommates who wait on one another, offer sympathy and advice, and are generally sensitive and supporting.

Adult patients who are hospitalized have to adapt in some degree to the loss of status that comes from losing varying amounts of freedom of choice and of control over their environment. When and what one eats; when one sleeps and awakens; whether one is free to go to the bathroom, sit up in a chair, or return to bed; when visitors can come and have to leave—these are events relatively out of the patients' control and therefore more precious to the losers. Medical care personnel have the power to compensate for some of these losses and to prevent such loss when it is avoidable. Some preventive measures are calling patients by their full titles and surnames;* refraining from talking over patients' heads in terms that they do not understand or, what may be even more threatening, in terms deliberately chosen to be obscure; preserving as best one can the patient's privacy (although a completely private conversation is almost impossible in a multibed room, drawn curtains do help); and respecting fully that it is the patient, not personnel, who has privileged communication. Hospital staff frequently yield to the temptation to "talk cases" informally on the stairs, in the halls, in the elevators, in the cafeterias, and in the lounges. Such violations of privacy and confidentiality by personnel are within their control, and it is ironic that they occur (allowing for some unprofessional curiosity) out of the staff's interest and concern for the patient and sometimes out of their anxiety about a grave or unusual problem.

In varying degrees patients/families feel anxiety and apprehension, some very little and some in a great amount. The degree of distress does not always reflect the physician's estimate of the risk the patient is facing. The patient's private, individualized estimate may be of great importance, as it was in the instance of a patient's needing two months to decide to have a herniotomy, described by the bewildered surgeon as minor surgery.** There is also always the point that no patient enters the hospital with all uncertainties resolved—cure is not guaranteed, there could be unforeseen complications, and there is no way

---

* This recommendation does not necessarily apply to those adolescents and young adults whose preference seems to be to forgo entirely the use of surnames in either formal or informal social encounters.

** See p. 61.

of knowing when or if the patient will fall in with the 25% who do experience side effects. When a patient asks "Am I going to get well?" he or she may be saying on a deeper level, "I will never get out of bed" or "I have forever to live." One social worker, commenting that one must hear accurately what a patient wants to know and what the source of worry is, recalled a conversation with a man who had a brain tumor. Her first reaction was that his talk was bizarre. Later she realized he was asking about his life expectancy and regretting that he had not accomplished more. Fortunately, there was still time for the neurologist to discuss the patient's illness with him more specifically and for the social worker to listen to the patient's assessment of his life and to help him sort out the unfinished business he could hope to complete and the things that would give him pleasure in the time that was left to him.

One request patients make that may prove to be highly significant both on the surface and below is to talk with their family. It does, of course, imply some satisfying aspects of relationships among family members; but one has to understand also whether the patient is asking for protection from certain matters or whether the patient is giving up the struggle and telling others to make the decisions. In this context, as in many others, social workers say "explore with the patient/family, but don't guess or make assumptions if concerned inquiry is possible."

Hospitalized patients and their relatives who express negative attitudes and feelings about the hospital, patient care, procedures, and personnel tend to express such reactions to staff members who are not physicians. The remarks are frequently passed on by those staff members to the physicians so that in the end all of the patients' givers-of-service may participate in resolving the problem. If the negative comment or troublesome behavior is perceived as a response to stress, then personnel will read the patient and relatives as persons in trouble rather than as critical, attacking, uncooperative, or ungrateful. Some negative expressions are reactions to phenomena such as the patient/family's failure to understand what is happening, a psychological need to deny or distort, or anger that masks fear. Very frequently indeed the negative attitudes toward the hospital and personnel are misdirected; they are actually worried reactions to a problem that has developed at home—perhaps a strained marital relationship, socioeconomic pressures, a child's school problem, or an unforeseen development in the patient's regular place of employment.

Social workers are skilled in exploring and intervening promptly when reactions are revealed. Some of the reactions may have rational bases, as when another medical opinion is requested because the patient is discouraged about his or her progress. Other reactions may be logical yet inappropriate, as when the patient wants to leave the hospital against medical advice because her elderly mother needs her. It is not until she talks to the social worker that she learns that homemaker service is available for her mother until the patient is able to resume her responsibilities.

Most patients who are without private physicians and who are admitted to teaching hospitals are cared for by the residents, that is, the house staff. Many patients come to recognize "the big doctors" or "the professors" and "the young doctors" as having different kinds and amounts of experience and different functions in the hospital. Although some patients/families openly express their desire for one of the big doctors, many others respond confidently to professional knowledge and competence and to evidences of the physician's caring and respect for patients and their relatives, regardless of the physician's position in the hierarchical structure of the hospital. Social workers familiar with the many kinds of stress-producing events and conditions that may precede and accompany hospitalization believe that a patient's feeling of trust in his or her physician's competence and concern for patients are among the most effective antidotes against the patient's anxiety and fear. One social worker, noting that there are many people on staff to whom patients have to relate at the point of admission, observed that some social workers withdraw "in order to reduce the number of relationships demanded of the patient." She strongly advocated that instead the social worker stand by, actively strengthening the patient's relation to his or her physician, relieving the patient's anxiety, and developing his or her own collaborative relationship with the other staff members in preparation for social work intervention should it be needed.

Hospitals in New York City which are undistricted attract patients whose residence is far beyond the boundaries of the hospital's immediate neighborhood. Patients come from other cities in New York State, from states across the nation, and from other countries in the Western and Eastern hemispheres. World-renowned reputations for work in specialties, for newly developed techniques, for areas of experimentation and research, for rare equipment, and the like bring people to teaching hospitals thousands of miles removed from their homes. Some impacts of the geographical distance from medical care upon such patients/families are sharply delineated when the home community is a foreign country. The language barrier for these hospitalized patients can be unusually severe even when they have relatives in the city who serve as interpreters and try in other ways to ease the adjustment, but the stress normally produced by hospitalization can reach great heights when not only the institutional atmosphere but the land and city are alien.

Many of the foreign patients are urged to come to New York by relatives and friends who live in the City, and to some extent they plan in advance about such matters as transportation and living arrangements. However, few of the people are affluent, many have only modest incomes, and the costs of living and of medical care are high in a metropolitan area. The financial strains may assume large proportions for the patient/family, for the friends and relatives who live in the City, and for the hospital; third-party payments often are not available under these circumstances. Lack of money, crowded living conditions caused by the patient's immediate family moving in with members of the extended family, and strained relationships resulting from these worries and inconveniences are among the most stress-producing and distressing conditions. In addition, the adult patient who is accompanied by his or her spouse may have left young children behind, and concern for them as well as feelings of loneliness add to the patient's distress. A disruption of family life, no matter what form it takes or for what reason, is always significantly stress producing.

Because serious illness is in itself a devastating experience, people may make decisions in response to it that seem irrational to the uninvolved onlooker. An example will support these obervations. One family from Upstate New York was more fortunate than out-of-state patients/families in that they were eligible for a number of essential benefits. The entire patient/family of seven moved down to the City into the home of the patient's parents, an apartment of four rooms which already housed four people. The patient was almost immediately hospitalized; the remaining ten people went through the bruising experience of living literally on top of one another in the four crowded rooms. The social worker's efforts to obtain separate housing for the patient's wife and children were unsuccessful until months after the patient's death. These two family groups survived the strains, and their affectional relations were maintained, fundamentally because their feelings were sound and their need for one another surmounted the difficulties.

Cultural factors may have special significance for the hospitalized patient and relatives. For instance, the close connection between illness and the need for spiritual sustenance is recognized by the availability of clergymen of major religious groups to patients/families who wish their compassion and guidance and the administration of rites. There are times, however, when the patient's hospitalization threatens rather than permits observance of religious beliefs and ritual, as in the case of Jewish patients/families whose orthodoxy prohibits travel and the handling of money on the Sabbath and religious holidays and who adhere to strict dietary laws. The patients usually react less strongly to violations that they cannot control than do their relatives, in part because people are normally released from certain religious obligations when they are ill. The adult patient's relatives, on the other hand, may be in serious conflict when the patient is gravely ill and they wish to be at the hospital every day for long hours and at the same time obey the commandments of their religion. In hospitals that serve substantial numbers of Jewish in-patients various accommodations may be made: Kosher food is available; on the eve of the Sabbath or a holy day a close relative of a critically ill patient is permitted to sleep in the hospital in order to avoid traveling; if Kosher food is available for patients but not for visitors, the latter are permitted to bring their food and eat it on hospital premises; and sometimes the rabbi affiliated with the hospital calls on members of his local congregation to open their nearby homes to a patient's relatives.

Members of a religious sect may, on the other hand, have a religious prohibition that directly affects medical care itself, such as a prohibition against blood transfusion. In such case the adult patient who is competent is allowed to resolve the conflict for himself or herself, after being properly informed about the medical situation; society can intervene through the courts in behalf of minor children or helpless adults whose survival is at stake. Either way, social workers are concerned about the patient/family's need for help in arriving at their own decision or in accepting one that the courts may have made in regard to a minor child.

Religious belief in spiritualism or in occultism my be stress producing for in-patients who perceive the medical care they receive as dangerous; they may feel helpless without access to a medium they have faith in or to a physician who they know does not oppose or interfere with their practice of spiritualism or magic. There are other patients, however, to whom in-hospital care is a "wonderful magic." It is well known that patients may practice their belief in spiritualism or occultism while concurrently receiving psychiatric or medical services in ambulatory care facilities. Hospitalization may therefore be particularly frustrating or even seem "dangerous" because direct access to the healer of their cult is not possible.

Food patterns constitute another potential source of stress for the hospitalized patient/family. The kind of food regularly served in the hospital and the way it is cooked may be so alien to the patient/family as to seem tasteless or even unnutritious. When the patient is on a restricted diet required by his or her illness, the lack of gratification is still greater; in fact, patients and their relatives often worry whether anyone can get well eating food that they feel has no strength in it. This is the tenor of remarks made when people who are heavy meat-eaters, for example, are put on low-protein diets and when patients used to well-seasoned foods are put on a salt-free diet.

There is another aspect of food habits to be noted: a patient's diminished appetite which is in itself symptomatic of his or her illness. The patient's decreased desire for or pleasure derived from food may be a special source of worry to his or her relatives. They may want the patient to eat because eating symbolizes growing strong and well; they often deny that the change in the patient's eating habits is symptomatic of the disease and try to deal with the loss of appetite as if it were a deterrent to cure. For example, Puerto Rican and Jewish families frequently respond in this way. Sometimes their feeling is so intense and their belief in the curative power of food so strong that they disobey hospital regulations and smuggle in the kinds of food the patient customarily enjoys. Food, being fed, and eating have values that are fundamental to human beings throughout the course of life. A change in diet is among the most difficult demands for adaptation; social workers are particularly empathic on this point and uncondemning of the questionable means some patients/families use to cope with the stress of dietary deprivation. The irrational, emotional responses to being deprived of an old and valued food pattern are frequently much stronger than the intellectual response to the medical rationale for a change in diet: this is the point of view that informs the social workers' supportive efforts to help patients/families cope constructively with dietary restrictions. That is to say, the interdependence of the external realities of life in the hospital and the internal reality of intrapsychic pressures has to be understood and worked with.

Although many patients now have some form of health insurance, union benefits at time of illness, and so forth, there are nevertheless many other patients who suffer financial hardship. People who are proud of their financial independence but have no medical insurance find that their modest earnings and savings are insufficient to pay for the cost of hospitalization. The illness may not be "catastrophic" by official definition yet it may be disastrous to the financial status of the patient/family.* Recourse to Medicaid or to a local welfare department which provides financial assistance for day-by-day living represents an indignity to some of these patients/families; they have to be persuaded to accept a resource that to them is not a social provision to which they are entitled but a mark of personal failure. Investigation for proof of eligibility, that is, the means test, is even more difficult for people to accept when their sense of status is already eroded by other aspects of illness and hospitalization.** The social workers' observations pointed to patients/families' dislike of financial dependence rather than to a preference for the "welfare ethic."***

* In 1972 the catastrophic costs of specified diseases were recognized by amending the federal law: adults under 65 with these diseases and who meet specified eligibility requirements may receive reimbursement under Medicare.

** The writer's notes describe the disapproval expressed by foreign-born social workers whose native countries provide universal health insurance. They were in disbelief that people already under stress because of illness were subjected to worry about the cost of their medical care.

*** A term used by some as pejorative in contrast to "work ethic."

The preceding discussion of stress-producing events and conditions associated with hospitalization concerns those that are more or less common to large numbers of patients/families. Within the hospital walls there are other experiences that touch a smaller portion of the total in-patient population and their relatives but that may generate a high degree of stress. These experiences are related largely to procedures and equipment used to support life and which are frightening to the average layperson precisely because they are associated—often correctly—with a struggle for survival. For example, even though use of the recovery room and the reasons for it are explained to the patient/family while preparing them for surgery, the demands for coping may be severe. The patient anticipates a long period of unconsciousness or helplessness or both, that is, a number of hours characterized by his or her complete dependence on those who are providing surgical/medical care. The patient's relatives, even if they receive an immediate postoperative report of his or her condition, are unable to see for themselves or to have any contact until the patient is moved out of the recovery room, frequently hours after surgery. It is the waiting, apprehension, and uncertainty that are so stress producing for the patient's relatives, not the use of the recovery room per se; that is usually understood as an essential and assuring procedure.

The units for intensive care always imply a question of survival (which the recovery room often does not) and therefore are noted here as specific sources of stress. The monitoring instruments and life-supporting appliances to which the patient is attached, the constant attendance of professionals and technicians working together with scientific precision, the devices that protect against contagion and infection, the strict regulations about visiting—these environmental circumstances underscore the perception of danger to the patient's life. Moreover, many patients/families have had no preparation for this experience because the condition necessitating the patient's admittance to an intensive care unit, such as cardiac failure or trauma incurred· during an accident, was an unpredictable incident. In the words of one social worker, "The intensive care units are apt to have different meanings from care in regular beds. For example, a patient in the unit is frequently so ill that all his or her energy goes into the process of physical recovery. After leaving the unit or at times not until after discharge from the hospital, the patient begins to react emotionally to the dangers there actually were to his or her life." These delayed reactions may take different forms, but depression is not an unusual one. The depression may be in part due to physiological conditions of fatigue; the patient may also be emotionally "let down" as his or her family, relieved after the crisis, lessens its support; or, after returning home, the patient may become anxious because hospital personnel who provided 24-hour care are no longer available. Also, his or her energy is no longer going so completely into recovering, and some is now released to express emotional reactions. It should be realized that denying the expression of feelings earlier may well be a patient's constructive defense in the process of healing.[1]

One can expect variations on this general theme. Many patients do react emotionally and with confusion and disorientation while they are in the unit and use the services of the social worker to relieve themselves of worries and apprehensions that might otherwise retard recovery. Exceedingly sick patients often respond to the caring and concerned attitudes of others. At first social workers expected to play an important role with anxious and upset relatives but a lesser one with the patient in intensive care. Now it is clear that some of those patients want and can actively use the social worker's services and that many physicians and nurses in the units accept and encourage the social worker's direct services and collaborative efforts.

Another example of a specialized therapeutic instrumentality which makes heavy demands for adaptation to stress is the unit that isolates a peculiarly vulnerable patient from other people as protection against the risk of infection. The full impact of what is sometimes called the Life Island or reverse isolation can be understood only if the isolation is seen in connection with related factors. Under any circumstances, the isolation is a severe deprivation of the satisfactions derived from normal human interchange and companionship. The confined space is sometimes room-sized but sometimes only bed-sized; visual and auditory expressions can be exchanged, but physical closeness and touch are impossible. Many patients in the Life Island, their relatives, and friends know that the unit is being used to prolong life as long as possible but without expectation of cure. For them the deprivations involved may become inhumane because of the need people have for closeness with one another at times of crisis; thus the patient may be removed from the Life Island when it is no longer supportive to the patient/family. While it is in use, however, the feeling of isolation may develop into feelings of desertion and abandonment; professional personnel coordinate their efforts with special care to minimize for the patient/family the sense of being apart and alone. When the use of the Life Island is not a last resort but one step in treatment, the patient/family's suffering from the isolation is made tolerable by the expectation of the patient's survival.

Children, too, are treated in intensive care units, for example, after open-heart surgery, and in reverse isolation units, when, for example, they are born with faulty immunological systems or are receiving drug therapy that suppresses those systems. The potential effects of lengthy isolation on the psychosocial development of young children and on their status of social-health sharply pits fundamental values against one another and forces people to make exceedingly difficult decisions. "What price survival?" is often the major issue.

Death comes to patients in all loci of the hospital, sometimes unexpectedly but frequently as the predicted outcome of an illness that is known to be potentially fatal. Death and the process of dying that may precede it are life-tasks that must be coped with by three groups of involved human beings: the patient; persons close to the patient, both relatives and significant others; and health care personnel. The fact of death and dying is universal; its meaning and the ways in which people cope with threatened and actual separation and loss differ enormously.[2,3,4] In the last few years both professional and lay authors have contributed greatly to the literature that informs and educates readers about death and dying. It responds to an already awakened public which now tends to remove the end phase of life from the list of forbidden subjects and dares to consider it a human experience worthy of conscious emotional and intellectual understanding.

This literature offers generalizations about people's reactions to dying and death, sometimes describes patterns of sequential reactions, suggests interpretations of their meaning, and provides insights into the motivations behind people's responses and attitudes when they are confronted with the terminal stage of life. These ideas are helpful guides which alert concerned persons to the knowledge needed for understanding, assessing, and dealing with the impacts of dying and death on individual patients and people in various relationships with them. Generalized knowledge about the psychosocial aspects of human life always has to a be applied cautiously to avoid stereotyping and making unwarranted assumptions.

Adult patients in the terminal phase of illness may show their awareness by expressing a variety of emotions "in all directions," as one social worker put it. Frustration, anger, depression, and grief may prevail in successive waves, not necessarily focused on a particular person or event. Some aware patients express emotions freely but also wish to talk about their feelings and their attempts to accept and resign themselves to the end of life and to discuss and plan what they wish to do in the time that remains. Some patients need and want human contact, support, and comfort to the end, while others sooner or later withdraw from all but the few closest to them.

Some patients give at least the appearance of total unawareness of the approach of death, and presumably in self-protection from the fear and pain of separation and loss their overt behavior conforms to the expectation of a long life ahead. Physicians may have to weaken a patient's strong defenses if, for example, informed consent is needed for certain diagnostic or therapeutic procedures or the patient's family and business responsibilities require that the patient put his or her affairs in order.

Some new medical knowledge and many new techniques contribute to the controversial issues of the right to die, death with dignity, and dying peacefully. They are not clear-cut issues in that they juxtapose values reflected in professional ethics and legal restraints, which in some instances are in conflict and in other instances reinforce one another. There is not now total agreement on the definition of death, on what constitute unjustifiable procedures for the prolongation of life, or on whether a professional and legal distinction can and should be made between allowing death to occur by the physician's taking active or passive measures.

Members of the health professions—physicians in particular—are currently besieged by an increasing number of malpractice suits and the soaring costs of malpractice insurance. It has become palpably difficult for them to exercise professional judgment about the use of medical procedures without considering possible consequences such as legal actions, jeopardized reputations, and high financial costs. Detached concern for the patient becomes closely intertwined with a compelling self-interest.

The death of another person is usually a reminder of one's own mortality, and for this reason alone those who give direct services to the dying patient may be tempted to turn away. This common human reaction may be intensified when the giver-of-service is, by profession, committed to save and prolong life and reduce human suffering. When a member of the health and health-related professions makes less frequent bedside visits to the patient who is dying or for whom he or she has no further effective interventions, the giver-of-service is protected from pain but at the cost to the patient/family of the support and comfort they need from the health care staff.

What is perhaps not sufficiently realized is that intraprofessional and interprofessional discussion—open acknowledgment among the professionals caring for a dying patient of the turmoil and distress experienced by them—can be highly effective in draining off and coping with emotions that, if acted upon directly, might result in depriving the patient/family of their physical presence and psychological strength.[5]

Leaving the hospital may be a simple process requiring the physician's notation of the patient's discharge, payment of the hospital's bill, and the patient's being called for by a relative or friend and driven happily home. For many patients, however, there is a problematic period preceding discharge which is marked by worry and conflict, dilemmas, and difficult choices. Most patients/families work out over time the anxiety and apprehensions they have had during hospitalization, and this process of coping usually extends into the period following discharge. The amount and kind of anxiety depend on many factors, such as the nature of the illness, the immediate and future expectations for the patient's social rehabilitation, the natural resources—personal, socioeconomic, and cultural—that the patient, relatives, and significant others can draw on; and the resources the community provides that will meet the short and long-term needs of the patient/family.

Implicit in the following recital of stress-producing conditions associated with leaving the hospital is the social workers' conviction that discharge planning involves medical, social, and emotional factors that need to be identified, discussed, and evaluated; that consideration of discharge should start as early as possible; and that there should be an opportunity for the participation of the patient and relatives (or those friends who stand for family), as well as for the collaborative pooling and coordination of information and ideas among the givers-of-services. The need for careful planning for discharge may exist even when patients are under the care of private physicians, live in comfortable and roomy quarters, and have the financial means to purchase required services. Ignorance about such practical matters as where to obtain services or the availability of benefits from the patient/family's insurance can be troublesome to people at any income level. The emotion-laden questions of "Where should I go?"; "Who will take care of me at home?"; and "What will happen to me in a nursing home?" can cause worry, guilt, confusion, and grief regardless of people's educational and socioeconomic status.

Social workers play an important part in making discharge plans, largely because they are the accepted professional link between hospital and patient/ family on the one hand and patient/family and the community on the other. Their knowledge of appropriate resources and how they can be obtained and their ability to explore problematic concerns with the patients/families and institutional personnel within and outside the hospital are constantly called on in the service of discharge planning. Social workers are often asked by physicians to make plans for a patient's discharge "practically overnight." Such sudden requests on behalf of patients whom social workers have not known before are usually due to lack of understanding of two major essentials. First, discharge planning must consider social and emotional as well as medical and nursing needs; it is a collaborative process that should take place among medical care personnel, the patient/family, and, when required, persons in the community who can provide needed services. Discharge planning may therefore take more time than the originator of the request realizes. Agreements have to be arrived at among persons with dissenting views about what are desirable and what are feasible plans. Environmental and financial factors may also create problems. Second, many health-related resources are in extremely short supply.

Some may not be obtainable at all. The waiting list for a needed resource may be so long that a second-best plan has to be accepted.

For example, facilities for the care of the chronically ill, and especially the terminally ill, have become unbelievably scarce in many communities; many institutions have changed their function in order to become eligible for federal reimbursement as extended care facilities. However, some extended care facilities refuse admission of patients dependent on third-party payments because of the long delay in receiving reimbursements. If a patient who is discharged home can make his or her own financial payments for homemaker or housekeeping services, they are usually available when needed. If a patient is unable to pay for them, the waiting period for service available through third-party providers may be so long as to make application impractical. Situations vary from community to community and change, for better or for worse, as policies and appropriations change in the public and voluntary sectors of society. Some problems of this kind can be avoided in hospitals that provide progressive care within their own walls. At present there are few such facilities, so patients who cannot return home immediately upon discharge have to be helped to find a place to which they can be tranferred for fuller recovery, rehabilitative services, and the like. The comparative lack of programs for comprehensive home health care is particularly unfortunate in that patients have to enter convalescent facilities even when being cared for at home is therapeutically preferable, feasible and far less expensive.

Accurate determination of what an in-patient's needs will be upon discharge and how they can best be provided for depends heavily on the kind of and degree of interplay among physicians, nurses, and social workers. They observe and inquire into the patient/family's life-and-illness-situation, each from his or her own professional perspective. They share the information each has obtained within the framework of his or her understanding of the data's significance. They join in collaborative participation to assess the interacting data as a cohesive whole on which they can base a plan for postdischarge services. Interprofessional coordination and collaboration vary from institution to institution and from service unit to service unit within an institution. Such interplay is perceived by some professionals as a necessary element in all health care programs of high quality. Others see it as selectively important, for example, for patients at exceedingly high risk. There are professionals who were introduced to the idea of interprofessional practice while they were students and take such practice for granted. To others, it is not only a new idea but one that threatens the values they attach to attributes such as authority, responsibility, accountability, and status. These and many other variables will influence the prevalence and success of professional interplay in health care.

The social worker needs time with the patient/family to determine their psychosocial needs, wants, preferences, and resources. Often he or she can begin early to acquire relevant information which will form part of the base for planning for discharge at a later date. To illustrate, a patient's illness may indicate at once that he or she will have special socioeconomic and psychological needs at the time of discharge. Does a cardiac patient have to climb steps to reach his or her living quarters? Has he or she been living alone? How close, emotionally and geographically, are relatives and friends whose help he or she might need? How attached is the patient to his or her present way and place of living?

The importance of exploring and assessing the relatives' wishes, apprehensions, attitudes, motives, and ability to cope with the patient's and their own
problem situations after the patient's discharge cannot be overemphasized. One
social worker said:

> *Family attitudes differ widely. Some relatives will not consider*
> *any plan except the patient's return home and will take care of*
> *him. Others are fearful of what may happen if the patient*
> *returning to live with them is left alone for any length of time—*
> *when they will be at work, for instance. Still others resist*
> *encroachment on their time and living space and do not want to*
> *get too involved. There are, on the other hand, patients without*
> *family or close friends who can manage in their own homes*
> *because of their drive to manage, although they may need*
> *services from community resources to minimize the danger of*
> *being alone.*

Because information about the psychosocial aspects of the patient's situation must be used in conjunction with his or her medical condition and needs, it
is clear that the professional givers-of-service should be well informed of the
strengths and lacks in the home situation and the kind and amount of responsibility members of the household can assume. In a collaborative effort the
physician and nurse and the social worker (who is usually the professional
source of the most detailed knowledge about the patient's day-by-day life) can
think together about the choices the patient/family have in regard to plans for
discharge and speculate on the potential impacts of these plans upon the
patient/family before they are discussed with the patient and his or her
relatives. The relatives will usually have their own plans to present, and strong
emotions may be evoked when compromises have to be made because of factors
such as medical and nursing requirements, limitations of available community
resources, family circumstances, and the like. For instance, while discharge
plans are being discussed, symptoms of depression may appear in the patient
and his or her relatives, or the patient may develop physical symptoms that may
be somatically expressed opposition to a plan or a wish to delay discharge.

Some distress occurs because of uncertainties about matters such as the
probable length of stay in an extended care facility or fears about the quality of
care in a nursing home, or because the discharge plan under consideration
represents a serious and permanent break with previous living arrangements
and manner of social functioning; that is, the plan demands a crisis-producing
process of adaptation. Undoubtedly, at the root of some arguments for and
against specific proposals for the period following discharge is the ability or
disability of the patient and those close to him or her to accept the patient's
altered states of psychological, physical, and social functioning.

The social worker's intent is that a plan for discharge sustain each family
member as an individual and maintain emotional equilibrium among the family
members. Social work values require that the patient not be sustained at the cost
of his or her relatives' well-being, nor should the reverse occur. For example, a
patient's treatment after leaving the hospital might depend on what relatives can
do for him or her, for example, changing a dressing, helping with prescribed
exercises, or giving injections of insulin. A family member may be capable of

following instructions and eager to be helpful yet emotionally unable to assume responsibilities that require, for example, exposing the patient's wound or sticking a needle into his or her arm.

A physician who has a strong preference for the plan he or she is proposing often yields to the patient's most hoped-for plan, realizing that the patient needs to test himself or herself and knowing that with an intense desire to succeed the patient's plan may be successful—at least for a time. The risks need to be identified and discussed and the way left open to an alternative plan should the patient's fail.

It is true that social workers take great responsibility in the process of preparing for, deciding upon, and making effective the discharge plan most suitable and feasible for a given patient/family. However, the total process is one of shared responsibility. Physicians and nurses have clearly allocated functions and tasks related to discharge, as do social workers and other health care personnel. For example, the physician explains the prescribed regimen to the patient and his or her relatives to provide guidelines for the patient's activity—what he or she should and should not be urged to do and can and cannot eat, what responses may be expected to medication, how the physician can be reached in an emergency, when the physician wishes to see the patient again, and so on. It may be necessary for a nutritionist to talk over the matter of diet or a public health nurse to give a relative instructions about giving medication or caring for the patient's wound. It is surprising how often such detailed procedures are omitted, although everyone would agree on their importance for the patient's recovery and the patient/family's peace of mind. For example, frequently discharge papers have not been signed by the physician or are mislaid, or there are too few copies of the documents required for transferring the patient to the nursing home, or the patient was not given sufficient medication to last until the next appointment with his or her physician. The possibilities for error and delay are endless when there are so many tasks to be done by so many different people. Just as there is no substitute for professional competence, there is no substitute for sound organization and structure to get things done in the right way at the right time. Social workers frequently assume an administrative, monitoring role to assure that the procedures essential to discharge are carried out in the best interests of the patient/family and the hospital.

In sum, leaving the hospital may be a simple matter requiring a few routine arrangements or, as the body of this section suggests, it may be a complex process requiring careful communication and many collaborative efforts on the part of the patient/family, multiprofessional givers-of-service, and persons outside the hospital who can make needed resources available. Decisions must be made on questions such as the following: Will the patient go home? Will a relative move in with the patient, or will the patient go to the home of a relative? Is an extended care facility preferable? If so, which one should it be, and will there be a bed available when the patient is discharged? Is home health care feasible? Is it available? Which of the possible plans is preferred by the patient/family and by health care personnel? Why? Before these decisions are made it is likely that careful consideration has been given to factors such as financial status and resources; housing arrangements, furnishings, and equipment; nuclear family relationships and those within the extended network of relatives and friends; medical and nursing needs and the resources for meeting them; and attitudes, emotional reactions, and cultural values that influence plans for discharge. It may be well to reemphasize that the professionals involved in the process of planning for discharge can be of more service to patients/families when they maintain an attitude of detached concern, that is, an attitude that does not underreact or overreact to patients/families and their problematic realities and that distinguishes between dissenting views and those that are unacceptable. This is a distinction particularly difficult to make when it hinges on differences in cultural values and customs.

Although planning the discharge of a hospitalized patient is often a complicated task that requires interprofessional collaboration, the task has come to have particularly negative meanings for some social workers. There are professional social workers who consider that practically all of the work connected with discharge planning can be carried out effectively by well-trained paraprofessionals in social service. There are other social workers who recognize, value, and use their special competence to handle problems of discharge which require their expertness in helping to resolve conflict among family members and between family members and health care personnel, and in reducing other emotional burdens that may arise in planning discharge because of demands to adapt to stressful conditions, such as separation and loss, reduced freedom to choose, or a changed self-image of decreased ability in social functioning. Many of these social workers do advocate the assignment of paraprofessionals to administrative details, such as locating resources required for an agreed-upon discharge plan, completing forms (e.g., application for home health care services or admission to a nursing home), or arranging for the transportation of a patient at the point of discharge.

A source of dissatisfaction for a considerable number of social workers who are hospital based is the tendency of some physicians to call on them for assistance with problems of discharge planning only; these physicians, the social workers believe, either ignore or are unfamiliar with the wide range of problems that their professional education and experience have equipped them to work with. Perhaps what troubles social workers even more than these perceptions of their roles is assigning solely to the physician the decision to adopt a specific plan and solely to the social worker the making of arrangements to carry it out.

It is hoped that this example of the need for interprofessional collaboration will be helpful in identifying other points in the course of health care when working together as professionals should supersede unilateral decision making and action.[7, 8]

Ambulatory care in hospital clinics[9] may be the only kind of medical care a patient experiences, but it often both precedes and follows in-patient care. For those patients who transfer back and forth between clinic care and hospitalization, there is a flow of experience, although the stress-producing events and conditions may make their impacts with differences in kind and degree. Under the rubric of ambulatory clinic care two kinds of setting will be considered: the traditional structure of general medical clinics with large numbers of specialty and subspecialty clinics to which ambulatory patients are referred from the general clinics, and the newer comprehensive care clinics which tend toward the elimination of the traditional medical clinics and of many specialty clinics. Specialists come to the comprehensive care clinics to consult with patients and their physicians, although when necessary patients are referred to those specialty clinics that have been maintained. A patient may also be transferred from a specialty clinic to a comprehensive care clinic when his or her condition has stabilized and involves no special risks.

[The Traditional Out-Patient Clinic]

In general, the traditional out-patient clinic follows the specialized model for tertiary care on a fee-for-service basis. In certain respects the established procedures are not suited to the needs of the patients who use the clinics most. These patients are poor and if employed, are bound by the demands of fixed working hours; if they are full-time housewives, they are seldom free of arduous duties during the day. Yet clinics are most often held during daytime work hours, with only a few in the evenings or on Saturdays. Another procedure requires patients to keep scheduled appointments—a procedure that is usually of benefit to both clinic personnel and patients. Yet in the cultural diversity of metropolitan areas there may always be a substantial number of newcomers to whom regard for time and being on time is an alien custom. It has been found desirable to make exceptions for such patients until they have accommodated themselves to the necessity for appointments. Thus not only will clinic cards with minimum information be available at all times, but a physician will be present to give essential treatment to patients who come to the clinic in which they are registered but on the wrong day or at the wrong time.*

There are particular hazards in the traditional structure due to the many clinics a patient may attend at a given time with no one clinic or physician responsible for his or her primary care or for coordinating the services of the specialty clinics the patient attends. The hospital can protect clinic patients from dangers such as being given drugs or other treatments that are incompatible. Adequate chart notations, prompt filing and retrieval of charts, and increased use of computerized data are among the measures the hospital can take. However, there are hazards for the ambulatory patient over which the hospital has much less or no control. The fact of being ambulatory puts most of the control in the hands of the participating patient, relatives, and friends. They are ordinarily responsible for following instructions about medication, exercise, diet, and other aspects of a prescribed regimen; for keeping clinic appointments; for reporting accurately to the physician about symptoms, unexpected effects of medication, tangible evidence of progress or lack of progress, and so on.[10] Being aware of people's differences in the ability to remember, in the power of observation and introspection, and in understanding the importance of reporting accurately, health care personnel need to estimtate the reliability of patients and relatives as informants quite apart from questions of compliance. The role of the patient/family as informants is but one illustration of communication as a major element in medical care.

Ambulatory patients whose medication may induce changes in mood or behavior are in special jeopardy when, for example, euphoria or depression leads them to break clinic appointments. Friends and relatives should be prepared for such possibilities and encouraged to alert the physician, nurse, or social worker when the patient is unable to take full responsibility for his or her judgments.

It needs to be reemphasized that patients and those close to them can be

---

* This substitute service is not to be confused with emergency service, which is described below.

successful participants in medical care only if they are well informed, understand the why's and wherefore's as well as the what's, have enabling attitudes and motivation, and have sufficiently positive feelings for one another to cope with incidents of discouragement and frustration. For example, do they have the information about the patient's illness or disability that they need? Do they understand the probable effects and outcomes of the prescribed interventions? Do they know what to do if unexpected symptoms occur? Do they understand why restrictions have been imposed, for example, on the patient's physical activity or diet, and what the consequences may be if the recommendations are ignored?

Perhaps it is pertinent to ask how widespread such patient/family education is across the nation and then to face the fact that it is spotty indeed and that physicians are seldom prepared for and practiced in assuming this educational role. Public health nurses and social workers, while they have their roles in the educational process, are not professionally qualified to assume totally the educator's role.

[A Model for comprehensive Medical Care[11]]

The material that follows describes the clinics of a voluntary hospital that began in 1966 to convert its traditional out-patient department and by 1970 had established comprehensive care clinics for adults, teenagers, and children. The change in structure and program was stimulated from both without and within the hospital. Many of its consumers were demanding an expansion of services, improved accountability, and recognition of patients' rights to dignity and privacy. Many of the professional personnel of the hospital had been making statements such as "In no single clinic in the Out-Patient Department could the total needs of a patient be met."[12] This awareness gave impetus for reorganizing ambulatory care "to achieve high quality total patient care, as family-centered as possible, under the supervision of a personal physician."[13, 14]

In this setting beneficial impacts on patients/families are noted resulting from the physical environment, the flexible procedures, the scope and purpose of the program, the staffing pattern, and professional collaboration. In general, group practice rather than solo practice more nearly describes the nature of the service. While families can readily be registered for medical care, adults, adolescents, and children receive care in different clinics, that is, the ideal of being family centered is partially achieved. Comprehensive care comes about in several dimensions. The inclusion of health education, diagnostic procedures, and treatment is one dimension. The multiprofessional character of the personnel assigned to each clinic is another dimension. Primary physicians (either internists or pediatricians), nurses, social workers, psychiatrists, and psychologists are available as needed by the patients/families or by the practitioners for consultation. Provision for preventive medicine as a major component of comprehensive care is still a future goal in most hospital-based programs.

Continuity of medical care becomes a more attainable goal here than under the conditions of traditional clinic care. Each patient has his or her own physician and public health nurse, with the nurse taking primary responsibility for health education; patients are encouraged to attend clinic for as long as is medically necessary and to return when symptoms recur or new symptoms appear. As an encouragement to positive attitudes toward health and medical care, patients' records and charts are closed only in a technical sense; the patients are not told their "cases" are closed. Importance is placed on motivating patients to follow through on medical care rather than drop out the moment they feel better. This aspect of health education reduces dropouts from medical care and helps reduce clogging of the hospital—and particularly the emergency service—with patients in crises. It is hoped that, in the end, comprehensive clinic care will provide health services with greater efficiency than is possible under the traditional structure.

Continuity of medical care is assured also by the patients' access by telephone to a public health nurse 24 hours a day. Unnecessary visits to the emergency service thus are often avoided and unfounded panic reactions handled with dispatch, sometimes by a simple question such as "Did you take your medicine?"

Because all physicians in the comprehensive care clinics are paid by the hospital, there is continuity of the physician-patient relationship over longer periods than is possible in the usual out-patient clinic. Some social workers have said that the idea of a "charity patient" is practically eliminated by this pattern of staffing. This observation seems related to a felt conflict between service and education, since the social workers emphasized that there were no resident house staff in the comprehensive care clinic for adults.

Observers have noted also the influence of the clinics' physical and social atmosphere on the patients' use of the clinic. Pleasing colors, air-conditioning, an informal grouping of chairs, a playroom for children, and the staff members' acceptance of the clinic's becoming a community meeting place—these attributes are frequently mentioned as contributing noticeably to the well-being of the patients and their concerned relatives.

Other advantages reported were that fewer specialty clinics and more consultations held in the comprehensive care clinics save the patient's energy, reduce the number of visits to the hospital, and lessen the confusion that patients feel while finding their way through the corridors of buildings that often seem forbidding and impenetrable.

There is also a side to this picture that is less bright; it falls under the shadow of conditions that are not controllable by the structure and scope of any program for ambulatory medical care. Most of the patients who attend the comprehensive care clinics in this particular hospital are very poor and have grossly inadequate resources in education and work experience. Adult patients who are foreign born sometimes have severe language barriers, and multilingual professionals are hard to come by. Many disadvantaged patients see no hope for a better future, their present is grim, and they do not readily see a relationship between health and the urgent needs of the moment for food, clothing, and shelter. One social worker, describing the difficulty some patients have in following a prescribed regimen, said, "For those who belong to the middle class it is easy to forget what these patients go home to, how little they have to work with. They are in a struggle with dust, rats and mice, inadequate income and food, and children to be cared for when they get back from clinic." These observations fit equally well the experience of many hospitalized patients who are discharged to their homes. Once more we see the convergence and interactions of the biological, psychological, and social aspects of human life and the urgent need for improved and coordinated services in many of the systems of care which should be better related to our systems of health care.

In the large urban area under consideration, the acute general teaching hospital tends to serve huge patient populations. In one hospital, the figures for a recent year were 36,000 in-patients, 59,000 clinic patients, and 50,000 patients in emergency services; in another hospital, for the same year, the figures were 6,500 in-patients, 12,000 clinic patients, and 21,000 patients in emergency services. The point of interest is not the absolute number in each group of patients, but the ratio of hospitalized patients to patients in clinic and emergency services. It is a figure that highlights the issues and problems connected with the deployment of social workers within a single hospital: which patients/families should be covered, for what problems and services, for how long, and in what location in the hospital. These are highly important administrative questions, especially when one considers the relatively small size of a social service department in an era of rising costs for health care and decreases in funding.*

However, patients/families cannot wait for the answers to these questions, and social workers offer individuals and groups of patients the help that their current deployment permits. As an example of both stress-producing conditions in ambulatory clinic care and the benefits of social work service to small groups of these patients, the following condensed description of one small-group meeting is offered. It illustrates the stress-producing factors three patients were struggling with; how the patients interacted; how the social worker intervened; and how the patients used her interventions. The group was composed of three women, each with carcinoma of the breast and each receiving chemotherapy at the time of the group session described below. The group had originated three months earlier, and this was its sixteenth session. However, Miss Davis was the only one who had been in the original group. Mrs. Brizzi had become a member two months ago. This was Mrs. Engel's first meeting.

Miss Davis, in her late fifties, lived alone but in the neighborhood of her two married brothers and a married sister. The family was Jewish with quite close ties. Miss Davis' carcinoma had been treated medically only. Mrs. Brizzi, of Italian descent, was in her early fifties. She and her husband lived in the city. Their daughter, a widow, lived with her children on the outskirts of the city. A married son who lived in another state was seldom in touch with the other family members. Recently Mrs. Brizzi had expressed unhappiness over her marital relationship. She had a mastectomy; her current treatment was for a metastatic condition. Mrs. Engel, Jewish and in her late fifties, lived with her husband. A married son, his wife, and their children lived nearby. Mr. Engel was said to rely heavily on his wife and to be exceedingly apprehensive about her illness.

Mrs. Frank, the social worker who had been with the group from its first session, worked regularly in the chemotherapy clinic. She was available to all of its staff and patients and was a familiar figure in the service unit.

* For example, in one hospital there were 58 professional social workers in a year when the total patient population was 140,000. In another hospital there were 14 professional social workers for a total patient population of approximately 50,000.

When Mrs. Frank entered the room the three women were talking intently. She asked, "What's going on?" and Mrs. Engel spoke up first. "We've been talking about Mrs. Winston. She looks terrible. I was sitting across from her in the waiting room and she upset me so I had to move. Her legs looked all red and swollen, like they were going to burst. I felt bad for her, but I had to move."

The three patients exchanged gossipy information about Mrs. Winston until Mrs. Frank remarked, "You know, it almost sounds as if you were putting yourselves in Mrs. Winston's place. Could that be?"

Miss Davis replied, "Oh, I don't know. When I was young my arms were heavy, but they certainly aren't swollen now like her legs."

Mrs. Engel took it up. "Well, she does look terrible, and I do feel sorry for her, and I had to move away. I don't know if I feel like Mrs. Frank said, but I do know that she upset me."

Mrs. Frank then pointed up their dilemma. "You know, you ladies are surely in a bind. You need treatment, and you want it. But then sometimes you see people who really upset you." All three patients nodded vigorously, and Mrs. Engel added, "It's scary to see someone like Mrs. Winston."

Mrs. Frank pushed for some specifics, and Mrs. Engel went to the heart of the matter. "Well, we all have cancer, and I guess we all know we're going to die someday. But nobody wants to be reminded. You're right, it is a bind. And you know nobody stops coming to this clinic because they got better or got cured."

Mrs. Brizzi asked, "Mrs. Frank, whatever happened to that heavy Puerto Rican lady who had trouble breathing and looked so sad?" When Mrs. Frank told them that Mrs. Testa had died a few weeks ago, they expressed sorrow and then tried to recall more vividly who she was and what she looked like. Soon they fell into a silence which Mrs. Frank broke. "I guess you all have a lot of feelings about Mrs. Testa's death." Mrs. Engel agreed, "It's like I said, no one ever stops coming because they got cured."

Mrs. Brizzi sounded more hopeful. "But some people can live a long time, you know. That's why we come to see the doctors even if it isn't always easy. Like when you think you're going to see people like Mrs. Winston."

Mrs. Engel underscored life's uncertainties: "You know, I had my breast removed about nine years ago, and the doctors all told me I had passed the dangerous period. So, when I started to get short of breath, the doctors thought it was pneumonia. It wasn't. They think now it has spread."

Miss Davis then said she hadn't wanted to know about her condition when her doctor told her; the disease would have told her anyway "in its own good time." Mrs. Engel, who wanted to know even if it made her "feel terrible," said she couldn't understand Miss Davis. Mrs. Frank explained that there were different ways of thinking about the illness, and each person has his or her own viewpoint.

Mrs. Engel turned immediately to Miss Davis. "Well, I respect your feeling your way. But I'd rather know what's what. I don't mean the doctor should tell me I have one year or two or three. I just want to be informed. If they take x-rays I want to know what they find and what they plan to do."

When Mrs. Frank encouraged Mrs. Brizzi to enter into the discussion, she related how she had moved in with her daughter last weekend because of Mr. Brizzi's drinking problem. Mrs. Engel thought that Mrs. Brizzi "should talk about that with Mrs. Frank outside the group," but Mrs. Brizzi ignored the remark and went on. Mr. Brizzi started drinking, according to Mrs. Brizzi, when her original diagnosis was established. He keeps telling her she is sick and shouldn't go out; it doesn't help her at all. Mrs. Engel and Miss Davis thought she needed someone to depend on, while his talk probably made her feel worse. Mrs. Brizzi became angry. "That's right. He's the sick one and look what he's doing to me." Suddenly, she put her head down and sobbed. Mrs. Frank put her hands on Mrs. Brizzi's shoulders, and the two other patients made clucking, comforting sounds. When Mrs. Brizzi stopped crying, she asked Mrs. Frank to talk with her husband "about what is happening to us." Mrs. Frank suggested that she and Mrs. Brizzi have a good talk first; Mrs. Brizzi said she'd like that.

Just then the clinic nurse announced the physicians' arrival, and Mrs. Frank closed the session with a brief summary of what had concerned them, noting their strength to talk openly about their difficulties. When she remarked also upon their helpful response to Mrs. Brizzi's intense emotion, Mrs. Brizzi said she felt better than she had when the session began.

In this abbreviated recording of an hour's discussion, there is clear evidence of stress-producing factors such as disfiguration; the risk of recurring symptoms; the knowledge that one's condition is incurable, medicine is fallible, and one's life span limited; and the failure of relatives to be understanding, supporting, and enabling.[15]

Perhaps the first fact to note is that open groups, which permit patients to join and discontinue as their respective situations dictate, may have restrictive influences on the social worker's interventions and on the patients' expression of ideas and feelings, especially during the first session of a new member's attendance. Although the impacts of Mrs. Engel's appearance on the other members of the group, on group behavior, and on the social worker cannot be assessed accurately, one may speculate that the mildness of Mrs. Frank's interpretive comments is one of the consequences.

The effect of one patient on another is a major factor in health care. The group session opens and closes on this note: first the hardship of observing how ill, disfigured, and disabled a particular disease may render a patient and wondering when this fate will befall them, and then the enabling effect of companions who are sympathetic and supportive.

In this one session, the patients' different ways of coping emerge with surprising clarity. Miss Davis leans toward the protection of denying—her arms have never been that swollen; she prefers her information to come from her body, not her physician. Mrs. Brizzi leads into and around the idea of cancer as a fatal disease—what happened to Mrs. Testa?—but can plunge into a revelation of the strains in her marriage. Mrs. Engel has the courage to face up to the name of their disease, to her physician's error in prognosis, and to the chronic nature of her condition, but she prefers not to be told when her life might end, and she seems unready to hear about Mrs. Brizzi's marital problem or, presumably, her own—that is too private for group discussion.

The social worker intervenes for a variety of reasons. She helps the group members put their cards on the table by asking what they are so concerned about when she enters the room. She redirects the patients' attention when they stray from a problem toward a cover-up; for example, she stops the gossipy exchange about Mrs. Winston, and a while later she urges the women to say what is scary. She lessens accumulated tension, as when she breaks the silence that follows the announcement of Mrs. Testa's death and thus makes possible Mrs. Engel's verbalization of what they must expect for themselves.

The social worker, who helps these patients realize the benefits derived from their common experiences, makes it clear also that there is no one way to cope; the acceptance of difference as well as of similarity is a powerful instrument in being of help to one's fellows. Mrs. Engel caught the meaning immediately when she declared her respect for Miss Davis' feeling and viewpoint. Respect was precisely what the social worker was demonstrating and advocating.

These three patients illustrate well how each has her way of coping with her own truth; and how clearly they can describe the boundaries of what they want and do not want to face. Two attributes are particularly worth noting: some degree of hope—not for cure, but for living and functioning as well as each can, and some degree of trust in the ability and willingness of other human beings to understand and to help.

Emergency Service*

Institutions and organizations and their subunits which offer professional services experience movement and change for both fortunate and unfortunate reasons. At face value, the fortunate reasons are connected with people's motivations to improve the quality and adequacy of professional services, while the unfortunate reasons seem to be connected with lacks and deprivation caused by environmental forces such as loss of funding and scarcity of resources, including manpower, to meet need and demand.

In looking at what is happening in emergency service units of a few large urban hospitals one is struck by the fact that on occasion, a phenomenon that appears to be highly undesirable can be turned into a force for good. Although real changes for the better are taking place, it is still valid to look closely at several problematic areas in emergency service: the huge volume of patients requesting it, their reasons for coming to the unit, and patterns of staffing.[16]

As befits this text the discussion that follows reflects the social worker's perspective more than it does the perspective of other professionals, but the comments have some significance for all health care personnel. Until the last few years it was customary for social workers to rotate being on call to come to emergency service during daytime working hours (9 AM to 5 PM);[17] the requests were largely from physicians and nurses assigned to the service. It was customary also for social workers to be available on the telephone at night and over the weekend. In these ways there was coverage, but as the social workers themseves said, the plan gave them almost no opportunity to develop collaborative relationships with physicians and nurses on the service. This staffing pattern is giving way to in-person, regular assignments of social workers to emergency service, and there are reports of such assignments being extended beyond the five o'clock closing time.

To help meet the greatly increased demand of recent years for emergency

* This section covers patients requiring medical/surgical services. Emergency psychiatric service is considered in Chapter 6 in the section devoted to psychiatric patients.

service,* the old pattern of staffing by physicians who volunteer their services is changing rather rapidly. Physicians are paid for their work; attending physicians are in both administrative and service positions; and house staff, too, are paid for their services in these units.

The reasons why people come to an emergency service, what they are seeking, and whether they have come to the best place to find it are significant issues in this time of change. A social work administrator described the fundamental problem in this way: "The service used to be seen as a life-saving, immediately urgent procedure. This is an outmoded concept, as it is not the way people across the country use emergency service. They tend to use it when they can't stand what is bothering them any longer."

At the operating level social workers describe the situation in specific terms which can easily be subsumed under the administrator's generalization. One social worker assigned to an allergy clinic was frequently called to emergency service. She found that some asthmatic patients who came in in an acute crisis were registered in clinic but did not attend sessions; others were not registered but came to emergency service recurrently in acute episodes. This social worker believed that many of the emergency visits could be eliminated if patients/families became convinced of the superiority of continuing care and if social conditions and psychological factors that interfered with their attending clinic were removed or alleviated through the help of social workers. It would take, she thought, regular coverage of emergency service by a social worker who could join with physicians and nurses in a program of health education and, in addition, provide direct social work services as needed.

A social worker in another hospital suggested that visits to emergency service could be reduced by referring potentially eligible patients to the home-care program. Her observation concerned patients who are in need of continuing medical care and do not need institutional care but are too incapacitated for regular attendance at ambulatory care clinics. These patients are apt to come to emergency service at times of crises and at excessive costs in energy, in psychological and physical distress, and in financial expenditure.

Though patients with serious trauma and illness do still come for emergency service, the foregoing comments support the view that many visits are no longer precipitated by the need for life-saving procedures. Instead, many of the patients are using emergency service as a substitute for primary medical care. If primary care were available, crises and related hardships could be avoided in many instances. Patient/family education would be a useful measure, but at the same time more available and accessible facilities in our various systems of health care and related services are an absolute necessity.

Hospital-Based Home-Care

Hospital-based home-care programs make it possible for patients to remain in their natural environment as long as possible. A wide range of services available for unlimited periods is essential to this purpose, for example, medical care; nursing care; physiotherapy; speech therapy; social work services; a variety of home health services from persons such as home health aides, homemakers, and housekeepers; and transportation between home and hospital

---

* Vorzimer and Katz note that there was an increase of 185 percent in the number of patients using the emergency service of Beth Israel Hospital in New York City between 1955 and 1965.

when required. In addition to comprehensive coverage of needs and availability of services for indeterminate periods, these programs should be characterized by flexibility, continuity of care, participation of family members, and a well-developed process of interprofessional and intraprofessional collaboration.

Flexibility is manifested in different ways. Patients can enter and leave the program as their medical-social situations require. They may have to transfer at intervals between home care and in-hospital care; others become able to attend clinic, perhaps for a short time only, perhaps for a long period; patients can be transferred from home care to nursing home care when their conditions demand it. Flexibility of another kind is provided, too. Patients need different services at different times or need a service more or less intensively. To illustrate, although medical care is basic to the program and uninterrupted, there will be times when the physician increases or decreases the number of house calls he or she makes to see a patient, or on occasion a special consultant will be called in. Visiting nurse services may be needed continuously or only at intervals. In situations of heightened tension in the home the social worker may visit once a week and telephone between visits. In other situations the social worker may visit regularly but infrequently, say, once a month. The fluid tailoring of services to the patient/family's needs is an outstanding benefit.

Continuity of care is another major advantage of these programs. The attributes of fragmentation and discontinuity so noticeable overall in our traditional systems of delivering medical care are considerably reduced by the comprehensive scope, unlimited periods of service, and flexible nature of the hospital-based home care programs. There are some home care programs offered by third-party providers, but they tend to be sharply limited in the kinds of services available and in the length of time services are available to a given patient. These programs are useful in meeting a limited scope of short-term needs, but the comprehensive, long-term programs—which are in exceedingly short supply nationwide—are the ones that are most needed.

A third important characteristic of these hospital-based programs is the encouragement they give and the opportunity they provide for the active participation of concerned family members in the patient's care. This characteristic recognizes the value our society places on the family as an institution (some subcultures in our society put more and some put less value on the family) and in particular recognizes the therapeutic effects of the patient's being restored to a familiar milieu with familiar faces. There may come a time when home care is no longer feasible, no matter how close the family bonds. But for a while, at least, the patient/family's desire can be fulfilled.

Last, there is the collaborative process which must take place among the professional and vocational personnel who provide the direct services of a home-care program to patients/families. Without this process, personnel who have access to the patient's home could convey contradictory messages about medicosocial plans, confuse patients and relatives, impair working relationships between personnel and family members, and create emotional strain within the family group. Not that inadequate collaboration within the hospital walls can be condoned either; it is, after all, a process that can be explicated and learned, and wherever it takes place its benefits are demonstrable.

The patients accepted for hospital-based home-care services are beneficiaries of the concept of coordinated, comprehensive, and continuing home care for the ill and disabled who do not require institutional care. The concept fits

well into the larger concept of progressive patient care.[18] There are comparative-
ly few such home care programs in the nation despite the great need for them.
As early as the middle 1960s it was estimated that there were "1.4 million
chronically ill non-institutionalized persons who are sufficiently incapacitated to
be confined to their homes. . . ."[19, 20]

An inquiry into the nature of the patient population in two home care
programs—one in a municipal and one in a voluntary hospital—showed a great
difference in numbers at a given time but no other significant distinctions. The
municipal hospital was serving 250 patients in its program, while the voluntary
hospital was caring for 35. In each program the majority of patients were elderly,
and there were more women than men. Their medical diagnoses covered a wide
range: cardiac diseases, cancer, orthopedic conditions, complications from diabetes, and blood disorders. Symptoms of mental confusion and deterioration
were not uncommon.

There were a number of younger adults, some still in their twenties, with
diseases such as multiple sclerosis, and occasionally there was a pediatric
patient with a chronic illness such as muscular dystrophy.

The composition of the family groups resembled that of the population at
large. Many of the older and middle-aged patients lived alone; others lived with
spouses or adult children. Sometimes the patient was a spouse and parent in a
relatively young nuclear family or a child in such a family. Family groups may
be composed of adult siblings (often elderly) and others of close friends who
have established themselves as a family. There may be more than one patient in
the household who has been admitted to the home care program.

In general, the patients/families in these home care programs lived on low
or marginal incomes, many of them either obtaining financial assistance from
public welfare agencies or maintaining themselves on Social Security benefits.
Occasionally a family was able to pay for a home service, such as the aid of a
homemaker, for a relatively short period of need. Patients in low-income
housing projects benefited not only from relatively adequate space and living
conditions but from the government subsidies that kept rents at reduced levels.

Programs for hospital-based home-care will be better understood if the
process of admission to home care programs and the experience of receiving
medical care at home are linked to experiences of hospitalization—especially in
regard to planning for discharge—and to experiences in units for ambulatory
care. The sequence in which these experiences occur will vary and form
different patterns, but an important fact is that the impact on the patient/family
of one set of experiences colors the impact of the next.

Since a patient's first admission to a hospital's home care program is apt to
follow immediately upon a period of hospitalization, the previous comments on
planning for discharge are all pertinent here. Then there are aspects of
determining the suitability of home care for patients with chronic or long-term
illness or disability which influence the intensiveness and extensiveness of
inquiry and exploration. The scope of the study of each patient/family em-
braces: (1) the expected medical and nursing needs of the patient, (2) the
resources and lacks in the patient/family's physical environment, (3) the
strengths and limitations in personal and human resources, and (4) the availability of needed community resources. While these are familiar criteria for
determining any plan for discharge, it is essential that the study in regard to
home care programs be made by a multiprofessional group; that the final
assessment and decision be collaboratively and interprofessionally arrived at

with the participation of the patient/family; and that the study always include visiting the home to which the patient will go, as well as talking with persons who will be living with him or her or coming in to care for the patient.

Usually the visits to the home during the period of exploration are made by a public health nurse and a social worker, and they are made with special concern for the patient/family's sensibilities. Inspection of equipment and living conditions is detailed, and inquiries may touch upon intimate and delicate situations. As one social worker put it, "It is very important not to seem nosy." The most effective way to conduct the visits is with the patient/family's full understanding of the reasons for the investigatory activities.

In general, the situation in the home has to be evaluated in relation to certain aspects of the patient's ability to function socially, for example, the ability to move about and to care for his or her personal needs, and requirements for care from others. The balance and kind of personal interdependence among family members and the resources that will make it possible for the patient/family to achieve a satisfying emotional equilibrium are prime matters for assessment.

Equally important is an assessment of the physical environment. There are numberless details that can be observed, so the process is selective, patient by patient, depending on what is most pertinent to his or her situation. A broad outline of the inquiry would include the following: (1) *adequacy of living space in general* (the number and size of the rooms, space that affords privacy when it is needed, a place for the patient/family and friends to gather for recreation, the accessibility of living space to the patient, when for example, rooms in a family house are on more than one floor or wide doorways are needed to accommodate a wheelchair or a person on crutches, or if thresholds, uneven floors, or holes in the carpet present hazards to safety); (2) *adequacy of bedroom, bathroom, and kitchen space and equipment* (the height of the patient's bed, space for a hospital bed, the height of the toilet seat, the need for bathroom rails and handholds, the height of cupboards and stove); (3) *adequacy of the building* (elevator service, safety measures against fire, ventilation, provision of heat and hot water); and (4) *adequacy of housekeeping* (cleanliness, orderliness).

A competent study and assessment will consider the welfare of the patient and all others significant to him or her. For example, in a household of adults a room given over to recreation may have minor importance. For a family in which there are growing children who should be able to have friends in or play their own brand of loud music, such a room may be essential to everyone's well-being. The height of a bed may be important because the patient should learn to move from bed to wheelchair and back to the bed. In another case the height of a bed may be of more importance to the patient's wife because she is the one who will have to bend over it to care for him.

Although public health nurses have the greater expertness in regard to most of these physical conditions, social workers also judge them. An exchange of observations leads to assessments jointly arrived at; there does not always have to be a hard and fast allocation of tasks. It is suggested that the reader relate this illustration of collaborative practice to other areas of inquiry; for example, although the social worker may have greater expertness in assessing family relationships, all members of the professional group will make their contributions to the final evaluation.

Human and institutional resources include the personal abilities and deficiencies, intellectual and emotional, which are reflected in people's capacity to cope with demands for adaptation; the strengths and limitations in human relationships within a family group and with their significant others; and socioeconomic resources, such as financial resources, already in use by the patient as well as resources in the community which can be drawn on to meet specific needs.

Along with the many benefits of a home care program, there exist a number of stress-producing conditions which can result in discomfort, frustration, and strain. For this reason social workers note that there must be a careful assessment of the persons' desire to have the services of a home-care program; of the kind and strength of their motivation to use such a program; and of their ability to deal with frustrations of various kinds. These inner strengths and limitations become known through both careful observation of nonverbal communication with hospital personnel and among family members and through the verbal communications personnel encourage and listen to for all their overt and hidden meanings. The process of exploration includes the task of making clear not only the reasons for the inquiry but such important matters as the details of the home care program—what it offers and does not offer and how it operates. The exploratory process is thus also preparatory and relies heavily on interaction, on a channel of communication between hospital staff members and patient/family. A daughter's desire to have a parent in her home for an indefinite period of care may be weak but become stronger when she realizes the kinds of service that will be available. A widow who is hemiplegic may be strongly motivated to return home to keep her family of children together but frightened and hopeless about coping with her limitations of speech and movement until she understands which services can be made available to her, how many days a week, and how many hours a day. Her children may be afraid that they may be placed with foster parents and equally frightened about caring for a strangely helpless mother. Understanding the nature and range of available services in the program and meeting the people who will share responsibility produce as much hope in the children as in their mother; everyone's potential to make a successful adaptation is enhanced.

Motivations to use or not use home-care services are varied. They may spring out of people's unqualified need for one another; out of seesawing ambivalence in family relationships; or out of painful guilt which impels the patient/family toward a plan that will assuage guilt but hold few other gratifications. Different members of a family may be differently motivated, so that the need for joint decisionmaking is urgent. The social worker may play a considerable role in helping people to weigh the pros and cons, in pointing out factors the family may not think of, and in facilitating the resolution of conflicting feelings and ideas.

Social workers make it clear that they do not look for ideal family relationships. People quarrel, may on occasion be punitive toward one another, reach points of tension that are explosive, are irritated by one another's foibles or compulsions—and yet may have learned to deal with their ups and downs and in some instances may have a need for such ups and downs as a way of life.

In the case of the many patients who wish to continue living alone, relationships with people outside the family are at times of more importance than relationships with members of the family. On whom can the patient count to help with household chores and shopping, to visit, and to maintain telephone contact? Are the patient's clergyman and members of the congregation actively interested in their housebound members? Is the patient congenial with these people? Does the patient prefer using institutional community resources for some essential tasks because he or she doesn't want everyone to know his business?

In coming to a decision about a patient's entering a home-care program there is a special need to look as far ahead as possible in order to estimate how the patient, relatives, and significant others may be able to cope with future stress-producing events and conditions. Despite the benefits inherent in a coordinated home-care program, there are always frustrations in the continuing life-and-illness-situation, and certain frustrations are associated with the program itself. For example, in a hospital-based home-care program the patient's physician is an employed staff member of the hospital. A patient faced with the requirement to give up his or her own physician may consider the loss too severe and decide not to enter the program. Patients who are alcoholic may be uncomfortable with the program—though they do not necessarily reject it— because, for example, they fear interference with their drinking and unconventional style of living or are ashamed and dread visitors. Patients with some mental impairment, such as failing memory and faulty judgment (signs usually found in elderly patients), may insist on trying the home-care program even though they will not have the 24-hour protection they need. They opt for risks such as forgetting to take their medicine in order to be in their own homes. Although hospital staff members are concerned about the physical safety and health of such patients, they tend to approve use of the home care program as long as possible. An important reason for this decision is that institutionalized patients run a greater risk of psychosocial deterioration than do patients living in the community.

However, whether a patient is living alone, with relatives, or with friends, the effects of chronicity may eventually take their toll; every human being has limits of tolerance for stress. Introduction of a new regimen in the patient's home or a complete change, such as transfer to a suitable health care facility, may be necessary.

SIGNIFICANT LACKS IN THE HEALTH-CARE SYSTEM

In order to appreciate fully the impacts of care in the various loci of the hospital, it is necessary to keep in mind what is not provided. Gaps and lacks have a way of influencing the utilization, function, and quality of what there is.

Much of the specialized tertiary medical care in current teaching hospitals is accurately called superb. At the same time there is a serious lack of programs for preventive intervention, for consumer and patient education, and for home health care. The lack of progressive care units within hospitals exaggerates the lack of patient education and increases the need for some form of institutional care after discharge from the hospital, or at least for better provision of home health care. Then there is the pervasive failure to provide universally accessible primary care. Another weak link in the chain of programs and services is the phenomenon of fragmented and uncoordinated but related systems of care—for example, for health care, income maintenance, housing, and education—which serves to underscore and increase the impacts of deficiencies within our health care systems.

For the most part the descriptive data in this chapter represent conditions and events in the hospital that have a direct and immediate impact. A step removed, but still vital to the experiences of patients/families and hospital personnel and also affecting the institution, are laws, policies, regulations, and procedures that originate in places of authority beyond the hospital walls.

The expansion of programs of medical care and of funding mechanisms has come about largely by way of legislation at the various levels of government. This use of public monies brings with it an obligation to assure the quality and volume of services and to monitor and control the efficiency and ethical conduct with which programs and services are administered and delivered. All such regulations affect the institutions, their personnel, and their patient populations.

Some of the most important of these regulations define the services that will be paid for and the professionals and types of institutions eligible for payments, and specify the maximum amounts of payment allowed for the respective services and the period of time for which payments may be made.[21]

Other significant controls concern such matters as the utilization of hospital beds, the development of Professional Standards Review Organizations, the establishment of Health Maintenance Organizations, and special legislation, as for catastrophic illness.

There are also important sources of impacts in medical practice, such as the status of group versus solo practice and the development of prepaid versus fee-for-service methods of payment. A rapidly increasing volume of malpractice suits, relatively uncontrolled costs of insurance against suits for malpractice, and increasingly large awards to plaintiffs also affect hospitals, personnel, and patients/families alike.

In the past decade there have been marked changes in labor-management relations manifested in the formation of unions and other kinds of bargaining units to which professionals and nonprofessionals belong. Negotiated or arbitrated settlements follow upon strikes which a short time ago seemed completely incompatible with the delivery of medical care. As in all big business, confrontations between management and labor affect the costs, the quality, and the volume of production—the product in this case being patient care in the various service units—and, in the last analysis, affect the success with which administrative and operational staff in their totality work toward common goals for the benefit of the patient population.

Recognition of gaps and deficits which are not easy to remedy must be complemented by recognition of the provision of many services; of advances in knowledge and technologies in the health care field; of efforts to redistribute and use professionals in new, more effective ways; and of more determined attempts by professionals to practice collaboratively among themselves and to encourage participation by patients/families and the general public.

REFERENCES

1. For a patient's account of her experience in intensive care, see Rachel McKenzie, Risk (New York: Viking Press, 1971). Available also in the New Yorker, November 21, 1970, p. 56.
2. Renee C. Fox, Experiment Perilous (New York: Free Press, 1959).
3. Elizabeth Kubler-Ross, On Death and Dying (New York: Macmillan, 1969).
4. Olga Knopf, Successful Aging (New York: Viking Press, 1975).
5. "Students Face Hard Questions on Death as They Move Through Their First Year," AAMC Education News, vol. 3, no. 5 (June 1976), p. 1.

6. Leslie J. Shellhase and Fern E. Shellhase, "Role of The Family in Rehabilitation," *Social Casework*, vol. 53, no. 9 (November 1972), pp. 544-550.

7. Katherine N. Olsen and Marvin E. Olsen, "Role Expectations and Perceptions for Social Workers in Medical Settings," *Journal of Social Work*, vol. 12, no. 3 (July 1967), pp. 70-78.

8. Helen Rehr, ed., Medicine and Social Work: An Exploration in Interprofessionalism (New York: Prodist, 1974).

9. Walter A. Morgan and Len Hughes Andrus, "Health Care System: Ambulatory Care," in *Encyclopedia of Social Work*, 17th ed. (Washington, D. C.: National Association of Social Workers, 1977), pp. 562-572.

10. Peter M. Lazes, "Health Education Project Guides Outpatients to Active Self-Care," *Hospitals*, vol. 51, no. 4 (February 1977), p. 81.

11. Jefferson J. Vorzimer and Gerald Katz, "Toward Comprehensive Ambulatory Care: A Case History of Decisive Change," *Medical Care*, vol. 8, no. 1 (January-February 1970), p. 76.

12. Ibid.

13. Ibid.

14. See also Paul J. Vogt, "Ambulatory Care," *Hospitals*, vol. 45, no. 24 (December 1971), pp. 59-61, for descriptions of primary care and comprehensive care.

15. Joan K. Parry and Nancy Kahn, "Group Work with Emphysema Patients," *Social Work in Health Care*, vol. 2, no. 1 (fall 1976), pp. 55-64.

16. Gerald W. Grumet and David L. Trachtman, "Psychiatric Social Workers in the Emergency Department," *Health and Social Work*, vol. 1, no. 3 (August 1976), pp. 113-131.

17. George I. Krell, "Hospital Social Work Should Be More Than a 9-5 Position," *Hospitals*, vol. 50, no. 10 (May 1976).

18. John D. Thompson, "Health Care System: General Hospital," in *Encyclopedia of Social Work*, 16th ed. (New York: National Association of Social Workers, 1971), pp. 530-537.

19. Harry T. Phillips, "Disability and Physical Handicap: Services for the Chronically Ill," in *Encyclopedia of Social Work*, 16th ed., op. cit., pp. 218-227.

20. "Home Health Care Conference," *Perspectives in Long-Term Care* (AMA Council on Medical Services), vol. 4, no. 2 (fall 1973), p. 2.

21. "Two-Year Study Provides Data on Costs of Home Health Care," *Visiting Nurse Service of New York Review*, vol. 5, no. 1 (winter 1977), pp. 1-2.

Chapter 6
Selected
Patient Groups:

PATIENTS IN PSYCHIATRIC SERVICE; PREGNANT WOMEN

In chapters 3 and 4 the focus was on adult patients requiring diagnostic, therapeutic, and rehabilitative measures associated primarily with medical and surgical services. The substance of this chapter concerns two groups of patients who fall outside this framework but within the function of most acute general hospitals in an urban area.

PATIENTS IN PSYCHIATRIC SERVICE

The first such group of patients consists of those whose problems are primarily psychiatric in nature. Over the past two decades acute general hospitals have become a major resource for these patients, some of whom need hospitalization for a limited period while others need ambulatory care.

The development of psychiatric services in general hospitals has taken place concurrently with other developments, such as a declining population in mental hospitals which in turn shows the influence of new therapeutic techniques, especially drug treatment, increased third-party funding, and expansion of transitional residential or day/night care.[1, 2]

Despite the establishment of psychiatric services within the walls of the general hospital, there remains much of the separateness that has existed for years between psychiatric and medical/surgical units of service and between the administrators and practitioners in these units. Anyone who questions whether there is a cleavage needs only to hear a physician, frustrated by the rebelliousness of a patient on the surgical floor, say, "he belongs on the other side of the house." Similarly, social workers who have been asked to continue contacts with a patient being transferred from psychiatric service to, say, an intensive coronary care unit have been known to respond with, "I don't know that much about medical problems." In light of that separateness this section will focus on the nature and impacts of psychiatric services per se. It will refer to age groups when they are pertinent, but the primary intent is to round out the three major categories of health care interventions: medical, surgical, and psychiatric.

Those who count the practice of physicians in each of the categories by centuries have to deal with the historical fact of a continuing, intraprofessional chasm: "Whether differences in ideology and method are at the base of the organizational and institutional split between physical and mental illness, it can be fairly said that the dominance of scientific thought in health organizational behavior has done little to make the mentally ill patient welcome in the general population of the ill or to unite the causes of physical and mental health."[3]

The material that follows describes two programs for patients with psychiatric problems. One program is an established part of a large voluntary acute general hospital; the other exists in a large municipal acute general hospital. The difference between the two hospitals in responsibility toward this group of patients, in the organization and structure of services, and in the rules and regulations that govern them are instructive. These differences show with unusual clarity how the nature of an institution's function, policy, and administration is related to the nature and quality of patient care.

There are several observations that are of general interest. First, social workers in both hospitals described the psychiatric patients in relation to symptoms and behavior, almost never using classical diagnoses; for example, they spoke of drug use or drug abuse, a confused sex identification, underachievement, a suicidal tendency, or school phobia. Second, many of the adult patients had long-standing disturbances, and they tended to return to the hospital when some external or internal pressure precipitated an acute episode. This circumstance is an interesting parallel in the population of the acute general hospital to the chronicity of medically ill patients who return for treatment when a period of remission terminates or symptoms become exacerbated. Third, the descriptive material that follows is subject to the shifts in policy, functions, structure, administration, regulations, and practices that inevitably occur in dynamic societies and their institutions. Such changes reinforce the intent of this section, that is, to illustrate how a health facility and its operation influence the nature, scope, and quality of patient care.

Many changes that occur within organizations are piecemeal responses to new or altered demands as they arise, rather than integral elements in a master plan for the growth and development of the institution. The learner in the health professions is thereby challenged to understand what patients/families and personnel experience and to become involved in thought and action to improve the remediable.

INSTITUTIONAL FUNCTIONS AND RESPONSIBILITIES

The municipal hospital was by law the admitting hospital for the borough of Queens (population just under 2 million); it had the only prison ward for the entire city. The hospital also maintained a mental hygiene clinic for adult and pediatric patients who could remain in the community, and an in-patient service for those who required in-hospital psychiatric observation or treatment for a period not to exceed three months.*

The voluntary hospital had a sharply contrasting program. It provided out-

---

* The acute general hospitals under discussion, both public and voluntary, require that psychiatric patients needing hospitalization beyond a period of three months be transferred to facilities for long-term care.

patient services for diagnosis and treatment, but psychiatric services to out-patients were given low priority. Greater attention was given to adolescent and adult patients who were in the hospital 24 hours a day and to patients in the day-night center, that is, those who were able to work or go to school during the day but needed the protection of the hospital at night, and those who needed the therapeutic services of the hospital during the day but could return to their homes for the night.

THE IMPACTS OF FUNCTION, POLICY, AND ADMINISTRATION

The municipal hospital had a tripartite responsibility—to the courts, to the correctional system, and to the residents of the community whom the hospital had a mandate to serve. The procedures established for one category of patients influenced the attention given to patients in the other categories. Patients suffering from one kind of emotional and behavioral disturbance could not always tolerate the different appearance and behavior of other patients. The comings and goings of ambulances and police officers frightened patients already anxious and upset. The inescapable questions seemed to be whether one general acute hospital could properly meet the needs of such diverse patient groups, and if no other course was feasible, how best could each function be carried out? Under then existing circumstances the procedures in the emergency service for registering, examining, and admitting patients into in- or out-patient psychiatric services were, as one social worker described them, "very hard on the extremes of the age range," a range that extended from "two to a hundred years of age."

Children for whom psychiatric service was sought were seen first in the emergency service, where as many as 30 or 40 children might be on the waiting list. At this point the design of the physical plant became an important factor: the mental hygiene clinic to which the examining psychiatric resident referred most of the children was at a distance of over two city streets from the emergency service. Once arrived at the clinic, the patient and whoever accompanied him or her waited again to see another psychiatrist and then waited to be escorted back to the emergency service. The entire process took from three to four hours, and because some persons could not tolerate the waiting or the surroundings or both, some patients were "lost," that is, left the hospital premises before any disposition could be recommended. The social workers urged two remedial measures: establishing criteria for granting priority to selected patients and providing an admitting room for children who are prospective psychiatric patients.

When during the examining process and prior to admission a medical problem was identified, the patient was referred to the medical emergency service, and the process was started from the beginning. The separation of psychiatry from medicine and surgery illustrated in this procedure was evidenced during the period of treatment as well. The psychiatrists treating adults and children did not follow their patients who had to be transferred to medical or surgical services, and, of course, nursing personnel changed too; the social workers could offer continuity of service and usually did.

As a municipal admitting hospital, the institution could not close intake to applicants for psychiatric service, although it could refer elsewhere patients who were clearly unsuited for the time-limited service available for hospitalized psychiatric patients. It was often difficult to make such a prognostication, especially when relatively inexperienced residents in psychiatry had to make the judgment. Rather ironically, one group of patients whose need for long-term care was easily determined could not be referred to a state mental hospital; elderly patients were admitted to state hospitals only if they were actively psychotic. The nonpsychotic elderly with marked behavioral disturbances were not eligible even when they could not be adequately cared for at home.

When patients were admitted for in-hospital psychiatric care, their relatives were asked to sign consent for transfer to a state hospital if needed. This was a step that was too much for most families to take when they were deeply upset, did not understand well enough what they were signing, were unsophisticated about the patient's psychiatric condition, and were often too fearful of authority to ask questions. The immediate request for consent was considered by the social workers on this service to be a convenience for staff but a hardship for patients' relatives. Their need for adequate preparation is obvious.

Patients referred by the courts and houses of detention for admission to the prison ward arrived at the emergency service in all degrees of agitation, handcuffed, and accompanied by police who were "apt to be angry" and impatient to return to their posts. In fact, these patients were usually given priority so that the correction officers could leave the hospital promptly. One questions these patients' exposure to the reactions of other patients and the exposure of patients with normal civilian status to the manacled patients. The question may be raised why these patients—whom the hospital was obligated to admit to the prison ward—had to go through the emergency service at all, since their immediate disposition was certain.

Social workers were on call, and the psychiatrists, with few exceptions, considered social workers' participation essential when patients were hospitalized for psychiatric care. The social workers preferred in-person rather than on-call assignments to the emergency service. They hoped thus to take more initiative in identifying patients/families in need of social work services and to provide a more complete range of service as well.*

The voluntary hospital operated within an administrative structure and according to regulations and procedures established largely by the institution itself—largely, not entirely, because institutions receiving funds from any level of government have to operate within specified guide lines established by the governmental agency for essential controls and accountability.

Whereas the description of the municipal hospital highlighted multiple and perhaps incompatible functions and an administrative structure, the concern most emphasized in the voluntary hospital was about the working relationship between psychiatrists and social workers. First, there were various aspects of the professional hierarchy that had adverse effects on patients/families and personnel. The organizational structure was such that the patients and relatives sensed that the psychiatrists had the highest status; yet they were the least available. The most available staff members had the lesser status and authority but carried a heavy burden of responsibility for patient care.

Then there was the rigid regulation whereby the psychiatrists were always responsible for the direct treatment of the patient and the social workers were assigned to give service to the patients' relatives. There was an important

---

* It is reassuring to note that current deployment of the social workers in the municipal hospital calls for in-person assignments to emergency service.

potential for error in this policy: the family member who is brought to the hospital as the patient is not necessarily the person most in need of psychiatric care. They may be the victim of someone's disturbed character and behavior rather than the agent. The well-known phenomenon of making a member of the family group a scapegoat is a case in point. It would have been preferable for the decision about who gives professional service to whom to rest on a full interprofessional assessment of the patient/family's total life-situation. Strict enforcement of the policy too often resulted in the patient's relatives having no or too infrequent contact with the psychiatrist. This separation was not an inevitable consequence of the policy of assigning patients and relatives for treatment, but the policy did lend itself to the psychiatrists' desire not to be besieged by anxious relatives and to their fears that contact with relatives would jeopardize their relations with patients, especially the maintenance of confidentiality.

Parents of young patients suffered peculiarly from these "side effects" of the policy; they had a justifiable need—legal, social, and emotional—to know about their child directly from the person treating him or her, and they needed enough contact to build up a feeling of trust in the physician's competence and concern.

A close observer of the professional hierarchy would have noted also that personnel other than psychiatrists did not always use their best judgment but were inhibited in the actions they took for fear of overstepping their authority. This description of staff behavior fits the old, classic idea of a team rather than the current idea of a collaborating professional group.

On the other hand, there were psychiatrists who accepted violations of rules that they had not made or that they disapproved of. They seemed not to realize that a ripple effect was possible which might result in people's breaking rules that the psychiatrists wanted kept. A good example concerns hospitalized adolescent patients. They were expected to wear night clothes except when they attended school or were in the gymnasium. They were constantly changing clothes, and when they tired of it and the staff grew tired of trying to enforce the regulation it was dropped—until the policy was reinstated.

At times two policies were inconsistent with each other. For instance, in an attempt to lessen the distance between staff and patients and between life within and outside the hospital, staff assigned to the day-night center ate their meals with the patients and did not wear uniforms. These procedures did not obtain in other sections of the psychiatric services, although they might well have been beneficial for all in-patients. The question may be asked, too, whether the policy of lessening distance between the hospital and the world outside was consistent with the adolescents' having to wear night clothes a good part of the day.

In the voluntary as in the municipal hospital, the influence of architectural design on staff and patients was significant. One social worker, for example, questioned the effectiveness of a floor plan that was identical for both medical/-surgical and psychiatric services. The in-patients in psychiatric service were isolated from one another and from the nursing station, although it was important to stimulate interaction among patients and draw the nursing staff into the life of the floor. The hospital milieu, physically and socially, can become a potent factor in the therapeutic process.

A feature of the floor that did stimulate personal contacts and a form of group living were the floor kitchens, available to patients and staff alike. The availability of food and drink during the evening hours lessened the impact of an early supper and encouraged the patients' creation of evening entertainment. These helpful activities contrasted markedly with the long, unrelieved evening hours bemoaned by so many adult patients on the medical and surgical services.

Regulations, procedures, and practices are changing from those just described. One factor accounting for the changes is the trend toward increasing biomedical research into mental and emotional disturbances and the trend toward enlarging the volume of services and the number of patients served in out-patient psychiatric units. Accompanying these changes there is in many facilities serving the mentally ill and the emotionally disturbed an interesting development in the working relationship between psychiatrists and social workers: social workers are being given more responsibility in the period of diagnosis and assessment, as well as primary or shared responsibility for the treatment of selected patients and patients/families.

An understanding of the latter trend requires an historical perspective. A demonstrable "common body of knowledge and techniques" exists and has existed for decades between social workers and psychiatrists. In principle, this mutuality in professional education and practice forms a sound base for productive, effective collaboration. In actuality, as a single factor the common base does not guarantee satisfactory collaborative efforts. For some members of the two professions the common base has greatly facilitated their learning to work together; for others, the common base has been a force for competitiveness and rivalry to such a degree that the old hierarchical structure remains rigidly in place. A third consequence of having a common base is that members of each profession develop some similar and some distinctive ways of using it in their respective practices. The differing opinions and attitudes that accompany differences in practice can at best lead to mutual learning and professional growth and can at worst deepen the existing split and further impede the attainment of professional collaboration. However, the fact that attitudinal and structural change comes slowly must not obscure the fact that in many institutional settings there is an evolutionary trend to use more fully the social worker's knowledge and competence. Thus there may be some acceptance of the concept that "a social model is more appropriate as the organizing theme for dealing with the problems of mental health and disease," though, as Dana points out, psychiatrists have made no clear choice as yet between a medical and a social model.[5]

Whatever the future brings in the way of progressive or regressive developments, the variables, mentioned above, in psychiatric service will serve to point up a given and stable phenomenon: the interaction among sponsorship, policy, administration, and patient care; the importance of understanding and evaluating functions, programs, and regulations in an institutional setting; and the desirability for personnel who are not administrators to have a voice in instituting needed change.

FAMILY RELATIONSHIPS AND BEHAVIOR CONTRIBUTING AND REACTING TO MENTAL AND EMOTIONAL DISORDERS

The material that follows is highly selective. These are the family structures and relationships that were found repeatedly among the hospital population of psychiatric patients. These are the parents and children who, given their circumstances, could not cope.

Factors contributing to the need for psychiatric care of children and adolescents are not confined to elements in the family structure: society plays its own part. However, as the basic unit in our society, the family is understandably believed to have great influence on its members' mental and emotional health.

In regard to the patients/families under consideration, a major contributing factor to the psychological disorders of young children and adolescents was believed to be a close symbiotic tie between the patient and his or her mother. This kind of tie was seen as the opposite of growth-producing individuation of the infant and gradual separation from the mother. When the tie persists past infancy, failure to achieve in school and to develop social relationships with peers is attributed also to the unmodified symbiosis. Since the tie binds the mother as severely as it does the child, an unfortunate negative effect occurs when the mother, finding it too painful to allow the child to become a separate person, withdraws him or her prematurely from treatment.

Parents may impose various other unhealthy pressures, such as an insistence on high scholastic achievement or great prowess in sports or social popularity. The children who react to such pressures with failure are apt to be among the patient population in substantial numbers. Many of the parents of these children are seeking their own achievement and gratification vicariously but are destined to fail through their children. The homes in these families are often organized around the children—"to give them everything"—but instead of being motivated positively from within, the children are provoked to resist what they perceive as pressure from without. Cultural factors seem to account for a number of pressures; for example, strong pressure for scholastic achievement of their children was observed more often in middle-class Jewish families than in other ethnic groups.

There are occasional instances of too-strong pressures being exerted on children to compensate their parents for unsatisfactory marital relationships. Illustrations of what occurs in these families come mostly from one-parent households; the selection may well reflect cultural conditions in a particular neighborhood. The following are some observations about the son or daughter whose father is out of the home.

The son whose mother's behavior toward him is sexually seductive becomes confused about his distorted relationship: Is he child or adult, son or father-husband substitute? These boys at times fall into the role thrust upon them; for example, they become overprotective of their mothers and may stay home from school to escort them to clinic. When the son's confusion and guilt-ridden conflict become intolerable, there may be outbreaks of socially unacceptable behavior, emotional withdrawal, and depression. Practically the same pattern can be observed when the father is in the home but lives in psychological and social isolation from the other members of the family.

The most often-cited effect on girls whose mothers head the households is their misperception of a man as a person who impregnates the woman and leaves her. These are frequently the girls who seek and respond to men who will treat them as their fathers treated their mothers.

In some families headed by one parent the children are shifted from relative to relative to live for periods of time. Social workers and other professionals differ in their opinions about the consequences of such an arrangement. Some think that the negative impacts outweigh any advantages. For example, the maternal grandmother often assumes a mother's authority and responsibility and may pit the children against their mother and create severe conflict which the mother and children cannot resolve. Other practitioners believe that experiencing care and affection from a large, extended family group in which there are substitute mothers and fathers is a distinct benefit to many children.

It is generally agreed that when siblings are separated to live with different relatives instead of being kept together they are seriously disadvantaged. Another agreement among professionals is that a succession of men in the home, appearing and disappearing, each visiting his own children, is undisputably a confusing and distorting experience for the children in that home. It is more profoundly agitating, they think, than for children to live with a series of relatives.

In any of the family structures that vary from a stable two-parent home children are apt to experience adverse effects. A child may be inappropriately forced to assume some of the tasks and relationships of an absent parent; a child may have to take unusual responsibility for the household and for younger siblings because the parent in the home is incapable of assuming his or her traditional duties. Pushed prematurely into such responsibilities, some of these children eventually come to the hospital with a regressive symptom, such as bedwetting, or with overt, rebellious symptoms, such as truancy, staying out all night, or being generally unmanageable. These are often the oldest children in the family, and when they develop behavior problems the younger ones, for whom the older children are models, develop similar problems—all of them rooted basically in a climate of psychosocial deprivation.

Reactions to mental and emotional disorders vary among families and among members of an individual family. Perhaps more important to professionals in the field of health care are the differences between these reactions and the reactions of people to physical illness and disability. The reader is urged to keep in mind that the statements below are descriptive of the same selected group of patients/families that were considered in the foregoing sections on family relationships and behavior.

Parents' recognition and acknowledgment of a child's emotional and behavioral disturbance tend to vary with the child's age and sex. Young children are more often perceived to be in need of psychiatric help if the symptom is sleep disturbance. It is common also for parents to consider boys' aggressive behavior normal as long as they can tolerate it. In contrast, parents are more alert to signs that their older and adolescent children are psychologically and emotionally disturbed. Adolescents who appeal to a school guidance counselor for help are often referred to the hospital; they come in a crisis, stay in treatment for a while, and drop out but return on the occasion of another crisis. The parents of these self-referred adolescents are likely to give consent to the young person's treatment but seldom participate actively in the process. Their relative passivity is unfortuntate in that those young patients can be expected to live at home, dependent upon their parents, for some years to come. Without their parents' involvement in treatment, the children bear the major burden of adjustment and accommodation.

The impact of a child's disturbance upon his parents seemed most severe when the child was hospitalized. To most parents a child's hospitalization for mental or emotional illness was viewed as a punishment for which they suffer shame and guilt, although in times of great upheaval the hospitalization can be felt by the parents and other members of the family as a relief. In any case, parents reacted to the very need for a child's hospitalization as traumatic. They feared what others in their social milieu would think. They feared the long-term effects on the patient and on the parent-child relationship: what would happen when the patient returned home? Will he or she ever be able to return home? These questions are not immediately and openly raised, parents sometimes mask them by asking about the treatment process when it is the consequences and far-reaching effects of the process that concern them the most.

Many parents react to their own feelings of guilt by expressing anger. Thus, while they are suffering from a belief that they have made the child sick, their overt reaction is anger toward the hospital or the doctor or both, because their rulings and instructions were perceived as punishments. For example, restrictions on visiting the patient were translated to mean "you are so bad you must keep away." On occasion, anger so directed delflected anger really felt toward the patient and left him or her freer to respond effectively to the psychiatrist's treatment.

One of the strongest and most fearful reactions experienced by relatives who have had a patient hospitalized is to his or her being admitted to a locked ward. No matter how carefully they and the patient have been prepared, the patient feels he or she is being imprisoned, and the relatives' reactions may mount to hysteria.

Hospitalized adolescents have their characteristic ways of behaving. They tend more than adult patients to show overt aggressive acts of rebellion toward rules and regulations. They tend to elope from the hospital more frequently than the older patients. They have tantrums and episodes of screaming, but, also characteristically, they are not consistently aggressive and difficult; a day of tantrums may be followed by a day of calm and acquiescence. On occasion the adolescents's aggression turns inward, and the patient cuts his or her wrists on a broken bottle or smashed windowpane. The adolescents who were drug users were adept at getting drugs into the hospital and would at time traffic in drugs. One social worker warned, "Do not underestimate these patients' capacity to manipulate, lie, and scheme to get drugs into the hospital."

The social workers' professional approach to an adolescent's disturbed behavior was to ask, "What is he or she telling us?" Some of the more frequent messages were "I can't control myself"; "How far can I go with you", and "I need more protection." It is also significant whether the adolescent misbehaves when alone or in the companionship of others, when within the walls of the institution or outside on a pass.

Adolescent and adult patients in need of greater protection, more controls, and a longer period of care than the acute general hospital can provide have to be transferred to institutions better equipped to meet their needs. It is difficult for patients/families to acknowledge the need for and accept such transfers; all the original reactions to the patient's hospitalization for emotional or mental disturbance are reactivated and intensified by the sterner realities that must now be faced.

SOME SOCIOCULTURAL FACTORS

Sociocultural factors play a variety of roles. They may contribute to the development of mental and emotional problems; they may help to prevent such disorders. They influence people's atttitudes toward these disorders and toward interpretation and treatment of them; the influence may be favorable or unfavorable. In other words, sociocultural factors in our diverse society are important, but it takes careful assessment to know in just what ways.

The influx of Spanish-speaking familes into the New York metropolitan area has for some years created a need for many more multilingual staff members than are available. It is a need felt most acutely by patients, relatives, and staff in regard to emotional and mental problems. Social workers think it ill-advised to use children or neighbors as interpreters when intensely personal and private matters have to be discussed.*[6] Requests for bilingual social workers have sometimes been denied for budgetary reasons or cannot be met because of the scarcity of qualified persons.

Relatives who bring patients to the hospital—and especially the parents of children and adolescents—are fearful of seeing the psychiatrists but for a variety of reasons. People who are financially and socially deprived tend to fear the physician's authority; they may have a language problem which makes communication difficult; and they are often unaccustomed to talking about personal matters to anyone outside the family group and consequently "clam up."

In contrast, relatives who are middle class and somewhat more sophisticated tend to fear what the physicians will tell them about the patient's condition; in particular, the young patient's parents fear they will be blamed for their child's illness.

Patients from deprived families and neighborhoods are like their parents, relatively unsophisticated, not readily verbal, and apt to reveal their inner disturbance through aggressive behavior toward others. Patients reared to believe in spiritualism or occultism tend to express their mental or emotional disturbances in ways appropriate to their beliefs; consequently, it is difficult to distinguish between a patient's paranoid thoughts or an episode of hysteria on the one hand and acts of retaliation or fearful anxiety reactive to a religious belief on the other.

Such beliefs influence in different ways patients/families' responses to psychological explanations of emotional disturbance and to both psychological treatment and drug therapy. In the same neighborhood persons from the same Latin American country differ widely in the strength of their belief in supernatural forces. The more educated persons may be more accepting of the abstract idea that symptoms may have a psychogenic origin and may yield to psychological treatment.

When relatively unsophisticated persons attribute symptoms to adverse, concrete circumstances of life or to supernatural forces, the idea of verbal communication as a means of treatment is frequently unacceptable. The concreteness of electrodes, for example, is more reassuring even if the patient/family is in fear of electricity—itself an invisible and potent element of nature. Among these family groups, even when the disturbed member becomes a patient in psychiatric service relatives may seek help from people in the community whose power and advice they believe in; sometimes medication prescribed by the psychiatrist is thrown out on a neighbor's suggestion; family members may fail to report the side effects of medication upon the patient as they have been instructed to do; or they decide that a change of scene will be the

---

* See the section on communication, p. 20.

best medicine and take the patient away from the city—often to the country of his or her family's origin.

TREATMENT OF PATIENTS IN PSYCHIATRIC SERVICE UNITS

Three significant and entangled themes appear in relation to treatment: methods and technologies; the behavior of patients/families as participants; relationships (1) between patients/families and professionals and (2) among professionals.

Medication and psychotherapy are, in this transitional era, contested modalities. Leaving aside the polarized positions which would exclude entirely one or the other modality, several noteworthy issues emerge. One is whether medication should not be used more selectively and with more adequate follow-up regarding its results.

Another issue concerns the conclusion that may be prematurely drawn in certain instances that "psychotherapy is not possible." Critics observe that some patients with a language barrier break through it with remarkable success as they gain trust in the therapist. Others who are at first uncommunicative for reasons such as fear, shame, guilt, or an inbred cultural inhibition, for instance, eventually dare to engage in real interchange.

Limited time is seen as another issue. Patients on medication in one hospital tend "to be seen briefly every three or four months; if there are no negative signs, the medication is renewed for another interval." Social workers are concerned with this exclusive use of medication when it might be combined effectively with an appropriate level of psychotherapy.

The fragmented treatment of patients who were drug addicted was a particular cause for concern on some services: paranoid or hallucinatory symptoms were cleared up, and the patients were discharged. The social workers then did their best to connect the patients promptly with a treatment center in the community, but the discontinuity in time, treatment processes, and personnel was paid for heavily by the patients' loss of motivation, renewed craving, and uncontrolled exposure to drug pushers, users, and abusers.

One cannot pass over the expressions of dissenting opinions between social workers and psychiatrists which can legitimately arise from possession of a common body of knowledge and techniques. It is outstanding that social workers' questions about physicians on medical/surgical services did not concern the latters' choice of interventions but focused primarily on the physicians' relative unfamilarity with psychosocial factors and problems in the field of health care. In other words, the social workers seemed to be hoping for a more serviceable common base with medical and surgical physicians.

The participation of family members in treatment—its planning and its processes—is considered esessential in some situations and most always desirable in the remainder.

"The younger the patient, the more involved his or her parents need to be" was a frequently stated generalization, but differences in degree of involvement seem less the issue than appropriate differences in purpose and kind of involvement. For example, young adult patients are often in need of social, psychological, and financial support from their families. Although many patients in this age group live apart from their nuclear families, supportive familial relations are important to their progress in treatment and to improved social functioning within the family group and in the community. It is not uncommon for parents of young adult patients to be antagonistic when approached about paying for treatment; yet it is often possible to enlist their supportive involvement because they are fundamentally concerned and the patient is in real need of their caring and attention. Many of these young adult patients are quite alone and lonely, out of work and without a place to live.

In conformity with the times and changing conventions, "family" has to be construed broadly to fit the way in which the young adult patient has been living and relating to others. In some instances, the only available people are friends who can be encouraged and assisted to be helpful to the patient. In other instances, the patient's most significant friends must be viewed as extensions of the family group, with an important influence on and meaning to the patient.

What these comments imply is the necessity for helping patients, their relatives, and their significant others (who are often surrogate family members) to work toward a mutually satisfying interdependence commensurate with the age and responsibilities of the persons involved. This objective leads directly to a closer look at relationships, the third theme in this discussion of treatment in psychiatric service.

Relationships—always important when human problems and human services are the focus of attention—play a special part when the giver of direct service has to use himself or herself as the primary medium for helping and healing. In this context the relationships to be discussed are (1) those between patient/family and givers of psychiatric service and (2) those among the givers of psychiatric service, who are usually in the hospital a multiprofessional staff which may or may not have developed into an interprofessional, collaborating unit.

When the use of oneself in a helping relationship with another human being is the basic instrument of treatment, the givers-of-service in psychiatric units—even when drug therapy is a major component in the total plan of treatment—are required to develop self-awareness, self-understanding, and self-discipline as prerequisites for helping others with mental or emotional problems. These are complex tasks. They take time and concentrated effort, and frequently the giver-of-service who is relatively inexperienced seeks help in healing himself or herself in order to become more effective in helping others.

There are several problematic areas that appear to be common among multiprofessional staff members. The resemblance between their very human problems and the problems many of their patients have complicates the development of professional objectivity and requisite therapeutic skills. A most important problem area is working with patients' relatives, particularly their parents. The easiest pitfall for staff members is to become the patient's ally against his or her family, whereas the helpful strategy in most instances is to engage the patient's relatives as allies of the hospital as an institution and of the people in direct service roles.

From the beginning of their professional education in the classroom and in the field (i.e., the practicum) social workers are required to consider a client in his or her natural milieu and to have concern for all family members—their relationships, their needs and wants, and the meaning of their behavior. This perspective is fundamental to their practice; it does not make social workers family therapists, although gradually now they are learning to work—as social workers—with groups of family members rather than solely with individual key members seriatim. However, the knowledge and skills the social workers do have have enabled them to observe closely and to break into component factors the large, vague area of relationships between givers-of-service and patients/families.

For one thing, the young psychiatrist in residence who leans toward strong identification with a young patient may feel little or no compassion for the patient's relatives. But that psychiatrist may shift radically when the patient is elderly; then the really strong identification may be with the patient's adult children. This is a transparent maneuver which maintains a therapist's sympathies with children in a family and places blame on the parents even when the children are grown—or perhaps *because* they are grown and presage a situation that may occur some day in the therapist's life.

A therapist's unresolved problems with his or her own parents are manifested also in other ways; for example, the therapists may fear contact and communication with a patient's parents, and the prospect of coping with a group of emotional relatives may be frightening indeed. When it is obvious that parents are angry, staff members may interpret the expression of anger as a personal attack when it is an indicator of anxiety, fear, or guilt.

The therapist's personal concept of family is of great importance. If the concept places the patient in relative isolation, with the family as a backdrop instead of a dynamic group that includes the patient, then there is a danger that the relatives are perceived as people who must accomodate themselves to the patient as though he or she were the only family member entitled to maximum feasible self-determination and self-realization.*

Privileged communication, which is the patient's right, is sometimes given by uneasy psychiatrists as the reason for the latter's infrequent contacts with a patient's relatives. The lack of contact may create hardship; contact is especially needed by family members during their periods of anger and guilt, when they require support and understanding as well as advice. There are ways to tell patients' relatives what they need to know without betraying the patient's confidentiality. When the psychiatrist does not realize the importance of knowing the emotional meaning of the patient's illness to his or her relatives but has only the patient in the focus of his or her attention, as one social worker put it, "he is prone to hold the family responsible and forever guilty about the illness."

Sociocultural differences and similarities between therapist and patient can have crucial consequences for mutual trust and the effectiveness of treatment. For example, when therapist and patient have grown up with a belief in the acceptability of drug use—and if the two are so close in age that the therapist begins to relive his or her adolescence in his or her mind's eye—the therapist may try to make a choice between two extremes or vacillate from one to the other; he or she may be exceedingly punitive toward the patient; or he or she may in effect subtly condone and encourage the patient's use of drugs. The preferred attitude of detached concern comes only when the therapist can distinguish clearly between his or her own situation and that of the patient. Biases and conflicts about other issues, such as homosexuality; conforming to authority; responsibility toward parents, spouses, and children; and militance and violence, may drastically interfere with a therapist's effectiveness, and especially so whenever the therapist's personal code of values and behavior is at odds with the expectations of his or her profession.

Many laypersons have the idea that professionals who serve patients

* See p. 5.

suffering from mental and emotional disturbances are as one social worker put it, "always working and making judgments. The idea develops into an expectation that makes people feel anxious, stiff, and unnatural. Everyone thinks he has emotional problems and takes readings of his emotional health." Less experienced givers of service often do feel self-conscious and somewhat unsure of themselves; these attitudes, which are natural enough, are likely to reinforce the layperson's expectations that he or she is constantly being judged.

Members of the multiprofessional staff in psychiatric service units of large urban teaching hospitals have varying opinions about the relationship between giving services to patients/families and to the community on the one hand and the function of education in health and health-related professions on the other. The issue is highly controversial, and the relationship between therapist and patient/family can be strongly influenced by the authority and responsibility that the institution allocates to the respective groups of learners. Resident psychiatrists—the house staff—in the kind of hospital under consideration have significant authority and power regarding the admission, treatment, and discharge of patients. Social workers on psychiatric service have noticed one consequence of this phenomenon with concern; as they see it, the residents' selection of patients with "rare diagnoses" and other "interesting conditions" not only limits the range of learning opportunities they should have but contributes to maintaining a dichotomy between the functions of service and teaching, because patients with the more common kinds of disturbances then fail to receive the amount and kind of attention they need. Social workers make similar comments in respect to residents on medical and surgical services, but less sharply. This dichotomy has to be seen in relation to the total professional/legal issue: Are residents primarily students or employees?* Are they to be recognized as members of a bargaining and negotiating unit? Do they have the right to strike? A full discussion of this problem is not appropriate to this text. It is mentioned because of its impact on patients/families and patient care. It will take a lengthy period of carefully directed effort to dissolve the notion of separateness, if not antagonism, between service on the one hand and teaching and learning on the other. Acceptance of the effectiveness of experiential learning, that is learning by doing, will do much toward perceiving the potentially close and positive relationship between the two functions.

There are aspects of interprofessional and intraprofessional relationships that affect patients/families—aspects that are of special importance in psychiatric service. For example, personnel on the floor may react to a patient's behavior with such strong emotion and so diversely as to cause divisiveness among staff. For example, a large, strong, and potentially abusive patient frightens the nurses, who express both fear and anger and request the removal of the patient from the hospital. The physicians want the patient to stay. There is an impasse until the staff members come to an agreement on the best approach to the difficult patient, who may not be ready for discharge or in need of a different kind of treatment facility. Social workers, who are not exposed to the patient eight hours at a time as are the nurses and who do not have ultimate professional and legal responsibility for the patient as do the psychiatrists, are frequently less beset emotionally than their colleagues and therefore are freer psychologically to help resolve the conflict between the nurses and physicians. The social worker's

---

* Recent decisions made by the courts and the Internal Revenue Service give residents the status of employees.

expertness in helping people to disentangle stressful personal relationships and to cope with socioenvironmental realities combined with the ability to practice in a collective setting equips him or her to be an enabler or negotiator in multiprofessional disputes. Resolution of conflict, that is, working things out with others, implies compromise consciously arrived at and is therefore easily distinguished from a state of mere coexistence.

Another illustration of the importance of interprofessional relationships in psychiatric service concerns the use of a therapeutic milieu within the hospital. While a strict hierarchical structure persists, it at best impedes and at worst makes impossible the development of a collaborative interprofessional group. Each member of such a group is responsible for contributing to a common goal—in this case a therapeutic milieu. That means that each giver-of-service needs to be free to make instant judgments and decisions compatible with his or her professional functions and competence within the agreed-upon plan of treatment for an individual or group of patients. Fear of encroaching on another professional's territory or fear of being encroached upon by another professional can determine what is or is not done on behalf of a patient or patient population.

There are many schools of psychiatry, ranging from those whose theoretical orientation is entirely toward psychological therapy, to those whose theory and practice are rooted in the social aspects of mental disorder, to those whose conviction lies in orthomolecular psychiatry. Within any one of such groupings there are a number of variants. For example, psychiatrists using psychological therapy only may practice psychoanalysis in classical or modified form, or existential psychotherapy, or nondirective psychotherapy. Thus, while psychiatrists are generally considered the authoritative figures in the diagnosis and treatment of mental disorder, the great diversity among them results in significant differences in their own direct service to patients, in the structure and organization of psychiatric units in institutions, and in the way the psychiatrists regard and work with members of related professions and disciplines.

An increasing number of professionals in the health care field view the years of basic professional education as the time for students to become aware of and experience the differences between their conceptions of other professionals' functions and of their own functions. Since all of the professionals have the same obligation to be thus aware, they can work together to arrive at more accurate perceptions of themselves and of one another. One social worker noted that some psychiatrists who do not prescribe to the necessity for correcting conceptions and perceptions of other professionals are inclined to recommend that all staff members who work in the department be accountable solely to the chief of psychiatric service. Such an administrative move would no doubt remove a number of sources of friction and tension; but by removing people from their professional bases it would also diminish their standing as members of differentiated professions, each with a different contribution to make to the patient's care.[7]

PREGNANT WOMEN

The pregnancy of women is in itself a normal developmental phenomenon and experience. However, the biological processes that take place are capable of producing emotional crises and consequently problems in adaptation and social functioning. In addition, pregnancy can be complicated by illness, injury, and stress-producing psychosocial factors. Any of these problem situations which affect the pregnant woman may have an effect also on the fetus she is bearing. Thus the well, pregnant woman is encouraged to take advantage of what is largely preventive medical care to keep herself and the fetus at lowest possible risk. In conformity with current usage in medicine, in law, and by the general public, "woman" refers to a female over 16 years of age. The discussion of pregnant women that follows includes both married and unmarried patients.*

PREGNANT WOMEN CARRYING TO TERM

The condition and experience of pregnant women is subject to three-pronged scrutiny, as are the situations of all patients: biological, psychological, and socioenvironmental factors, their interactions, and their combined contribution to the patient's status of social-health. As the social worker sees the general picture, the pregnant woman may fall into one of three groups: (1) the woman whose pregnancy does not disturb normal functioning, (2) the woman whose pregnancy upsets normal functioning, and (3) the woman whose reactions to pregnancy are part of her usual dysfunctioning. It is in the nature of the social worker's functions in the hospital that his or her professional experience is concentrated on the second two groups.

Significant factors in, and reactions to pregnancy cover a wide range of events and conditions, patients' ways of dealing with their impacts, and interventive measures that may be employed by givers-of-service. Insofar as patients' experiences have consequences for their relatives, significant others, and givers of direct service, these impacts too will be noted.

Commonly, pregnant women experience some anxiety, but it is expressed about different eventualities, for example: Will I carry to term? Will it be a healthy baby? How will I bear the pain? What kind of anesthetic will I have? A woman's first pregnancy in particular is apt to arouse many fears which need to be explored to determine which are normal or pathological emotional reactions to an unknown situation, which are due to ignorance, and which spring from myths and old wives' tales.

Many of the women whose normal functioning is disturbed by their pregnancy react with some degree of regressive—for example, immature and overly dependent—behavior. Women who find that pregnancy is critically stress producing do not always react with open anxiety. Some will attempt to master their problem by disregarding the pregnancy even after they have registered for obstetrical care. The behavior that reveals their inner distress takes various forms. For example, the woman may try to do everything as usual, may diet to keep her weight down and her figure slim, and may fail to keep her medical appointments. Other women's distress is expressed in symptoms of depression, such as continually feeling unwell or not sleeping. There is at times such strong resistance to the idea of a coming baby that some women with sufficient income do not buy clothes or supplies for the expected infant. In all such instances it is essential that the physician know about the woman's

---

* Discussion of the pregnant adolescent girl 16 years old or younger, married and unmarried, is included in Chapter 7.

attitudes toward the baby; her feelings and behavior may create risks to her health and to that of the fetus.*

FAMILY RELATIONSHIPS.

One useful way to view the phenomenon of pregnancy is as an event in a family situation in which all family members are involved. The relation between the woman and her husband or nonlegal partner affects and is affected by the course of her pregnancy and by the reactions of each to the pregnancy. When there are growing children in the family they too will have reactions to the pregnancy which may affect their relations with the woman and man and which may precipitate changes in the children's behavior and their social functioning in general.

The pregnant woman frequently uses the services of a social worker to help her find a satisfactory way to explain her pregnancy to the children already in the household; to help her handle any disturbed feelings and relationships of her own, especially those that affect her male partner; and sometimes to help by giving direct social work service to family members under unusual stress because of her pregnancy.

It is useful for all givers-of-service to families in which the patient is a pregnant woman to keep in mind that enlargement of the family group will always create demands for adaptation: there may be changes in the balance of interdependence among family members, in the quality of personal relations, in the sufficiency of income and living space, and so on. If these demands sound familiar, it is because they are similar to those suggested earlier, when the enlargement of the group occurred not via the birth of a baby, but via the discharge of a patient to the home of relatives in which he or she has not lived before.

The unmarried pregnant woman and the married woman who is bearing a child by a man other than her husband are inclined to feelings of guilt and fear of dying in childbirth rather more frequently than are other pregnant women. Some of these women who want help from a social worker find it easier when the social worker leads a group of women in similar predicaments. Talking with a social worker in a one-to-one relationship is apparently too difficult for them— they need the alleviation of feelings such as shame, guilt, and fear of ostracism that can result from experiences shared with and by one's peers.

Some unmarried women feel better for themselves and for their babies if they can obtain affidavits of paternity even when they do not expect to have a continuing relation with the putative father.

A final comment on the factor of family relationships has to do with the presence of a woman's relative in the labor room. In some hospitals only husbands are allowed into the labor room with their wives. Neither the nonlegal male partner, even in a stable union, nor the woman's mother may be present. Some patients are deprived by this ruling of a supportive presence; but not all patients want someone with them, nor do all male partners wish to share the women's experience. Husbands need preparation for being with their wives in the labor room. Of course, when the patient is delivering by natural childbirth

* The reader may remark that in these comments there is no clear distinction between the condition of pregnancy and the child who will be delivered. The literature, however, does make a distinction and takes note of the anxiety that frequently creates a crisis situation when the infant becomes an actuality, and an accession to the family.

her husband is apt to be well prepared, since both usually have been enrolled in the educational program, and he has helped her with the breathing exercises and other preparatory measures.

BODILY CHANGES.

The changes that take place in the body of the pregnant woman have a psychosocial impact upon her whether they occur in a first or subsequent pregnancy. Most women find the changes in body image significant. They talk of their bodies as being unwieldy or emphasize their difficulty in obtaining clothing or in keeping to a prescribed diet.

Women's knowledge of their bodies and of the development of the fetus is so imperfect even when they have good educational backgrounds that many social workers recommend giving full explanations to women each time they are pregnant. It is of special importance that the patient understand the medical examinations, tests, and procedures related to pregnancy and in particular those connected with the start and course of labor pains. The patients frequently have complaints, anxieties, and questions that call first for authentic response from their physicians before social workers and nurses make their responses.

SOCIOECONOMIC CONDITIONS.

Numerous demands for adaptation spring from socioeconomic conditions which are for many clinic patients marginal or only slightly above. First is the problem of housing, characterized by insufficient space, heating, hot water, ventilation, and so on, which may impair the health of a pregnant woman and impose an especially heavy burden upon one who has a medical problem such as asthma or a cardiac condition. One of the terrifying aspects of bad housing is the presence of vermin. Pregnant women with young children often get little sleep; they keep themselves awake to protect the children from rat bites. Attempts to obtain better housing are not often successful; the Housing Authority in New York City, for example, is said to respond slowly even in cases of medically complicated pregnancies, and the private housing sector is a poor resource for the low-income family.

A period of bed rest is sometimes prescribed for a pregnant woman with low income who lives alone with her children, does all her own work, and occupies a fourth-floor apartment in a walk-up tenement. In principle, home-maker service is available under these circumstances, but in actuality there may be a long delay before it is obtainable.

Low income makes it almost impossible for some patients to buy sufficient clothing designed for the comfort and convenience of pregnant women or to follow instructions for the patient's special dietary needs. Another problem may arise in regard to sleeping arrangements; some women who have always shared a bed find that they need one to themselves during pregnancy. A bed is a disproportionately expensive item for a family with little money; and a family currently receiving financial assistance from the New York City Department of Social Services, for example, cannot hope for a special allowance for such household equipment or other special needs connected with pregnancy. The state of the family's finances will also affect the preparations they can make for a new baby. Parents with low income find it difficult to purchase items such as clothing, toilet articles, or a crib for the newborn. One notes rather sadly that the infant-sized "box" the hospital provides when the baby is taken home often serves as his or her sleeping place until it is outgrown.

SOCIAL, MEDICAL, AND LEGAL FACTORS.

The decision whether to keep or surrender her baby is a crucial one for most adult women who are pregnant out of wedlock. The decision is influenced by a variety of social, medical, and legal factors. Women tend more than formerly to keep their babies. There is evidence of a national trend in this direction: "Practitioners' observations [are] that unmarried pregnant women including those who contact an adoption agency have increasingly been keeping their children."[9] The reader may wish to view this trend in relation to some significant implications: "Although fewer children are now surrendered for adoption, it cannot be assumed that they are living with their parents. Many of the young, unmarried parents have neither the ability nor the facilities to care for [their illegitimate children]. Consequently, far too many children are placed in foster care where they remain indefinitely."[10]

One must be particularly concerned with the scarce social resources for the adoption of black babies and those of other minorities and the potentially unfavorable implications. There are black mothers who keep their babies because they know well that adoptive homes are rare, and their concern for their babies influences them in their decision. If the woman's decision is to surrender the baby despite scarce resources, her well baby may remain in a hospital environment for a very long time, while simultaneously there is great pressure (usually on the social worker) to find a place for the baby. The lack of coordination between the health care systems and the social welfare systems creates a jeopardy to the social and psychological health of these infants and their mothers which neither the physician nor the social worker as individuals can prevent.

PREVENTIVE AND INTERVENTIVE MEASURES.

Matters concerning contraception are frequently an integral part of a pregnant woman's concerns and of her male partner's, too. Some women who have stopped taking an oral contraceptive for fear of its possible adverse consequences become pregnant while changing to another method. Both the woman and her partner will at best have ambivalent reactions to the accidental pregnancy during its early period. In the desire to avoid another unwanted pregnancy some women ask for a tubal ligation, and some men decide to have a vasectomy.

These requests for interventive mesasures may in themselves become a source of stress if the woman and her partner have dissenting opinions and attitudes toward the intervention one of them has requested. Hospitals establish their own regulations for carrying out these medical procedures. The regulations change, conforming to changes in society's attitudes; they in turn are reflected in leglislation and judicial decisions. Givers of direct services need to keep their information up-to-date not only because such changes may have an influence on their opinions and attitudes as well as on their procedures, but because patients/families are directly affected by new policies and new ways of putting them into effect.

For the most part, changes are currrently directed toward liberalization, although open and sometimes strong opposition is expressed by special interest groups. An informative example of change occurred within recent years in a large voluntary medical center. For many years ligation was approved in that center's hospital for women under 30 who had at least four children and for women over 30 who had at least three children. Exceptions were made only with the approval of a psychiatrist. In all husband-wife partnerships the written consent of the legal husband had to be obtained in the physician's presence. Social workers were of the opinion that relatively few husbands had sufficient opportunity at that time to discuss with the physicians the exact nature of ligation and its consequences. Some women had difficulty in obtaining a ligation, sometimes because they had to wait for a psychiatrist's approval but frequently because their husbands refused to consent. In either case, the marital relationship became strained, and often the women took it out on their husbands. Approximately three years ago the hospital removed the requirements relating to size of family. The new regulations put heavy emphasis on the patient's understanding fully the consequences of ligation and on her legal husband's giving consent that is fully informed.

One must be alert also to changes that are regressive. After many years during which unmarried girls and women dropped out of school after becoming pregnant, New York City established special schools which they could attend with less embarrassment and fear of censure than their regular elementary and high schools exposed them to. It is considered most unfortunate by many concerned citizens that in the city's fiscal crisis of the 1970s these schools fell victim to the curtailment of funds. Thus a coordinated attempt to meet a sociomedical problem could not survive in a period of shrunken financial resources. There is a strong element of values in the determination of priorities for maintaining or abandoning social programs and services. In this instance, official data are needed on the social, educational, and vocational careers of those young pregnant women who do and do not complete their schooling as one of the bases for evaluating present policy and determining amended or new policy.

POSTPARTUM PRESSURES.

Postpartum depression occurs in some patients who have lived through the prenatal period without incident. When the depression appears while the patient is in the hospital, it is observed more often by the nurse than by the physician. The nurse usually asks a social worker to stop into the situation, and the social worker in turn is apt to call in a consulting psychiatrist immediately.

A delayed depression may appear after the patient has returned home. Social workers identify a few precipitating causes: the mother finds that the responsibility for the baby is more than she can cope with or has held an illusory expectation that "everything will be all right after the baby is born;" an unmarried mother may have been counting unrealistically on the putative father's returning to her; an unmarried mother living alone with her baby may be deeply oppressed by a feeling of abandonment and the weight of having sole responsibility for the child. Many of these mothers find partial relief both in the practical help that a visiting nurse can give in her role as educator and in the social and psychological support provided by her interest and concern.

Another kind of postpartum pressure comes into play when the mother delivers an infant with a visible birth defect.* Having to talk with parents about the defect and the possible reason for it, about how much correction can be

---

* Defects in the infant's heritage may manifest themselves months or years after birth, as in the case of Tay-Sachs disease and juvenile diabetes.

expected and by what means, about the potential impact of the defect upon the child and the immediate emotional impact upon the parents, is also having to acknowledge and having to cope—tasks difficult indeed for all the professionals involved and in particular for the obstetrician. The desire that givers-of-service may feel to avoid or at least to delay assuming these professional duties is entirely understandable. The desire to turn away may be precipitated by feelings such as guilt, sorrow, loss of self-regard, and a sense of futility. When the infant is severely damaged, there may also be a series of medical, legal and moral questions about sustaining and prolonging the infant's biological functioning. Who has the right to raise these questions? Who has the authority to answer them? Does or should our society sanction a choice at all?

The infant's parents react with emotions similar in kind to those of the professinonals but different in intensity, in source, in consequences, and in continuance. The woman who feels guilty because her body nurtured and produced an impaired infant may suffer from a deep sense of personal inadequacy which differs from a physician's feelings of guilt and inadequacy in reaction to his or her profession's limitations in knowledge and skill rather than to his or her individual negligence and incompetence. Parents may have to live through a prolonged period of fear and psychological recovery before daring to plan another conception.* The givers-of-service, on the other hand, can look forward to serving the parents of many healthy, well-formed infants and can hope for the fruits of experiments and research that in time will reduce the hazards and risks of procreation and enhance their professional competence and gratification. The professional's initial moments of sorrowful identification with the parents of an impaired newborn has to give way to the detached concern of the compassionate giver-of-service.

Pregnant Women and Abortion

The data presented in this section are descriptive of women who seek and obtain abortions. The data also afford an unusual opportunity to compare the nature and consequences of two public sociomedical policies; an old and highly restrictive policy has been followed by a much more permissive one, but one that has created a lively state of controversy. The issue remains unresolved in politics, in the courts, in medicine, in religion, in ethics, and in social philosophy. The issue has so many dimensions and the multiplicity of perspectives is so great that agreement on a national policy may be a long-term goal indeed.

It is an issue that touches all professionals in the health care field and personnel in the most closely related systems of services, such as income maintenance, financial assistance to individuals for health care, third-party payments to hospitals, nursing homes, other health facilities, and institutions for professional and technical education in the health care field. This is an issue that illustrates the complexities in formulating policy and the need for professional and technical personnel to keep their information current, to be aware of the impacts of existing circumstances, to anticipate the potential significance of proposed changes, and to develop a point of view of his or her own—to be responsible for taking a position and acting upon it.**

* For detailed discussion of congenital and familial impairments, see Chapter 7 on pediatric and adolescent patients and Appendix A.

** See the section on improving and expanding resources and systems of care, p. 41.

Two laws, two programs also covers two sets of procedures and their respective impacts upon patients/families and givers-of-service in cases of abortion performed in one acute general voluntary hospital.

Under the law in New York State until April 1970, the only legal abortions were those considered essential to the physical or mental health of a pregnant woman. Furthermore, if the woman was married and her husband was the father of the expected child, an abortion could be performed legally only with her husband's consent.

The prescribed procedures extended over a span of weeks for each patient. A pregnant woman receiving clinic care in the hospital who requested an abortion was examined by a gynecologist and referred promptly to a social worker for an interview. A pregnant woman cared for by a private physician who requested an abortion was examined by her own physician; it was not regular procedure for these patients to be referred to a social worker.

When gynecological examination did not reveal a medical reason for an abortion, the woman was referred for an interview with two psychiatrists. There was usually a waiting period for this interview and a second waiting period until the Committee on Therapeutic Abortions made its decision.

There was a third waiting period if the request for an abortion was approved. Under the law a dilation and curettage was performed if the patient was pregnant less than 12 weeks; no medical intervention took place between the twelfth and eighteenth weeks of pregnancy; after the eighteenth week the procedure was salting-out. The medical procedure, whether D and C or salting-out, necessitated hospitalization. A D and C was performed on the gynecological service, and there was usually a delay in obtaining a bed. A bed in the obstetrical service, where salting-out was performed, was available more quickly.

The patients seeking therapeutic abortions under the old law were mostly unmarried or separated from their husbands and pregnant by another man. The few married women were pregnant by their husbands, usually because birth control measures had failed. Following an abortion, in all instances contraception was discussed with the patient, contraceptive advice was given, and the inadvisability of using abortion as a means of birth control was emphasized.

Although the hospital honored the provisions of the new law from the time of enactment in April 1970, the new structure and organization of services that the law required took several months to put into operation. At the point when data covering a 6-months' period under the new law were being examined by the social work staff there were already some useful observations.[11] The new law greatly simplified the procedures in that the decision to have an abortion was made by the woman in consultation with her physician, and a married woman pregnant by her husband did not need his consent.

The patient telephoned or came to the abortion clinic for an appointment to register. When she registered she was seen by a social worker for a first assessment of her psychosocial situation. However, if she had a private physician, she had an interview with a social worker only if she (the patient) or her physician requested it. At the time of registration x-rays were taken, the patient's blood was typed, and, if there had been an interview with a social worker, he or she and the patient decided together on the advisability of future contacts.

On a day of the week set aside for the purpose, the patient was examined by a physician, but only after the physician explained to the group of patients present that day the three possible medical procedures: (1) suction, if the patient was pregnant 10 to 12 weeks or less; this procedure would take place in the clinic; (2) D and C, if the pregnancy was advanced 12 to 14 or 12 to 16 weeks; the patient would be hospitalized on the gynecologic service; (3) salting-out, at about the fourteenth but preferably the sixteenth week, if the pregnancy was beyond the twelfth week. For somewhat over two years the salting-out process was started in the clinic, and the patient returned home. She was admitted as an in-patient on obstetrics service when labor began. In July 1973 the city's health code was changed, and patients were accordingly hospitalized for the entire salting-out process.

The hospital considered a waiting period of more than a week or two undesirable because of both physical and emotional risks. Therefore patients were referred to other qualified facilities at the time of registration if the waiting period would be excessive.

The significant similiarity between the two programs has to do with the availability of contact with a social worker. Under the new law, the program in this hospital again did not routinely provide a psychosocial assessment of a private patient's situation.

The significant differences between the two programs were the simpler legal requirements that the patient had to meet; the greater responsibility the patient had to take for her decision; the probability of fewer and shorter waiting periods; and the greater possibility of obtaining an abortion as an out-patient during the early weeks of pregnancy.

Significant impacts of abortion on patients/families and others, as observed in the early days of the new law and program, were attributed by social workers more often to the patient's making her own decision than to any other single circumstance: "No longer are an obstetrician and two psychiatrists involved in the decision. We are seeing patients who have to face their own guilt and responsibility for the action to be taken." Reference to the woman's guilt ran like a theme, whether social workers were talking about the old or the new liberalized law—a commentary, no doubt, on the difference in meaning to individuals between legality and morality.

One social worker said, speaking of the patients she knew under the old law, "The guilt a woman feels about having an abortion is not necessarily the product of a specific religious culture alone. It is usual for the woman to think she will be punished [after the abortion], to wonder whether the punishment will be death or sterility, and so on." These women explained their guilt in various ways. Some said they had a sense of killing the fetus. Some were ashamed because the cultural group they belonged to did not countenance pregnancy out of wedlock or disapproved strongly of abortion or frowned upon sex relations outside marriage. Some of the women voiced fear that the physicians would be critical of them. There were women receiving public assistance who were afraid their welfare workers would "cut them off" even though the law forbade it. "In all," a social worker said, "it is a highly emotional time for the woman. She may look stoic, but she isn't."

Another social worker observing patients in the early months of the new law and program emphasized that "the impact of moral and religious convictions is strong, and the later in pregnancy the more likely the patient is to feel 'this is killing; this wrong.' . . . Her conflicts may never be resolved, she may continue to ponder 'did I do right?'" The social worker noted as a natural consequence of these patients' general state of upset that "the display of tension and anxiety is greater now than [under the old law] for all patients who use the operating room [for an abortion]."

Women in severe conflict are likely to seek help from a social worker both before and after the abortion is performed. One social worker with long experience and much practice wisdom thought it important not to open up the patient's emotional reactions unless one is prepared to follow through with as much time and attention as are necessary. If the social work service has to be brief and the patient is openly upset, the social worker should respond supportively but without probing; if the patient denies being upset, the social worker should accept the denial. Some patients have a way of protecting themselves against overwhelming guilt by forgetting their appointments and finally not having an abortion at all.

When a woman has strong and painful emotional reactions to seeking or having obtained an abortion, her feelings will spill over into the various aspects of her life, particularly affecting her family relations. Under the old law, which required the husband's consent, there were married couples who were in agreement about an abortion before they came to the clinic; in these instances, the marital relationship usually appeared not to be at risk. However, when married partners were not in agreement, a social worker saw the spouses together—and separately, too, if necessary—to explore the situation and help the couple to come to terms. In some of these instances, the wife had to grapple with the potential consequences to the marriage if her husband felt she was forcing him to give consent. Similar conditions obtained in nonlegal unions, especially in stable, long-term partnerships, when both the man and the woman wanted to be in agreement about the abortion.

Speaking from early experience with the new law, social workers noted that husbands usually knew about and agreed to their wives' abortions. The woman either had told her husband directly or let him know in a more roundabout way that she wanted an abortion. Unmarried women in stable unions were observed to act similarly in respect to long-time nonlegal partners. It was not to comply with a legal technicality that both partners became involved in the decision to request an abortion but to preserve the strength and quality of a relationship.

In addition, there are associations with those other than the woman's partner—with her parents, siblings, and close friends, for instance—which must be considered, if for no other reason than that concealment of an emotion-laden event can undermine or even destroy a once comfortable and mutually satisfying relationship.

Although in the end it is easier for many adult patients to tell their parents than to conceal that they are seeking or have had an abortion, they may encounter some special problems. If, for example, defiance toward her parents had been a factor in the patient's having had sexual experience, or if for other reasons she has knowingly violated or is about to violate their standards of behavior, telling them of her decision may be a formidable undertaking. To illustrate, a number of unmarried women who seek abortions are somewhat alienated from their parents but nevertheless hope for their emotional support in a time of crisis. Social workers are called upon to assist patients who want to make their problem known to their parents but are afraid or ashamed, or failing that, to some other relative or at least to a friend. It is not only emotional support that the patient needs at this time. There are also practical reasons for sharing knowledge of her condition. Each patient is given instructions to have a responsible person with her when she comes for the actual medical procedure.

If the procedure requires hospitalization, it is seldom feasible or desirable for a patient to hide her whereabouts or the reason for hospitalization from everyone in her social milieu. It is particularly hard if the patient has tried to conceal her pregnancy from her young children; making arrangements for someone to care for them may add to the patient's difficulty, since, as a rule, several persons have to be involved in making plans and some explanation has to be made to each one. These conditions are problematic for the married and unmarried patient alike. Then there are the awkward questions that people ask, such as "Why are you going to the hospital?"; "How long will you be there?"; and "May I visit you?"

These questions cannot be divorced from the impact upon the patient of the service unit in which she will be hospitalized. When she is on the gynecological service for a D and C, she is not often confronted with painful situations. In the first months of the new program, however, when the patient was on the obstetrical service for salting-out, both she and her fellow patients experienced moments of considerable distress. The patient having an abortion was among other women who had had, or were waiting to have, their babies. The nursery was in full view; the babies were brought to their mothers for feeding; the fathers visited to hold and fondle the infants. Subsequently, arrangements were made to separate the women obtaining abortions from the other obstetrical patients and from the site of the nursery. This rearrangement of space also spared the women who were terminating their pregnancies from the unpleasant, hostile reactions which the other women often expressed openly and sometimes obliquely.

Physicians have their individual reactions to abortion, and these too affect the patient. If a physician believes that unmarried women should have abortions, he or she may miss clues that indicate that a patient really wants her baby. An exceedingly upset patient may be trying to say that she is asking for an abortion she does not want. Repeated requests for abortions may mean the failure of a contraceptive method, but it can also reflect a wish to have a baby. If a physician opposes abortions except for therapeutic reasons, he or she is legally and professionally free to refuse to perform them, but under current law the patient may still seek the service she wants elsewhere. The physician's right to a dissenting opinion is also the right of nurses and other givers-of-service. We should know more about how the pregnant woman wanting an abortion reacts to and copes with the knowledge of such dissenting opinions among health professionals and about the consequences of her ways of coping. In the absence of a single and stable legal, social, and medical policy, these may be questions worth answering.

Financial status may be a major factor in a pregnant woman's search for an abortion. Women with financial means had little difficulty under the old law in New York State in obtaining abortions under safe, medically adequate conditions, although they were technically illegal; women with limited incomes were sometimes entitled to therapeutic abortions, but far too often they had to resort to unsafe, illegal procedures or to dangerous self-induced abortions; still others bore their unwanted children.

Although the new law of 1970 made it possible for women receiving public assistance or who were certified for Medicaid to obtain third-party payments for abortions, women who were neither wealthy enough to pay for the service nor poor enough to be eligible for Medicaid or who were not protected by private medical insurance still had to turn to unsafe as well as illegal resources for an abortion. Even women with some form of coverage may have had to make financial sacrifices because the available payments did not cover all of the costs.

The continuing controversy over the ethics and social and moral attitudes concerned with legalized abortion on request was exemplified in 1977 in congressional and judicial attempts to forbid the use of federal funds to pay for nontherapeutic abortions, while other courts declared such restriction to be discriminatory against the poor. It is indeed difficult—perhaps impossible—to legislate issues that so many people believe are matters of individual, philosophical choice.*

There are social embarrassments a woman may experience, connected not with money but created by disapproving and ambivalent attitudes within herself which still exist among the general public in respect to children born out of wedlock, abortions for nontherapeutic reasons, the one-parent family, and so on. For example, a woman receiving public assistance is not able to obtain homemaker service to care for her children while she is in the hospital unless the diagnosis is stated in her application to the New York City Department of Social Services. Might it not suffice to affirm that no one in the family has a contagious or infectious disease? Another example: since even with the best planning the patient may miss some classes at school or a few days of work, she may be extremely apprehensive when the physician has to complete an official form or sign a letter of explanation to a school or place of employment. Could not the patient participate in planning with the doctor what he or she will say in official reports to persons outside the hospital?

COMMON FORCES IN DIVERSE SITUATIONS

Although each of these two groups of patients—those in psychiatric service and the adult pregnant woman whose condition is medically uncomplicated—is of intrinsic professional interest and has its own biopsychosocial significance, the patients in both groups serve to illustrate some of the common characteristics of patient populations in hospital-based service.

In each group the interaction of biopsychosocial elements in human life is clearly manifested. The impacts of socioenvironmental conditions on patients/ families and givers-of-service are particularly notable at the level of an individual institution and at various governmental levels; the influence of factors such as administrative regulations or procedures, deployment of staff, allocation of functions and tasks, and financial status and funding is discernible throughout.

Another cluster of significant forces can be identified as attitudinal, again at several levels of expression. Society's ideas about emotional and mental disturbances, professional understanding and interpretation of changes in mani-

* Halfway through 1978 the situation remains chaotic. Congressional legislation now forbids the use of federal funds for abortions except under a few specified circumstances. Many states have followed suit in respect to state funds, although a few states, New York among them, will use state funds in the case of those women who request abortions but are unable to pay for them.

fest behavior among youths and adults, what society expects and will tolerate as young people's physical maturation is attained earlier and earlier, the changes taking place in family roles, responsibility, and authority even while the family is deeply rooted in our social systems—all of these areas and aspects of life can be seen in one form or another in these two dissimilar groups of patients.

A third constellation of factors—one that affects directly the quality of service provided—concerns intrarelations and interrelations among hospital personnel. The need for, and potentially constructive consequences of, professional collaboration emerge continually in regard to all phases of health care. Many of the barriers to achieving adequate collaboration are attitudinal; many of the impeding attitudes are habitual, customary and barely conscious, but exceedingly influential. Overcoming inertia and developing mutual understanding and mutual professional respect and trust are among the most significant issues. But no amount of talk, no matter how well intentioned and sincere, can substitute for the actual doing—the demonstration of collaborative effort and action in the practice of the health and health-related professions.

REFERENCES

1. Ruth D. Knee and Warren C. Lamson, "Mental Health Services," in *Encyclopedia of Social Work*, 16th ed. (New York: National Association of Social Workers, 1971), pp. 802-812.
2. Philip M. Margolis and Armando R. Fawazza, "Mental Health and Illness," in *Encyclopedia of Social Work*, 17th ed. (Washington, D.C.: National Association of Social Workers, 1977), pp. 849-860.
3. Bess Dana, "Health, Social Work and Social Justice," in *Social Work Practice and Social Justice*, Bernard Ross and Charles Shireman (Washington, D. C.: National Association of Social Workers, 1973).
4. Ibid., p. 124.
5. Ibid., p. 116.
6. Vincente Abad, Juan Ramos, and Elizabeth Boyce, "A Model for Delivery of Mental Health Services to Spanish-Speaking Minorities," *American Journal of Orthopsychiatry*, vol. 44, no. 4 (July 1974), p. 584.
7. Helen Rehr, ed., *Medicine and Social Work: An Exploration in Interprofessionalism* (New York: Prodist, 1974).
8. E. E. LeMasters, "Parenthood as Crisis," in *Crisis Intervention*, ed. Howard J. Parad (New York: Family Service Association of America, 1965), p. 111.
9. Trudy Bradley Festinger, "Unmarried Mothers and Their Decision to Keep or Surrender Children," *Child Welfare*, vol. 50, no. 5 (May 1971), pp. 253-263.
10. *Louise Wise Services Annual Report, 1970-1971* (New York).
11. Alma T. Young, Barbara Berkman, and Helen Rehr, "Women Who Seek Abortions: A Study," *Social Work*, vol. 18, no. 3 (May 1973), pp. 60-65.

Chapter 7
Selected
Patient Groups:

PEDIATRIC AND ADOLESCENT PATIENTS

To supplement the discussion of adult patients in Chapters 3 and 4, this chapter and the one that follows are concerned with patients in four developmental/age groups: pediatric and adolescent patients in this chapter, and young adult and geriatric patients in Chapter 8.* Under the stress-producing impact of long-term or lifetime diseases, bodily defects, and anomalies, patients in these significant phases of the lifecycle are faced with obstacles to achieving their full potential for social-health and sometimes are confronted with threats to survival itself. The forms and consequences of these impacts and their meanings to patients/families, to others significant in their everyday lives, and to hospital personnel who serve them constitute the central concern of these two chapters.

In a text meant to be suggestive rather than conclusive, there will be omissions disappointing to readers with certain special interests. In this chapter, for example, there is little about sick infants, children in intensive care units, or children who are fatally ill. Also, references to short-term, transitory illness are made usually in the context of long-term conditions. To illustrate, it may be noted that a child with diabetes can be affected seriously by an infection that other children easily overcome, or that an infant with a cleft palate is especially vulnerable to upper respiratory illnesses. An important exception concerns abused and neglected children, who are apt to present both acute conditions such as fractures and burns and long-term health problems such as malnutrition and retarded development.

The material in this chapter focuses first on the pediatric patient and then on the adolescent patient. Each developmental group has characteristics, tasks,

---

* The age ranges adopted for each of the four phases are as follows: pediatric patients, from birth through 12 years of age; adolescent patients, 13 through 17 years of age; young adult patients 18 through 20 years of age; and elderly patients, 65 years of age and over. (Adult patients, treated in earlier chapters, were from 21 through 64 years of age.)

and conflicts which interact with situations of illness, affecting and being affected by the course of a disease or deficiency, its treatment and its outcome.*

In chapter VIII the illustration of young adult patients is atypical in the severity and harshness of physical disability, but for that very reason it throws a strong light on the meaning of social-health status. Discussion of the elderly patient rounds out the phases of the life cycle. By now the term *elderly* is vague, and many persons differentiate the "young old" from the "old" and the "old old." But the division into age groups alone obscures the differences that exist in people's rate or tempo of aging, in the diverse ways in which aging is revealed, and in the areas of social functioning which show or do not show the onset and effects of aging. So the elderly patients will differ from one another as do members of each of the younger groups.

The Pediatric Patient: Some Common Characteristics and Themes

Common threads run through the observations about the meanings, the impacts, and the demands for adaptation resulting from a variety of biological conditions that affect children, their relatives, their significant others, and hospital personnel. Observations about adult patients are, in their broadest terms, relevant to pediatric patients; but translated into specific terms relevant to children at risk, the details of the observations differ. For example, the patient's illness no matter what his or her age affects the family group, but the form and consequences of the impacts, meanings, and demands for adaptation are discernibly different for patients at various stages of the life cycle. These differences are associated with such interacting factors as an individual's developmental processes and maturational status, his or her opportunities for biopsychosocial growth, his or her experiences of biopsychosocial deprivation, and the expectations that society has in regard to the social functioning of persons in a specified phase of the life cycle.

The child's logic is a significant determinant of the meaning of an illness, defect, or injury to the pediatric patient; it is shaped by fantasies which are usually more punitive and nearer the surface of consciousness than the fantasies of adult patients. Children, to whom family relationships are still paramount, who normally have some ambivalent feelings toward parents and siblings, and who also normally have done or wanted to do things their parents consider bad, often perceive their deviant physical conditions and the treatment they have to undergo as punishments and evidence of parental disapproval and sometimes as withdrawal of love. The same ideas are easily carried over to the physicians whose examinations and treatment cause conditions such as pain, discomfort, or restriction of movement. The pediatric patient's incompletely developed sense of reality and time make certain distinctions difficult if not impossible to make. The pain is here and now, and feeling better later is very far away. The doctor to whom his or her mother takes the patient is another powerful adult whose stated desire to help does not seem consistent with the pain of an injection, the discomfort of a brace, or a taboo on sweets.

The meaning of hospitalization as an abandonment is the child's reasoning carried to its extreme. Very young children may not understand separation any other way; to them people who disappear are gone forever. Long and flexible

---

* Appendix A contains two examples of the flow of life-and-illness in interaction during the continuum of childhood and adolescence.

visiting hours, allowing parents to care for and feed a hospitalized child when it is medically permissible, and permitting siblings to visit are among the measures that make hospitalization less traumatic for the pediatric patient. The balance of interdependence on the people he or she knows is kept in better equilibrium, and this helps to deal with the demands for adaptation that cannot be eliminated.

The child's sense of reality can be strengthened by giving him or her explanations, forewarnings, and honest assurances at the time and in the language most suitable to his or her age and development. Preparation for a procedure given a week in advance may be too late for one child and too early for another. A diabetic child of preschool age may find explanation enough in "If mommy gives you this medicine every day, you won't be so thirsty all the time"; but later, when it comes time to inject himself or herself, he or she will need to understand that: "the medicine makes up for something your body doesn't produce." In other words, as the child develops in the understanding of cause and effect, in the grasp of time and time intervals, in the ability to distinguish inner and outer reality, and in self-reliance, the meaning and significance of his or her disease, defect, or disability develop also.

The pediatric patient/family constellation plays an indispensable role. The child is heavily dependent on his or her parents for recognizing signs and symptoms of illness, impairment, or injury; for obtaining medical care when it is needed; and for carrying treatment through to completion. Since parents assume these responsibilities in different ways and since the patient's siblings and members of the extended family are almost always active participants in the life of the family, it is essential to assess the family in relation to the projected medical care of the pediatric patient. Parental attitudes toward illness and parental behavior when children in the family are ill can be understood in contexts such as cultural background; educational, financial, and occupational status; the psychological and emotional characteristics of individual family members; the nature of family relationships; and the functioning of the family unit.

The emotional and physical impacts of illness upon the pediatric patient/family have the potential for either strengthening or disrupting the family's structure and relationships. Many of these impacts are strains which result from the young patient's need for unusual kinds and amounts of attention. Mothers and fathers suffer from physical fatigue, often compounded by worry and anxiety; long visits to the hospitalized child and lengthy travel time take their toll. When parents return home, there may be other children who want and should have attention, and the mother may have to cook supper when she needs to rest. When the pediatric patient is home-bound or bed-bound for long periods, the mother has less leisure than she needs and often more and heavier household chores than usual.[1]

When the family is a strong, cohesive unit to start with, available members of the patient's nuclear and extended family find ways to relieve the parents of some of their usual responsibilities. The reallocation of tasks is in some families spontaneous and in others a response to suggestions—often from a social worker. When family ties are weak at best, the needs of the pediatric patient may be disruptive; conditions in the home become chaotic, children develop behavioral problems at school, and spouses quarrel. Reassessing responsibilities is no longer a relieving measure but a provocative, controversial idea. Social workers have to give psychological support, encourage communication among family members, offer suggestions for problem solving, and call on community resources when they are available.

In the instance of hospitalized children who are not in serious condition, it is often possible to persuade the parents—and especially the mother—that a hospital recreation worker, a volunteer visitor, the public school teacher assigned to the hospital, and a social worker will arrange to keep the patient busy and reasonably content so that the parents can redistribute the frequency and length of their visits. Concern for the other children in the family is one factor in this recommendation; it is not unusual for siblings to resent the time and attention their parents give to the patient, and the other children's capacity for sharing should not be stretched too far. This situation illustrates again the social worker's commitment to preserve family equilibrium and protect each member's well-being insofar as possible. It has to be kept in mind that these are situations in which the illness extends over long periods of time, as does its treatment; what the patient's siblings might tolerate well for a short period may become a crisis-producing condition over a prolonged interval.

The personality characteristics of the young patient's parents have special bearing on a child's medical care. In this regard, one is concerned with tendencies toward traits such as rigidity, permissiveness, and flexibility. Rigidity and permissiveness are potentially harmful to the pediatric patient, the former holding the patient too tightly to his or her prescribed regimen and the latter being too casual to afford the patient the protection he or she needs. From the standpoint of the patient's safety and comfort, many givers-of-service seem to agree that flexibility on the part of parents is preferable; social workers read into this trait good judgment and only a useful degree of anxiety. For instance, flexible parents can allow the diabetic child a little sweet on rare occasions and will increase the dosage of insulin accordingly. However, since physicians differ in their flexibility, it is recognized that professional authority will influence the way in which people exercise their parental authority.

Social workers note also the different ways in which parents respond to the unexpected, such as a new symptom or other sign of trouble. One needs to know whether the adults in the home, and especially the mother, who customarily has major responsibility for the care of the children, lose their heads in an emergency or can control their anxiety enough to take necessary steps.

In the event that the child's illness, deficiency, or other notable deviance is congenital or familial, it is usual for parents to feel responsible and rather cruelly threatened. Parental reactions take such various forms as shame, fear, repulsion, guilt, or an overwhelming need to do everything for and give everything to the damaged child. It is usual for parents to search for reasons: What did they do wrong? Does it run in the family? Was the baby injured during delivery? Parents are subjected not only to their own reactions but to critical questioning and curious stares on the part of others. Parents' fears regarding a child with serious defects are from one standpoint entirely justifiable. What parent might not be fearful of feeding a newborn infant with a cleft palate or of taking care of a nine-year-old with a colostomy? It is important that physicians, nurses, social workers, and other personnel who may be involved collaborate in enabling parents to adapt to the new tasks and responsibilities demanded by a child's unusual medicosocial needs.

When treatment procedures are being contemplated that would put the pediatric patient at high risk, the parents need a preparatory period in which to work with key professional personnel *before* they are requested to give formal, signed consent.* They can use this period to understand what is being recommended, why, and what the expected outcome is; to express and master emotional reactions; to come to a reasoned decision; and to plan how they will prepare the young patient for whatever will take place next.

A similar period of preparation is needed by the patient/family when a child who will require special care is discharged from the hospital to his or her parents. Frequently they will have to tend to the child's special physical problem once the patient returns home and simultaneously foster the child's psychological and social growth lest it fall victim to the extended period of physical dependence.

A good example is a nine-year-old child with a colostomy. Her mother was the most apprehensive member of the family, but the physician, nurse, and social worker collaborating in the preparatory period included the young patient's father and siblings in the sphere of their concern. In terms that everyone could understand, the professionals explained the patient's physical condition, how her colostomy functioned, what the patient could do for herself, and what someone else had to help her with. These were very important points to make; the patient must be perceived not as helpless but as needing specific kinds of care and attention at home and at school. With the signed consent of the parents and a verbal agreement with the patient, the social worker undertook to prepare the child's teacher and school principal for the kind of help she would need. The three members of the hospital staff continued to work with the patient/family in frequent contacts at first and at longer intervals thereafter. In this particular instance, in which every family member, including the patient, made an adaptation to the little girl's unusual bodily functioning and its consequences, the process of adjustment took approximately a year.

The impact on professionals of a child's serious illness, severe suffering, threatened survival, and similar stress-producing conditions may be so strong as to arouse powerful defensive mechanisms or, at the other extreme, break down the professional's customarily useful defenses. For the very reason that the patient is a helpless infant or child given into their hands, the givers of direct services have to deal frequently with their own emotional responses. They are thrust to a considerable extent into a surrogate parental role with a variety of possible consequences. They may defensively deny some of the patient/family's anxieties and fears; they may become strongly identified with the parents and suffer with them; or they may become intensely protective of the young patient, especially if they do not understand or approve of the parents' attitudes and child-rearing practices. There is always the knowledge, too, that in the process of treating a sick child there are interventions that inflict physical pain or cause psychological discomfort, and these experiences may precipitate distortion in normally professional behavior. For example, one kindly physician was so distressed by a little girl's frightened screaming that he slapped her, much as a parent might who is as upset as the child but gives vent to fear through anger.

Normally, the professionals take some responsibility for allaying the pediatric patient's anxiety, while at the same time they recognize that over the long haul this is the parents' task. As one social worker said, "If the parents'

* See the section on anticipatory and preparatory activity, p. 30.

anxiety is taken care of by the physician, they can care for much of the child's anxiety and do it better at the child's level." In other words, it is preferable to enable parents to carry out their roles in their own way rather than to substitute for them or give them "how-to" instructions.

THE MALTREATED AND ABUSED CHILD*

It is one of the great misfortunes of our current era that in a society which is often described as child centered there exists an unbelievably large number of abused and maltreated children.

Up to this point the discussion of the pediatric patient/family has described parents who are capable of providing their children with at least the minimum of nurturing, love, and protection needed to promote growth and development. These parents can be said to have a socially acceptable quality of caring, though such factors as ignorance and anxieties caused by life's crises may impair the quality of their child rearing.

We have now to turn to those other parents who can neither care about nor care for their children sufficiently well to assure even the minimal opportunities essential to a child's achieving an acceptable status of social-health. These parents are primarily maltreating or abusive, and the children, in manner, behavior, and emotional and physical condition, are the products of parental maltreatment or abuse. It has taken this country an inexplicable length of time to provide even minimal legal provisions for the protection of children against abuse and maltreatment and for the prevention of maltreatment and abuse.[2]

Practitioners in the human services have to be familiar with their respective state and local laws and regulations concerning maltreated and abused children. Taking New York State as an example, the law currently mandates the reporting of known and suspected cases of abused children (under 16 years of age) and maltreated children (under 18 years of age). In New York City two agencies are authorized to receive such reports: the society for the Prevention of Cruelty to Children and a Special Services for Children unit of the Bureau of Child Welfare of the New York City Department of Social Services. As one would expect, a large volume of reporting comes from the city's municipal and voluntary hospitals. Children may be admitted to and detained in a reporting hospital until adequate plans are made for their protection, and personnel who report the children have immunity from liability if they act in good faith.

Early in 1974 the federal government officially recognized the problem of child abuse and maltreatment. Legislation was passed which established a national center, located in the Department of Health, Education and Welfare, to promote programs and projects for the prevention and treatment of child abuse and maltreatment. It was impossible to ignore any longer the "evidence that the problem affects tens of thousands of children throughout the nation."[3,4]

A designation of child abuse or maltreatment requires an assessment of the child's total life experience and in particular a comprehensive appraisal of the people responsible for the young patient's care.** But the physicians, nurses, and social workers who attend the children when they are brought to the hospital are alerted first by signs and signals of possible abuse or maltreatment.

---

* In the New York Family Court Act, 1012(f), the word maltreated is used to designate what is often termed neglected.

** These people may be parents, other adult relatives, babysitters, siblings, and so on.

Examples of these in the child are malnutrition, fractures, bruises, irritability, obvious neglect of physical care, psychotic behavior, subdural hematomas, retarded growth and development, x-rays of bones showing periosteal reaction, and trauma and burns of suspicious origin.

Of great importance also are the signals the social workers hear and see because of their expert knowledge of the ways in which people express themselves: a mother who sits apathetically waiting in the clinic when the child on her lap is found to be comatose; the woman who says, "Some mothers tie their children with a rope, but I never do that," when her child has a suspected rope burn all around the wrist; the parents who argue furiously about which one of them let the child climb on the window ledge; the passive man in the house who has no idea how the two-year-old got into a tub of scalding water; the 18-month-old girl who buried her head in the pillow when her mother came to visit and shouted "no."

Finally, there are the recurring visits to the emergency service or clinic which eventually give rise to the suspicion that the child's injuries are not accidental. It is more difficult than one might think to note these recurring episodes, because abusive parents in particular tend to go from hospital to hospital and use false identifying data to throw officials off the trail. In an effort to combat this kind of concealment, information in the New York City Registry of reported cases is made available to prescribed or authorized persons. The subject of such a report may have access to the information about him or her and has the right to a hearing, and disproved allegations are expunged from the registry.

It is a complicating fact that acts of abuse or maltreatment may occur during a parent's absence. The parent who brings the sick or injured child to the hospital may in truth not know what happened while someone else was in charge, or perhaps while no one was in charge. The reported absence of the parent from the scene of the action always raises difficult questions when there is suspicion of abuse or maltreatment. For example, has the parent unknowingly and unintentionally allowed an abusive or maltreating person to take care of the child? Does the parent openly or subtly sanction or provoke maltreatment or abuse of the child by others? Is the child's condition the result of a genuine accident? Or is the child habitually left without the protection of a responsible adult—a situation that may spell maltreatment rather than point to abuse?

Differentiations between abuse and maltreatment are important not only because they figure so strongly in medical-social assessments and interventions but also because of their legal implications should a situation get to the courts. The differences are not always sharply drawn, but in broad terms, as presented below, they are useful benchmarks for those who have to make the first tentative determination about the accidental or nonaccidental nature of a child's condition.

A *composite picture of maltreating parents* and the family situations they create starts with the marked disorganization of their lives. Their homes are neglected and apt to be dirty. Meals may be irregular and are sometimes skipped entirely. The home is likely to be in commotion, the living space chaotic and disordered. The young children in these families are often left at home without adult supervision. The parents, many of whom are deeply deprived socially, economically, and emotionally, are prone to be without personal or family goals, isolated, childlike, and unable to respond as one expects an adult parent to respond. They have difficulty dealing with frustration, and, consequently when gratification is delayed they often act out their impulses.

Parents who maltreat their children may have bursts of anger more to be rid of the children's demands than out of a desire to harm the children. Maltreatment, many observers believe, arises more from indifference than from hatred. Maltreated children are often deserted—left without care and protection. Their parents, so often immature and isolated, have little feeling of "possessing" their children. As one social worker described it, "if the children are placed [outside their natural homes,] just as the parents did nothing about the neglect so they do nothing about the children being returned to them."

Because children tend to learn their parents' patterns of behavior, maltreated children tend to become maltreating parents. It is possible to break this chain of deprivation and negligence if social workers and other helping professionals reach out to maltreating parents over a long period of time, consistently, patiently, and with compassion. The parents and children who form these deprived and depriving families have great need for a wide range of services, as many of which as possible should be provided under the aegis of one social agency. The point is to make the assistance the family members need as available as possible; people who are by temperament immature, essentially unrelated to other human beings, and isolated from their communities cannot be expected to go from agency to agency, to relate to any number of helping people, to maintain numerous contacts, and to keep countless appointments with many different people over extended periods of time. One must infer from these comments that these parents and children have need for a long-term, continuous contact with one social worker—one person who will help make services available, help to coordinate the services, and be the primary source of help, whether indirectly or directly through others. Someone must be in that role for this group of needful families since, as the social workers know well, services for social welfare, health care, and related needs are not structured in our society to provide one-stop resources. It is a demanding role because these patients/families for a long time cannot deal constructively with frustration or assume responsibility with comfort or success.

A description of abusing parents starts with a fact difficult to believe: The injuries they inflict upon children are intentional rather than impulsive and spring from a hatred which may have the power to destroy. "Physical abuse of children is the intentional, non-accidental use of physical force, or intentional non-accidental acts of omission on the part of a parent or other caretaker interacting with a child in his care, aimed at hurting, injuring, or destroying that child."[5] Abusing parents are found at all economic, educational, and financial levels of society, another fact which seems unlikely to many people. These parents may be unskilled laborers or professionals, intellectually dull or brilliant, barely literate or holders of postgraduate degrees. They may live in what one social worker described as "substandard, messy homes or well-kept clean homes." The physical appearance of an abused child may be deceptive, for he or she is often clean, adequately clothed, and well-fed, just as his or her home may be well ordered and well cared for.

Abusing parents suffer from a wide range of emotional disorders, and an individual's attitude may swing widely and wildly from indifference to hostility. Since these parents from their own accounts rarely feel that their parents loved them, one has a clue to one of their outstanding characteristics: they tend to expect and demand from their infants and young children (often only one child in the family is singled out consistently as the victim) love, attention, help, reassurance, and comforting that the child is totally unable to provide; since the child is incapable of assuming a nurturing role and is a source of enormous frustration, the child becomes in effect the target of his or her parents' revenge upon their parents.

An abusive parent may not feel guilt about his or her behavior or assume responsibility for it. While it is rather common for only one of the child's parents to be actively abusive, a frequent characteristic of the nonabusing parent is that he or she may give tacit, or even provocative, support to the actions of the abusing parent. Similar behavior occurs in the marital relationship of other psychologically disturbed people and is particularly familiar to those who work with alcoholic patients and their spouses.

Abusing parents in general have respect for power, play on fear, sneer at weakness, and are suspicious, angry, and surly. They may be skilled in the use of words and convincing in saying what they believe an investigator wants to hear. Abused children themselves are almost never a source of direct, verbalized information; they are too afraid and mistrustful to tell their miserable stories. Close observation of their nonverbal behavior does provide clues, as in the instance cited earlier of the young child who buried her head in the pillow and cried "no" when she saw her mother.

Some abused children grow up to become abusive like their parents; others become extremely withdrawn. Few manage to become well-functioning adults. Again, professionals try to break the chain of pathological adult behavior. They find it essential to take the initiative with abusing parents, going to their homes, repeatedly accepting the rebuff of unopened doors, and making frequent efforts to reach the parents, psychologically speaking. Because the parents can be so elusive, sometimes the only hope for the child is when the abusing parent leaves the home or the child is removed from his or her parents' home usually through court action.

Despite the uncertain outcome, it is desirable that attempts be made to help parents provide, at least minimally, for the child's nurturing and protection before an abused child is removed from the home. There are three major reasons for taking this position. First, there is in our society a strong commitment to parental rights, and this is likely to have a decided influence in the courts which may have to rule on separating a child from his or her family. Second, but basically unacceptable to the helping professions, resources are scarce for the placement of children in adequate substitute homes, and children are known to have been badly treated by unsuitable foster parents. Also, because abused children may have unusual difficulty adapting to their new families, they may be moved from one foster home to another, thus experiencing no more security than they had in their own homes. Third, and the most telling argument, is the child's own need to stay with his or her family. Separation from the biological family creates conflict even in the child who has been abused by his or her parents. Separation anxiety is one of the most painful emotions to endure; one should not assume that the abused or maltreated child will welcome separation from the family he or she considers his or her own—the one he or she belongs to by birth and blood kinship.

How can one approach the parents of a child who is suspected by hospital personnel of being maltreated or abused or both? When physical signs and significant behavior add up to possible maltreatment or abuse of a child who is known to the hospital, the social worker becomes a major collaborator in exploring and assessing the patient/family situation. The immediate objective is to obtain as much and as accurate evidence as possible of what actually occurred to account for the child's current condition.

In order to achieve this goal the exploration should be conducted as benignly as possible. To create a benign climate requires that the attitude, manner, and tone of the investigator be free of accusation, blame, or vindictiveness. Otherwise the person interviewed will defensively close himself or herself off as a source of believable evidence. Then no judgment can be made of the circumstances behind the child's condition, and the patient/family could be deprived of the services and opportunities they need to correct or alleviate a dangerous life-situation. Interviews of this kind impose severe demands upon interviewers for control of their emotions and biases against persons suspected of maltreating, and especially of abusing, children.

Hospital-based professionals in the human services are faced with a problem of ethics in that they are seeking information from parents (or surrogates) who may as a consequence be exposed to official investigation and eventually in some instances to legal separation from their children. With all the care, caution, and expert skill interviewers can muster, it may never be possible to obtain accurate or complete accounts of what took place in some of these family situations. However, evidence in the form of laboratory and clinical findings and in the form of careful observations and appraisals of both verbal and nonverbal messages is frequently an adequate base for the decision that the hospital has to make—either to detain the child in the hospital until the situation is further clarified by the authorities legally responsible for the welfare of children or to permit the child to go home with the parent who brought him or her. In the latter case, hospital personnel may not be certain that the family situation is adequate for child rearing, but neither do they have sufficient evidence to the contrary. In either case, however, the patient/family is reported to the registry, because there are questions about parental fitness.

From then on, responsibility lies with authorities outside the hospital to pursue investigation further and make the final decision.*However, this responsibility is not to be interpreted rigidly. The reporting institution, for example, may maintain a working relationship with the child's parents in the hope of effecting some desirable change during the period of official investigation and prior to the court's making a definite decision about the patient/family's disposition. These interim services may be multiprofessional, involving a psychiatrist, psychologist, social worker, and so on.

Perhaps the most telling and chilling implication of the foregoing comments is the vulnerability of a child to extreme social and emotional deficits in the parents' capacity for nurturing and protecting and for meeting a child's normal need for dependency. The balance of a child's interdependence is normally on the side of dependence upon his or her parents. This text has described some family situations in which the practices of child rearing are within the range of socially acceptable behavior and others in which the practices fall so short of meeting minimal expectations that intervention on behalf of the patient/family is deemed socially and legally imperative.

---

* These are the procedures currently required by New York State and New York City. Procedures vary from place to place.

Socioeconomic Factors

Financial status bears a strong relation to parental attitudes and behavior in regard to medical care when the struggle for survival is so difficult and discouraging that food and housing are the primary concerns; then health is not perceived as an integral part of one's current and future life. For instance, when families have migrated to New York in the hope of higher earnings and a better education for their children, the gap between expectations and reality creates confusion and hopelessness. These distresses may push health and medical care far down on the family's list of priorities. When the hopelessness expresses itself in passivity, parents may be apathetic in regard to health care for themselves and their children. Noncompliance should not be considered pejorative when low income, unemployment, and partial, fragmented third-party payments are the real issues. Financial problems connected, for example, with the cost of medication and prostheses, of transportation, and of arranging for the care of the patient's siblings at home often account for the failure to follow a prescribed regimen, broken clinic appointments, and the like. One is forced to recognize the lack of coordination among our various social welfare and medical systems and the incomplete coverage of need in all of them.

Housing and neighborhood conditions are closely allied to financial status. When parents are fearful of the range and rate of criminal behavior where they live, some are more concerned about the specific dangers of drug pushers and rapists than about the general dangers of ill health. With all their worries, these people do not necessarily want to leave their neighborhoods. Those who have their origins in other regions of the country or the world may not want to move from the place where they have begun to feel at home. Ties of friendship and the use of their own language make it preferable to stay where they are. Receiving care at the same hospital that their neighbors attend is a bond for some families, especially if they begin to use the clinic as a community meeting place in the same way that they drop into the corner grocery store to chat. Thus the gratifications experienced by a family may outweigh the deprivations inherent in a poor and dangerous neighborhood. Even this kind of neighborhood may contain resources to promote the residents' social welfare—adults and children alike. Social workers have a prime obligation to know or find out about these resources, and they frequently urge physicians to consult with them before giving "social prescriptions" to a pediatric patient's parents. For instance, a physician recommends allowing an orthopedically handicapped child to play with children on the street. This is advice that the mother who lives in a crowded, rough-and-tumble urban community will not follow; her reality is the child's need for protection, and unlike the physician, she will not see keeping him in the house as overprotection. In this kind of situation, the social worker does not merely supply a list of neighborhood recreation centers; the real task is to enable the mother to consider and accept an alternative to watching over her son at home. An implicit problem of a too-close relationship may emerge as a highly complicating factor in what first seemed to the physician a simple matter of making a helpful recommendation.

Intervention: Participants and Resources

Although the section of this chapter that deals with the pediatric patient/family constellation implies that parents are active participants in their children's health care, it will be useful to spell out this role in further detail before turning to other participants.

The pediatric patients are by definition too immature, too inexperienced, and too dependent on their parents for nurturing and protection either to take the initiative in seeking medical care or to complete diagnostic and treatment mesures without their guidance and support. Their natural developmental incapacity to fend for themselves and their parents' obligation to meet various needs for care are, in fact, recognized—although imperfectly—in laws and statutes established for the children's protection.* Legislation also clearly asserts rights, such as giving consent for a minor child's medical care; at the same time some legislation permits access of authorized agents to court action in order to void parents' refusal to give such consent. Thus society formally acknowledges both the affirmative and the negative aspects of parental participation in children's health care.

Parents of pediatric patients are called upon to participate with medical and related personnel throughout the course of a child's illness and its treatment. They are prime sources for obtaining a family's social and medical history and prime partners with personnel in carrying through diagnostic, treatment, and rehabilitative procedures. Directly or indirectly, they are responsible for matters such as the child's keeping appointments, taking medication, staying on a diet, and wearing a brace. In practical terms, however, the young patient's participation is as essential as that of the parents, especially when active rather than passive behavior is an important element in the child's medical care.

The participation of the child, parents, and other caretakers in the patient's natural milieu takes many forms, which change with the course of the illness or disability and its treatment, with the increasing or decreasing ability of the pediatric patient to participate, and sometimes with the tolerance the child's caretakers have for bearing and coping with conditions of stress, strain, or hardship. Lest their importance be overlooked, it may be well to identify a few forms of participation that may be undertaken by a pediatric patient or his or her responsible elders or both. First is answering all the questions: How do you feel bad? Where does it hurt? When do you have a pain? What did you have for breakfast? How many times did you take your medicine yesterday? Second is demonstrating how the child does his or her prescribed exercises, puts on his or her prosthesis, tests his or her urine, or walks up and down stairs. Third is listening to the physician's explanations and instructions and asking for clarification, carrying out a recommended daily regimen, and so on.

The pediatric patient should be free to express fears, frustrations, and hopes—not only to his or her parents but to the professional people who give him or her care. In the hospital setting it is often the physician who has the least time to develop a relationship of trust with the pediatric patient, and this is a great pity. The physician is the authority who becomes associated with restrictions, discomfort, and pain. His or her other side—kindliness, gentleness, concern, interest—should have its day to balance the inevitable negatives.

As an act of participation, listening is of particular importance when connected with the patient/family's preparation for the next step, the next phase of treatment, and the like. There is a limit to how far ahead a patient of any age can be prepared. The pediatric patient's ability to gauge time, to wait, and to

* Regulations of New York State and New York City are again used illustratively.

endure apprehension is relatively slight; thus he or she is apt to go through many periods of preparation in the course of one long-term illness, as do his or her parents and siblings.

There is one more aspect of a child's participation that is relatively new and cannot be ignored: participation in decision making about his or her health care. Currently childhood seems to develop into adolescence at a younger age than was true a decade ago. Biological maturation tends to take place earlier, as does sophistication about sexual behavior; it is a question, however, whether these developments inevitably spell social maturity and the wisdom to make sound judgments. Nevertheless, as long as the young person's impulses precipitate inner turmoil and a search for his or her own brand of independence and autonomy, one must reckon with the patient's desire to have a say about his or her health care even earlier than the law permits access to this care without parental consent.

To answer the question of when a child should participate in deciding on steps and procedures requires assessment of numerous interacting factors, such as age, intelligence, biological and social maturity, whether there are medical options, and the probable outcomes of alternative procedures. Some individual circumstances need consideration too, such as how able the pediatric patient is at a given time to adapt to one more stress-producing experience or conversely, whether the patient's request for a specific intervention should be carried out because of its potential for significant benefits.

In sum, the pediatric patient's developmental needs put a premium on the people who can help to nurture, support, and protect him or her, while concurrently the patient's ability to perform in his or her own behalf is encouraged to improve his or her status of social health.

MULTIFACETED PEDIATRIC HEALTH CARE

When it comes to the institutionalized resources in the community, the pediatric patient/family needs in particular highly effective, coordinated, and collaborative relations among the systems for health care, education, income maintenance, and transportation. No doubt, in any region of the country there is a mixed bag of adequate, inadequate, and unavailable services and programs in these aspects of human need.

Each community has to make its own blueprint, but many communities will have to find answers to the same problems and issues. When social workers talk about the neighborhoods and populations from which a number of hospitals in New York City draw their pediatric patients, the pattern formed by their questions and comments goes like this: (1) What is the structural and functional relationship between the elementary and secondary school systems? What does each system do, or not do, in regard to the screening and detection of health problems and the referral of children to resources for health care? These broadly phrased questions may eventually come down to specific ones, such as the following: How many doctors and nurses are assigned to the public schools? For how many children are they responsible? Who employs them? How often and for how many hours during the school week are medical personnel in attendance? What are their functions? How effective is the mechanism for referral for health care outside the school system? Is the program oriented to the family unit? In what ways? (2) When children are home-bound or hospital-bound for long-term medical care, what provisions are there for the children's formal education? For example, are qualified teachers and a sufficient number of them assigned to work with children in the home or hospital setting? Are there supplementary means, such as closed-circuit programs on radio and television? (3) Is an appropriate educational program provided for every handicapped child? For example, are there special schools or special classes with special teachers as needed; transfers between regular and special classes when the children's situations require such flexibility; teachers in regular classrooms adequately prepared to teach children who may have occasional acute episodes of a chronic illness for which emergency measures are needed or whose condition requires extra protection or unusual privilege? (4) What do the current systems of income maintenance provide for children's health care and how adequate is that provision? What is provided, and how completely, by supplemental programs of payment or reimbursement? In regard to the pediatric patient, which social-health needs are unprovided for or provided for in fragmented and discontinuous programs? (5) How does the local system of transportation affect access of the pediatric patient to the health care and educational facilities he or she needs to use? This factor can be an important one in large urban areas where public transportation is expensive, is sparse in some areas, requires several changes, and is often too crowded for sick or handicapped children; where traveling by taxi is even more expensive and requires complicated procedures for reimbursement; and where possessing one's own car is a rarity.

A special point should be made about procedures that professionals have to follow to obtain a specific service for a specific patient. Few if any professional givers-of-service will complain about preparing patients for events and conditions in order to facilitate adjustment and reduce stress or about having similar therapeutic in-person contacts with a patient's relative. But there is frequent evidence of reactions such as grumbling, delaying tactics, and attempts to transfer responsibility when forms have to be filled out, reports have to be sent, and requests made in writing in order to make specific resources available to a patient. When these resources are related to health certain of the information must come from the authentic medical source, which is the physician. The most interesting and gratifying professional work requires some chores and routines; paper work is one of the most disliked and resented. This is frankly a plea that students in the health professions learn early to perceive the paper work as an integral part of helping and healing, an instrument for achieving specific professional goals, and a symbol of the social responsibility that is part of the practitioner's function no matter what his or her profession may be. From the standpoint of the pediatric patient, the paper work leads to rehabilitative services to admittance to a special educational program or to a residential treatment center, to third-party payments, and the like. No one can substitute for the professional whose knowledge, skill, and opinion have firsthand, authoritative significance. It is not too much to hope, however, that forms be intelligible, as brief and simple as possible, and relevant to their purpose.

The Adolescent Patient: Some Common Characteristics and Themes
The adolescent patient, aged 13 through 17, is in a far more complex and unstable phase of biopsychosocial development than is the pediatric patient. In our society adolescence is in itself crisis producing, and the impact may be

exacerbated by or may exacerbate a situation of physical illness or disability or of behavioral deviance. The unmarried pregnant teen-aged girl, who will be discussed later, illustrates such deviance.

Perhaps the major task of adolescents is to find themselves—to discover who they are and what their "thing" is and to forge the freedom to pursue it. Whether one uses these phrases or more technical terms such as ego identity and emancipation, adolescents' behavior is rather obviously dual in nature— they form tight ties with their peers, demonstrating the essence of conformity in respect to conduct, language, morality, and physical appearance, for example, while at the same time they struggle to loosen and eventually restructure their relations with figures of authority, beginning naturally enough with their parents.

The adolescent's psychosocial conflicts, problems, and tasks are made all the more difficult and bewildering by genital maturation and its accompanying physiological changes which in themselves demand critical adaptations to a changing self-image and to new desires and impulses. It becomes necessary to understand how these characteristics of adolescents are manifested in situations of illness, deficiency, or disability. The data that describe adolescents indicate dramatically the significance of maturational phases and developmental tasks in understanding the interrelatedness of the course of a disease, the course of medical care, and the psychosocial experiences of the human beings involved in the adolescent's life-and-illness-situation. But however accurately the generalities about adolescents may be stated, one needs to guard against stereotyping them as human beings. They mature at different rates, differ in native endowment and sociocultural background, and are exposed to vastly different opportunities and deprivations.

The *legal and social status* of adolescents in the United States varies from state to state. The professional practitioner needs to be informed about significant differences among states and to be kept fully up to date about changes from year to year in the state in which he or she practices and in which his or her adolescent patients reside. As the developmental period that marks the transition from childhood to adulthood, adolescence always seems to be in flux, whether it is seen from the perspective of the individual youth or of the community in which he or she lives.

For example, in New York State in 1970 an adolescent was defined legally as a youth between 13 and 21 years of age. He or she would have fallen into either of two categories: adolescent minor or emancipated minor. If an adolescent minor, he or she might have been either a protected minor—that is, living with parents or parental surrogates who were responsible for him or her—or an unprotected minor—that is, not living with responsible adults, although perhaps at times in touch with his or her parents, and without a legally recognized means of support. If an emancipated minor, he or she would have been self-maintaining, either because he or she or a spouse was of legal age to work and was self-supporting or because he or she or a spouse had met eligibility requirements for obtaining public assistance in his or her own name.

In the context of medical care, the significance of the adolescent's legal status in New York State in 1970 lay in whether he or she had the right to seek and obtain medical care without parental consent. An adolescent minor, whether protected or unprotected, had to have a parent's consent; but consent given in broad or general terms usually did not cover measures such as surgery, hospitalization, contraceptive advice, or abortion. The requirement for parental consent to each of these specific measures—especially those that concerned the adolescent's sexual interests and activity—tended to create grave social, legal, and ethical dilemmas for the patient, physician, and other hospital personnel as well. Moreover payment for the adolescent minor's medical care had to be through his or her parents' resources—earnings, insurance, or Medicaid. In contrast, the emancipated minor could receive medical care in his or her own right, and payment could be made through his or her own resources, which might be the same as any adult's.

Concurrently, many physicians practicing in the clinics of hospitals and in their private offices were keenly aware of the confrontation between such tortuous and convoluted sociomedical policies and laws on the one hand and the perception that their adolescent patients had of themselves and of persons in authority on the other. Members of the New York Chapter of the Society of Adolescent Medicine were deeply involved in efforts to obtain legislative change "to permit minors in serious health risk to receive restitutive and/or preventive services in the absence of parental consent when the rendering of such treatment stands in jeopardy because of this prerequisite."[6] The state's public health law was amended in 1972 and 1973 to allow "emancipated minors" (those 16 or younger who were married, were parents, or were not supported by parents or guardians) to obtain medical care without parental consent.

The adolescent patient/family constellation and relationships are inextricably bound to the patient's legal rights to medical care and financial benefits. The other side of the coin is equally important, namely, the desires and rights of the adolescent patient's parents to be informed about their child's health problems and health care.

Since the adolescent's perception of self and his or her striving to become a self apart from his or her parents may not coincide with his or her official status, there are always the makings of a conflict and struggle which may influence the adolescent's search for and use of medical care and affect its consequences. Whether the young person is technically an adolescent minor or an emancipated minor, his or her family relationships tend to be intricate, ambivalent, and unstable. The emancipated minor may fancy himself or herself far freer of parental ties and of the need for parental psychological support and protection than he or she really is. In the course of the adolescent's ambivalent struggle to get out from under figures of authority, the young patient is prone to make access to his or her parents difficult for physicians, social workers, and other personnel. The adolescent's feeling of privacy about his or her body, behavior, feelings, and thoughts is strong. If the adolescent's relationship with his or her parents has been consistently and fundamentally poor, the desire to conceal his or her medical condition is all the more understandable. Often there exists a mutual caring and affection; but differences in beliefs and values are surfacing, and the parents and the adolescent patient feel a diminution of confidence and trust in one another. For example, the parents' culture may turn to nonmedical sources, such as spiritualism, for treatment of illness, or the parents' religion may forbid the use of certain medical and surgical procedures. If the patient is seeking something that his or her parents are known to disapprove of, the adolescent may build quite an obstacle course to his or her parents, even when it is clear that their consent to medical care is needed. In general, the values of parents and adolescent patients are most likely to run counter to each other in regard to sexual behavior and the use of drugs.

The adolescent's loss of confidence and trust in his or her parents and other adults occurs at that very time in life when he or she feels least self-assured—in a word, at a time when he or she needs to be able to trust others. In consequence, he or she tends to test out repeatedly the honesty and trustworthiness of people in authority, such as physicians, nurses, teachers, and social workers, before he or she can be open and honest with them. For their part, while the adolescent strives more and more toward identity as a young adult, his or her parents may become increasingly worried about the youth's behavior and less and less able to communicate with him or her. All these contradictions create large and small crises for the adolescent patient during this turbulent period of life.

Reciprocal to the adolescent's struggles is the demand upon his or her parents to change the nature of their relationship to the adolescent. They have to learn new ways of behaving and of discharging their parental responsibilities. There is no single point of view among professionals about the axis of parent-adolescent relationships. However, many who are committed to the value and significance of the family unit—and a large number of social workers fall into this group—believe firmly that it is both possible and necessary to understand and work with the adolescent and his or her parents with the objective of preserving the family unit while developing a new balance of interdependence among family members.

During the transitional period of adolescence when all family members experience the impact of the adolescent's fluctuations in mood, feeling, and behavior, hospital personnel have to find their ways to respond constructively and helpfully to both the adolescent patient and his or her parents. Social workers who regularly walk this tightrope have a fundamental rule that complete honesty and openness on the part of hospital personnel are essential to working with adolescent patients. As one social worker said, "Adolescents will not forgive you for lying or concealing the truth." One of the most troublesome problems encountered by givers-of-service in the hospital centers on the adolescent's ideas about what his or her parents should be told. While the professional giver-of-service acts on the belief that the adolescent patient still has some need for his or her parents, with rare exceptions, the practitioner has a complementary belief that parents have a part to play in their child's health care, again with rare exceptions, and therefore a right to know what is or may be endangering to the adolescent patient and to others in his or her milieu.

Based on these beliefs, social workers may fulfill their obligations to adolescent patients and their parents by making an open, deliberated agreement with an individual patient in this general vein: the social workers will not promise to conceal anything from the adolescents' parents but do promise to discuss with each patient in advance what they (the social workers) believe they have to tell his or her parents and why. The social workers make clear from the beginning that the information to be shared with the patient's parents will pertain to situations injurious to the patient or to others. The social workers also make it clear that sharing such information is free of punitive intent. Even if the adolescent dislikes some aspects of this mode of professional behavior, the social worker's frankness about what he or she will and will not do is a potentially good base for an effective working relationship between him or her and the adolescent.

Important also is the timing of contacts between hospital personnel and adolescent patients. Some social workers think it best for the adolescent patients to make their contacts first—with the physician and social worker in particular—before their parents have their initial interviews. It is thought that being first helps to establish the adolescent as the patient—the person of primary concern. Other social workers favor holding first interviews with a patient and parents together, so that their way of working is demonstrated for all to see at the same time. It is understood that timing cannot always be planned—the patient's medical condition or other uncontrollable factors may prevent it.

Although much of the adolescent's behavior is correctly attributed to a critical struggle with authority, conditions in society such as poverty, unemployment, inadequate educational and vocational programs, and uncontrolled access to drugs may in some instances have even more significance or serve to exaggerate and greatly heighten the usual signals of adolescent crises.

Since the use and abuse of drugs continues to be a major concern in respect to adolescents (and is becoming a more and more frightening concern in respect to young school-aged children), students and practitioners in programs for health care will want to know much more than this text is meant to convey about the problems and their treatment. Some salient observations made about adolescent patients in medical clinics (not in specialty units for treatment of drug problems) are more in keeping with the purpose of this book. First, there are many patterns of using drugs, different reasons for using drugs and different consequences. There seems always to be a range of drugs used, and the prevalence of one over others varies over time. The social consequences vary from getting into trouble with the law to dropping out of school to leaving home and living literally on the streets. Some users suffer none of these bad effects; many others contract infectious hepatitis. One has to consider also whether a young person's use of drugs is addictive, moderate and nonaddictive, or as yet merely experimental. Motivations vary from going along with one's peers to trying to ward off or relieve symptoms of mental illness. Where and with whom the use of drugs takes place and the climate in the family unit and in the immediate neighborhood in regard to drugs are social factors that have to be assessed.

Identification and evaluation of these components aid in understanding the meaning of a drug problem to an adolescent and aid in planning for its treatment. Within the hospital setting these are usually collaborative decisions which at best are arrived at through the active participation of the adolescent patient, the patient's parents, and a number of professionals. A medical physician, psychiatrist, and social worker are most often involved in such decisions, although not all of them necessarily become involved in the process and parents may become crucial partners in helping the adolescent.[7]

The adolescent patient's reactions to illness and medical care need to be understood and measured against conditions and concerns that characterize this phase of life. The adolescent has a deep concern for his or her body and whether it is developing normally; there is an intense need to keep his or her body private and unexposed to the eyes of others. The adolescent has a tendency to worry over physical symptoms that physicians attribute to anxiety, stress-producing experiences such as biological development, unfamiliar and uncontrollable feelings and impulses, and strained family relationships. The adolescent patient seldom connects his or her symptoms or complaints with social or emotional aspects of life unless helped to do so by physicians or other givers-of-service.

The adolescents who see themselves as centers of concern in hospital clinic settings act like adolescents, which usually poses some problems. The adolescent is a "here and now" person, crisis oriented, wanting and expecting to be seen "then and there" whenever he or she appears at the clinic. Custom and habit in the family or ethnic group may reinforce these attitudes and expectations, but they are more adolescent behaviors in any case. The adolescent patient's disregard of clinic schedules or of appointments may make sustained, consistent medical treatment difficult until the patient learns the advantages of the rules and regulations. The adolescent patients are inclined to be jealous of their scheduled time with hospital personnel and openly resent interruptions. They are equally sensitive to any impatience staff members may feel about the patients' capricious use of their professional time. This awareness often helps the patients realize that conformity to clinic regulations brings worthwhile benefits. However, because adolescent patients do find themselves in crisis situations, real or imagined, there has to be a way of accommodating special, unpredicted needs for help.

When adolescent patients carry the struggle with authority over to people in the medical setting, they may then disregard medical recommendations—behavior that is of course illogical in light of their concern and anxiety about themselves. Sometimes, though, the adolescent's failure to carry out instructions regarding exercise, eating, medication, and the like is less an expression of rebellion than of the need to conform to the ways of his or her peers who are not restricted or frustrated by medical recommendations.

Also to be understood are the possible impacts resulting from the organizational structure of hospitals. At some point in his or her life, the pediatric patient becomes an adolescent patient. He or she may be transferred to a clinic for adolescents, but it often happens that the transfer is directly to a clinic for adults. If the patient has been receiving medical care from a pediatrician in private practice, there is a point at which he or she is referred to a physician, the majority of whose patients are adults. Such transfers have some potentially stress-producing consequences. The recent development of a specialty in adolescent medicine may reduce some problematic conditions. For instance, adolescents may have chronic diseases that place them in the category of special risk. Thus when adolescent patients are in a waiting room with older patients with the same disease, when they observe the outward signs of their illness and disabilities and hear their elders exchange experiences, the adolescents usually learn much more about their own conditions and their possible consequences than they knew before. This new information, some of which may be distorted or misunderstood, suddenly confronts the younger patients for the first time with the possibility of a shortened life span, of loss of sensory functioning, of limited vocational choices, and of other deprivations.

These disclosures have grave significance if they come at a time when the adolescent is beginning to think about the future: More schooling? Training? For what carreer? Marriage? Children? Greater understanding of his or her own condition, the natural history of the disease he or she has, and the course of treatment it requires may force the patient and perhaps his or her parents as well into making some hard choices. In any case, this point of change may occur when the adolescent needs as much support and sound counseling as family, hospital personnel, and significant others can offer.

The adolescent reveals not only problems and problematic behavior; normally the adolescent also possesses a growing ability to cope. The adolescent patient ordinarily responds with pride and manifests a sense of responsibility when emphasis is placed on his or her participation in diagnostic and treatment procedures. The patient needs to acquire a working understanding of his or her condition, to learn to keep it under control, and to avoid what might send it out of control. Such participation requires self-discipline, self-denial, the ability to be aware of reactions and symptoms, and when necessary the development of skills needed to self-administer prescribed tests and medication. This account of responsible behavior is not incongruous with a propensity for acts of noncompliance and rebellion. The adolescent is capable of extremes, many fluctuations from day to day, many conflicting ideas and feelings; there may be turbulence and turmoil today, relative calm and quiet tomorrow.

In assessing the adolescent's response to medical recommendations, living arrangements may be an important factor. If the patient is with his or her family, the amount of living space, the sleeping arrangements, bathroom and cooking facilities, supplies, and equipment may be adequate and make compliance relatively easy, or they may be inadequate and stand in the way of following medical advice. There is the special plight of the unprotected adolescent minor who is living as a runaway or is in a commune and has practically no opportunity to follow a medically prescribed regimen. The unprotected minor adolescents, unlike the emancipated adolescents, have no means of legal support and therefore are at extremely high risk, socially and medically.

Impacts of the adolescent patient on hospital personnel, even on those whose natural response is understanding and helpful, at times have a negative effect on staff members and therefore on the patient's care. The patient's appearance, behavior, language, and values may conflict with those of personnel to a degree that impedes the establishment and maintenance of a sound working relationship. Some professional and nonprofessional staff members can tolerate sharp differences between the adolescent's way of life and their own and build a good relationship with them. Those who cannot tolerate the differences may become negatively reactive rather than positively responsive. For instance, a member of the staff may make audible, provocative remarks about an unusual or bizarre characteristic of the patient that the staff member frowns upon, may show intolerance for a young patient's low threshold for pain, and may take a retaliatory stance against an adolescent's pugnacious behavior or obscene language.

When components of the adolescent's beliefs and behavior coincide with those of a staff member, the latter's understanding of the patient may be sufficiently detached to facilitate the development of an effective relationship. But if there is sympathy without the degree of detachment that permits seeing the patient as he or she is, the resulting interactions may impair both the staff member's competence to help and the patient's capacity for being helped.

Givers-of-service who relate effectively to the adolescent patient are empathic and realistically aware that the patient needs limits and controls as much as he or she needs opportunities to make his or her own decisions. Adolescents do attempt to manipulate, maneuver, and provoke their elders. They also respect and feel the benefits of an older, more experienced person's supportive strength.

The pregnant teen-aged girl, 16 years old or younger, is rarely married in our society, and this circumstance places her in a social situation that has special risks. "As Erikson, Bowlby, and other clinical investigators have frequently pointed out, when a situational or accidental crisis—a stressful external event—is superimposed on a normal phase-of-development crisis, the combined impact of these simultaneous events can often lead to a crisis of major proportions."[8] The developmental crisis of adolescence is the normal one for girls of this age; to this crisis is added the crisis of pregnancy which socially and legally is not considered normal for these young patients, and in consequence they have to cope also with a critical psychosocial situation. An additional stress-producing condition which is not always sufficiently emphasized is that the young pregnant girl and the fetus are at special physical risk because of the girl's incomplete biological development. It is more accurate, then, to say that she is in a critical biopsychosocial situation.

The need of these young girls for health care services that are oriented toward their particular problems is self-evident. The number of young pregnant girls is increasing each year, and the problem is nationwide. Of the approximately 1 million pregnant young girls in the United States in 1976, perhaps two-thirds carried to term. There were spontaneous miscarriages and abortions, self-induced abortions, and medically induced abortions.

Concurrently with the large increase in the number of pregnant girls, the total birthrate is declining in this country. The reasons have to be sought in changes taking place that particularly affect women 17 years of age and older. In fact, the total picture of pregnancies, births, and abortions seems skewed and distorted when compared to the data of a decade or two ago.

To understand the changes that have taken place and anticipate those that will take place in the near future, students and practitioners in the health care field will be challenged to inquire into a constellation of interacting factors, for example, new medical information and techniques, overt and tacit social and medical policies, legislation at several levels of government, and the fiscal status and policies of individual institutions and systems for health care and related services and of federal, state, and local governments. Changes of a different order are part of the picture, too, such as changes in the age at which young people are attaining biological maturity and in values attached to single-parent families, marriage, and divorce.

The potential consequences of pregnancy in the unmarried teen-aged girl who receives hospital-based health care cover a wide range of biological, psychological, and social effects. Regardless of the legal status of the girl, professional givers-of-service—and in particular social workers—encourage the patient to tell her parents, or at least her mother, about the pregnancy. It takes a lot of helping, because most of these young people feel a mixture of considerable fear, shame, and rebellion. There is agreement among some professionals that despite the problematic aspects of confrontation between daughters and parents or parent surrogates, there are certain gains: valuable medical and family history is made available to clinic personnel, mainly from the girl's mother, and contact is established by personnel with an adult whose support is essential to the pregnant teen-ager. After all, many of these girls live at home and will continue to do so for some time. Many others who live apart are in touch with family members or feel a deep need to make contact again.

The financial situation of the pregnant girl and her parents is a frequent concern. A number of families are financially self-maintaining but often at a low level; the extra expense of the pregnant daughter's diet, clothing, transportation to and from clinic, and other special needs may strain both income and personal relations, especially if someone else in the family has to do without in order to provide for the patient. In some instances in New York City financial assistance from the municipal Department of Social Services will be available later for the baby, providing specified eligibility requirements have been met. Insofar as these requirements involve the putative father's responsibility for support of the baby, many of the young mothers face a difficult situation. Some wish to protect the boy, and some wish to ward off his and his family's angry reactions; these girls are apt to be hoping for an ongoing relation with the baby's father even when the hope has little base in reality. On the other hand, refusing to involve the putative father in order to become eligible for assistance could result in worsening relations with her own family if the financial burden of caring for her and her baby devolves upon her relatives or if the baby "has no name." Practitioners and students in the health care field have to be familiar with relevant changes in policy and procedure. For example, there is currently intensive search for putative fathers who should contribute financially to the rearing of their out-of-wedlock children. The issue is in part moral but is also largely created by the fiscal status of our states and municipalities and by pressures from the federal level of government which is similarly concerned with the social responsibility of individuals, the taxpayers' burdens, and the costs of providing for the social welfare.

Then there is the central issue of the girl's sexual behavior and resulting pregnancy which, contrary to some stereotyped notions, are considered by most family members to be deviations from accepted social standards. In consequence, significant emotional reactions are aroused in the patient, her parents, and other members of the family group which appreciably aggravate the stress-producing demands for adaptation made by even the usual extravagances of adolescence. Furthermore, attitudes toward pregnancy out of wedlock are more intense in some subcultures than in others, the emotional climate may reach a high pitch of tension, and the family drama may end in disaster. Social workers make special note, for example, of the values placed on virginity by families of Latin American and Oriental descent. Some girls from these families can never bring themselves to tell their parents about their pregnancy no matter how much support and encouragement physicians and social workers try to give them. In one such instance, when it was impossible for the patient to obtain an abortion without parental consent, she committed suicide. Another similar case ended more benignly because the physician and social worker succeeded in obtaining a court order for an abortion when parental consent was not obtainable.

Within the hospital itself arrangements are usually made that recognize the girl's special situation. The basic intent is to offer gynecological-obstetrical services separately to pregnant women and to unmarried teen-aged pregnant girls. For instance, the same clinic space and staff are used for both groups of patients, but the clinic hours for each group are different. This is the arrangement, for example, in a hospital that has established a comprehensive care clinic for adolescents 14 years and older; unmarried pregnant patients in the clinic are referred to the regular gynecological-obstetrical service but are seen at a time reserved for them. In another hospital there is a specialized unit for unmarried girls 16 years and younger and for married teen-agers with serious psychosocial problems.

Social workers in a specialized unit have an unusual opportunity to learn about and learn to help these girls. A few valuable observations from this experience follow. Some of these girls have access to special educational programs in the public schools directed toward their physical and psychosocial needs. Others attend regular classes for a while and then drop out, without having had any special instruction. Thus for quite a number of pregnant girls hospitals programs provide the most fruitful opportunity they will have to gain understanding of their bodily changes and of the development of the fetus and the onset and course of labor, and to gain some preparation for the practical tasks of motherhood. These opportunities are cut rather short because the young patient tends to register for care when she is already four or five months pregnant.

A specialized unit that sees its patients' problems in the round needs not only a multiprofessional staff but a stable staff offering continuity of direct services. If one considers educational services before and after delivery and perinatal medical services, which will always include contraceptive advice and services, the basic staff will consist of physicians, public health nurses, and social workers; the availability of psychologists and psychiatrists will, it is hoped, be assured. Continuity with the same staff members has particular significance for the young patients under consideration because of disapproving attitudes and emotions frequently expressed in our society toward pregnancy out of wedlock and because of the teen-agers' own fears and fantasies. Social workers and public health nurses are apt to remain constant figures during a patient's period of care. Residents, however, rotate on and off the service; in addition, if there is a small number of attending physicians and resident house staff on the service, it is all but impossible for a patient to have the same physician at each clinic visit.

Patients benefit from a minimum of scheduled appointments at the hospital (the minimum for optimum care, to be precise) so that they can attend school as regularly as possible. Also, offering programs of health education to groups of pregnant teen-agers works well in many instances; it provides a good climate for learning from an experienced professional and for the patients to help and support one another. Social workers and public health nurses cover some of the same areas of health and social need, but with a well-developed collaborative relationship the similarities can reinforce the patients' learning rather than create competitiveness among staff or boredom among patients. Effective service to groups of pregnant teen-agers is not a substitute for one-to-one relationships with professionals. Customarily social workers have contact with each individual patient concurrently with groups, and public health nurses provide a one-to-one relationship when it seems desirable.

There seems to be a gradually increasing concern among professionals about putative fathers, who have their own dilemmas and problems. Hospital-based personnel do not always seek out these boys, and the boys do not ordinarily become involved in the patients' care. When a putative father does accompany the patient on a clinic visit, as happens occasionally, his continued participation is encouraged.

The significance of the family to this group of patients needs special emphasis. Large numbers of girls live at home, will continue to after their babies are born, and are unprepared to support themselves. Many of the girls who do not live at home are in touch with their families; others who have a strong desire to resume contact need help to master the fear or shame that stands in the way. For a number of pregnant teen-agers, family participation has started before the girl registers at clinic; it has been observed by some social workers that more of these young patients come to clinic with their mothers than in years past. In some of these families the girl's father is not an active figure, but when he is he is encouraged to discuss his daughter's situation and to help in planning for her care and the baby's.

The mothers who meet in a group with a social worker as a leader have as a rule at least two objectives: (1) to acquire useful information from the social worker which will help not only the patient but other members of the family and the family unit as well and (2) to help one another by discussing their feelings about and behavior toward their daughters, their attitudes toward pregnancy out of wedlock, the mixture of emotions they feel about the coming babies and the putative fathers, and the numerous practical problems that face them now as well as those they anticipate will occur in the near future.

All professional efforts of this kind which help to make the family group a firmer base of support are of value to each family member in his or her own right. For the young patient, heightened support from her close relatives, in particular from her parents, will be one of the most important elements in her life during the crucial period of her pregnancy. Apart from the medical and legal requirements for parental involvement in the teen-ager's situation, the patient's need for personal security, for help in planning for herself and the coming child, and for coping with a not-always friendly world is in principle best met with the help of her parents. It is not always easy for parents to give their daughters the support they need, and they do not always respond positively to the professionals' efforts to elicit supporting attitudes and behavior. Common initial reactions of mothers and fathers are anger and disappointment; some parents are enraged. Social workers have observed that these first reactions tend to lessen in intensity for a while. During such a period social workers have noted that parents become more accepting of, or resigned to, their daughter's situation but seldom develop real sympathy. Closer to the time of the delivery some parents may show some empathic reactions. On the whole, the father's anger, hostility, and disappointment are thought to be more persistent than the mother's. It must be remembered, however, that most of this information comes from the girls and their mothers. A variant of the general pattern of emotions and family reactions seems to fit into the picture of the father's considerable anger. It was noted that in some families the pregnant teen-ager and her mother "bind together to keep the father ignorant of what is happening." For example, the mother may sign consent for an abortion but tells the girl's father a fabricated story. Another variant is the behavior of a mother who rejects the idea of abortion for her daughter and then forces the girl's marriage to the putative father.

When the mothers talk individually with social workers, "they almost never [have] any insight into their 'failure' as mothers or into any ways in which they may have been contributory [to their daughter's pregnancy]." For the most part, the mothers put responsibility on external circumstances; these women are "in fact overwhelmed by their household chores and care of the children" and sometimes by working outside the home as well. One social worker observed that the mother had "as a rule, little communication with the patient except on current matters such as money or sibling relationships in the family. Matters of survival are uppermost; there is not so much 'conversation' between mother and her pregnant daughter as 'hostile exchange.'" The social workers' general impression is that whatever negative relationship existed previously between mother and daughter is aggravated by the pregnancy of the unmarried teenager.

When the teen-aged mother returns home with her baby, her own mother is likely to revert to her original open hostility. No doubt the renewed expression of negative feelings is due in part to the demands made by the new realities: both the daughter and grandchild are in the home, requiring a place to sleep, bathing facilities for the infant, the usual supplies and clothing for its care and protection, and adequate diet for the teen-aged mother and her child. These essentials make large demands on low and marginal incomes and increase the discomfort and inconvenience of a home with too little space and a lack of equipment. In some families there will be relief from financial strain if the newborn infant is eligible for public assistance as a dependent child.

The return home of young mother and child can be seen in two contexts over and beyond that of financial status. One is the constellation of social conditions that in great measure influence the planning for the care of the child. The other is the tension created by the gap between the usual developmental and social tasks of an adolescent girl and the additional demands made by her premature motherhood.

First are conditions that lead a large number of teen-aged mothers to keep their babies: When these mothers are black or Puerto Rican, both adoptive opportunities and resources for foster home placement are exceedingly scarce. Thus for many of the young mothers who may prefer to have their babies adopted there is no real choice. Nevertheless, social workers initiate consideration of adoption or foster home placement of the baby when the psychosocial hazards of the teen-ager's total situation seem to warrant it. Some young mothers choose to keep their babies to gratify their own emotional needs. Some make the choice in the hope that with the baby they can maneuver an escape from home to join the putative father; failing that route to gratification, they hope at least that the baby will help them maintain contact with the putative father. In still other instances, the young mother keeps her baby because her family members do not sanction surrendering the child or evading responsibility for its care.

The varied motivations the teen-aged mother may have for keeping her infant seem logically connected with issues concerning her human relationships. For example, these girls frequently have tenuous relationships with the men in their lives, particularly with their fathers and with the putative fathers of their babies. Despite the weakness of their relationships, however, many of these young mothers have not been promiscuous; they have often dated the same boy for a year or longer. As one social worker said, the girls seem to have a strong need "to be with someone they care for and each one holds on to the boy regardless of the consequences. It is not certain how much the boys care for their girlfriends...." It is worth noting that the steadiness of their relationship seems not to be a mitigating factor in the eyes of the girl's parents.

The foregoing observations suggest that a broadly based inquiry into what happens in the unmarried teen-aged mother's family of origin and in her own one-parent nuclear family would yield data of significance for improving the kind and delivery of services needed. Some of the questions that should be answered are the following: What does the future hold for these people? How adequate is the provision of services they need? How effective are the services they obtain? What is, and what should be, the continuum of perinatal medical and social services in cases like these? If current laws governing abortions and the requirement for parental consent continue in effect or do not continue, what changes will occur in the human picture described here?[9] Many studies have been made that are relevant to these questions but do not necessarily answer them satisfactorily for the specific patient population of a specific medical setting. Mores, values, socioeconomic factors, community resources, and individual and family strengths and deficits are among the many variables that will influence the answers obtained.[10]

At the specific level of everyday living and functioning during the adolescent's pregnancy and early postpartum period, the following further observations apply. As young people of school age, their health care should be planned to interfere as little as possible with their schooling. Many of these girls wish to complete high school, which is normally a most acceptable and highly valued goal. But with pregnancy and eventually a baby to be considered, it can no longer be taken for granted that the adolescent girl will complete either grade school or high school. The baby's need for care precipitates changes in priorities and thus threatens the usual functions of family members. The accession of the baby to the family becomes a reality to be reckoned with; the reality has a double impact when the baby is neither wanted by the family members nor born in wedlock.[11] Some family situations force the young mother into choosing between going to work or continuing at school; some of the situations aggravate tensions between the young mother and her mother because the older woman wants to keep her own job rather than care for the baby while the teen-aged mother goes to school. Occasionally a girl solves this problem by completing high school at night. Day-care centers are in short supply, and there is also the controversial issue of whether substitute care for infants should be sanctioned.[12]

The pressures on the teen-aged mother to care for her infant are commonly in conflict with her internal pressure to pursue freedom. This is an expected desire for a teen-ager, but it is incompatible with the responsibility for mothering and nurturing another human being. In addition, each of these girls has been sexually active and used to going out with their boyfriends. This mode of life, which is in harmony with certain adolescent longings, conflicts strongly with the life that confronts many young unmarried mothers who take home their babies. Observations like these made by hospital-based social workers are echoed by their colleagues in the field of child welfare: "Many of these young people need help in finding and holding jobs, in getting back to school or into vocational training, in finding decent housing...."[13] "Practical assistance is needed in learning about child care...."[14]

On the whole, the foregoing description of the consequences of the teen-aged mother's return home with her baby—a description based on a selected patient group in selected hospitals—is implicitly substantiated for the national scene in the following statement: "It should be possible for [the unmarried mother] to have a choice of remaining with her own family, living in an apartment, in a foster family home, wage, or companion home, maternity residence, or in a group or group care facility."[15] Obviously, these options are available to very few unmarried mothers. There are extremely scarce social provisions for this patient group, whether the girl's decision is to keep or to surrender her baby.

Since drug use and abuse are pervasive problems among teen-agers, and the abuse of alcohol is an ever-increasing problem in this age group, it is important to establish whether the pregnant girl or the putative father or both have been or are taking drugs. They may be candidates for treatment, and everyone involved may have to be prepared for the shocking symptoms of withdrawal suffered by the newborn baby of an addicted mother. In New York State or New York City such a baby is officially considered maltreated and the procedures described previously in regard to abused and maltreated children are mandatory.*

It should not be surprising that there are members of hospital staffs, both professionals and nonprofessionals who feel hostile toward unmarried pregnant girls. There are among these staff members some who express their feelings in words and rather punitive behavior. It takes people, even sophisticated and professional adults, time and experience to develop compassionate attitudes toward gross violations of their codes of conduct. In any hospital or other institution offering human services there will be personnel struggling with the need to acknowledge and deal helpfully with the strange and different beliefs and behaviors of others. To accept—not approve, but merely accept—the existence of active sexual behavior on the part of teen-agers is difficult enough; to be empathic with the unmarried pregnant girl will be even more difficult for the adult who finds the adolescents' sex life abhorrent and alien. The fact that most contemporary adults have been brought up on a double standard does not ease their dilemma.

These crosscurrents are evident also when a girl asks for contraceptive devices. When the law requires parental consent, some physicians adhere to it because it reinforces their moral convictions that the girls should not be sexually active. Some physicians disregard the law because they hope at least to protect the girl from becoming pregnant, knowing they cannot dissuade her from intercourse.

It is to be recognized that the patients sense negative attitudes and correctly interpret unsympathetic behavior, all the more because they expect exactly this kind of reaction from most adults or, when they are from minority groups, are watchful for signs that people do not want to help them.

The patients react variously—sometimes with open anger, and sometimes with a retreat into passivity, which is a safe mask for the short run but not a desirable mechanism in the long run. These patients are sensitive to everyone in the hospital with whom they have contact, but they are particularly reactive to what they believe to be a physician's attitudes.

It is essential to understanding and helping these girls that health care personnel realize the strong element of fear and the great lack of knowledge and experience that characterize this patient population. Some of the patients do show their fears and doubts quite openly, but a larger number come to the hospital clinic armed with certain defensive-offensive behavior in reaction to their anxiety-producing situations—behavior that is instantly released against persons whom they perceive as punishing.

* Some procedures laid down by state laws are incompatible with recent federal legislation on the same problem. As of June 1977, the incompatibilities had not been resolved.

The framework within which pediatric and adolescent patients were described here does not differ materially for the two phases of the life cycle. In each instance one considers how the patients perceive themselves in relation to illness, how families and family members are affected by the patients' illnesses, how patients in each phase of life participate in their own care, and how givers of direct services are apt to react or respond to pediatric and adolescent patients receiving hospital-based health care. Over and beyond these immediate components in life-and-illness situations are the influences wielded by the institutions and systems that provide and deliver health care and related services.

What do differ enormously are the specific events, conditions, reactions, and responses of each of the people involved in these life-and-illness situations. The nature of these specific factors is shaped in part by the characteristics of the patient's disease or disability; the patient's biological and social development; the tasks, problems, and capacity to cope that normally mark the patient's place in the life cycle; and the opportunities and resources available for learning to adapt to and master the obstacles created by illness, developmental anomaly, dysfunction, or disability.

REFERENCES

1. For the confirming point of view of a pediatric nurse-clinician, see Truda R. Aufhauser and Diane Lesh, "Parents Need T.L.C., Too," *Hospitals*, vol. 47, no. 8 (April 1973), pp 88–91.
2. Robert Mulford, "Protective Services for Children," in *Encyclopedia of Social Work*, 16th ed. (New York, National Association of Social Workers, 1971), p.1007.
3. Ibid., p. 1010.
4. Philip Hayda, "Child Welfare: Child Abuse," in *Encyclopedia of Social Work*, *17th ed.* Washington, D.C.: National Association of Social Workers, 1977), pp. 125–129.
5. David G. Gil, *Violence Against Children: Physical Child Abuse in The United States* (Cambridge: Harvard University Press, 1970), p. 6.
6. "The Law and Health Care of the Adolescent in New York: Recommendations for Legislative Change," mimeographed, New York Chapter of the Society for Adolescent Medicine, undated (circa 1969).
7. Phyllis Caroff, Florence Lieberman, and Mary Gottesfeld, "The Drug Problem: Treating Preaddictive Adolescents," *Social Casework*, vol. 51, no. 9 (November 1970), pp. 527–532.
8. Howard J. Parad, ed., *Crisis Intervention: Selected Readings* (New York City: Family Service Association of America, 1965), p. 74.
9. Rose Bernstein, "Are We Still Stereotyping the Unmarried Mother?" in ibid., p. 100.
10. Elizabeth Navarre, "Illegitimacy," in *Encyclopedia of Social Work*, 16th ed., op. cit., p. 646.
11. Reuben Hill, "Generic Features of Families under Stress," in Parad, op. cit., p. 32.
12. Therese W. Lansburgh, "Child Welfare: Day Care of Children," in *Encyclopedia of Social Work*, 16th ed., op cit., p. 114.
13. *Louise Wise Services Annual Report, 1970–1971* (New York).
14. Brigadier Dorothy Purser and Joan L. Lindsay, "Clinic Serves Unwed Parents," *Hospitals*, vol. 48, no. 4 (February 1974), p. 58.
15. Child Welfare League of America, *Standards for Services for Unmarried Parents*, rev. ed., 1971 (New York).

Chapter 8
Selected
Patient Groups:

Young Adult and Elderly Patients

This chapter completes the descriptions of patients in phases of the life cycle. Chapters 3 and 4 on adult patients fill the gap between the young adults and the elderly.

A SPECIAL GROUP OF YOUNG ADULT PATIENTS

Young adulthood, as a developmental phase of the life cycle, is a recent concept. It designates the brief span between the end of adolescence at 18 years of age and the beginning of adulthood at the age of 21. There are both legal and social reasons for recognizing a category of young adults. These patients are at special risk when disease, bodily dysfunctioning, or disability seriously impairs achievement of the goals normally pursued in young adulthood.

Such impairment and some of its consequences were manifested in a group of paraplegic and quadruplegic men, most of whom at the time they entered the military hospital were 20 years of age or slightly younger. They were all victims of spinal cord injuries incurred in active military duty but were at various stages of treatment and rehabilitation. The discussion of these young men focuses on their reactions to their disabilities and to the hospital milieu, on the significance of the social work services to individuals and small groups, and on some of the significant influences of these young men's predicaments on their givers-of-service.

Not recorded here but deserving study are the effects of severe disability on the patients' close relatives and significant others and the influence of socioenvironmental factors on restorative and rehabilitative processes. However, the extraordinary nature of these patients' physical disabilities sharpens and dramatizes the meaning to a group of young adult men of severe, irreversible handicaps and severely restricted social functioning. Inquiries into the experiences of young adult patients of both sexes with less severe but still significant impairments should throw additional light on the impacts of such experiences and lead to increasingly effective ways of enabling patients to cope with problems of daily living.

Under ordinary circumstances these young adults would have entered the labor market or would be in educational or vocational training programs with the expectation of being financially self-maintaining. They would have become members of formal or informal groups of their peers for recreational purposes. They would have had young women friends, fallen in and out of love, wondered whether to commit themselves to one person in or outside of wedlock, and speculated on the responsibilities and gratifications of parenthood. What effects severe bodily injury, from which complete recovery is impossible, may have on the expected goals and experiences of men in young adulthood is the central focus of the discussion that follows.

Under the extraordinary circumstances of their hospitalization for spinal cord injuries, the patients' experiences in the military probably constituted some kind of bond among them. However, the concerns recorded here do not overtly reflect the nature and meaning of that bond or the way in which their common experiences in the immediate past influenced their potential power to cope with life's problems. Instead, these concerns have to do with their current predicaments and the management of the immediate future.

The hospital setting is apt to be a major stress-producing factor for these young men insofar as the pervading presence of medical authority augments the felt pressure of being in a military institution. Many patients have difficulty expressing their needs and wants to the physicians and nurses, as though their loss of control over their lives and bodies induces a kind of psychological paralysis; often young men such as these feel even more helpless than in truth they are.

Social workers who have been witness to this kind of reaction believe in encouraging the patients from the beginning of their hospitalization to make themselves, their feelings, their needs, and their desires known to those responsible for giving them care. To make such efforts is crucial to the patients' realization that they still have some power, influence, and control to exert in their own behalf. One is reminded of the point made in Chapter 4 that many actions directed toward social rehabilitation are taken by professionals during the early stages of diagnosis and treatment. By encouraging acts of self-help at the start of these patients' hospitalization, there is implanted in them the idea of self-respect and self-regard and a beginning belief that despite severe physical disability, they can maintain an effective degree of psychological and social self-reliance.

Worry over finances, which is such an important factor in the lives of many other severely disabled young men and women, is often not an immediate stress-producing factor for those whose disability is connected with military service. The assurance that medical care will be paid for by the federal government and that other related benefits will be available as needed cannot be overlooked as a factor that contributes positively to the outcome of treatment.

The physical helplessness of these young adult patients when they were admitted to the hospital was no fantasy. They felt most alone then, and their problems seemed insurmountable: deprivation of sexual activity, inability to move their bodies, and loss of friendships were to them the most threatening consequences of their injuries. The feelings of exclusion and inability to cope were joined to feelings of deep fear and dread of the future. At precisely the time when they should have felt eager to develop strong and intimate relationships they were despairing of the capacity and opportunity to form them.

The social workers identified three kinds of reactions such severely disabled patients frequently have. One is anger, which is a healthy reaction the patient has to his disability and its psychosocial consequences. Another is depression, which is a normal reaction to loss and a normal phase in the process of assimilating such a stark disability. The anger, when it is not understood by others, begets anger in response and often arouses a desire in those others to be rid of the angry patient. The depression, on the other hand, is apt to frighten people. They may then retreat from the patient who during his depression cannot talk to them and cannot explain himself but needs desperately not to feel abandoned. The third kind of reaction is a strong desire for privacy. The young patient who tends to feel that his damaged body "doesn't belong to me anymore, it's a mess, somebody is always working on it" may cherish and nourish privacy of mind and feelings. This striving to preserve integrity and identity is to be expected, as are many other defenses. There are so many areas of life in which the patient cannot exercise self-determination that strengthening his ability to mobilize himself psychologically is of primary importance. His strength grows largely through the enabling role of hospital personnel.

Social workers in the military hospital who gave services to the patients with spinal cord injuries sought out each patient on his first day of hospitalization. The relationship started on a one-to-one basis, but as soon as it seemed feasible each patient was offered a concurrent, supplementary experience with a small group of patients in the same unit. Occasionally a patient could respond only in a one-to-one relationship with his social worker. The reverse was true for some patients, and in these instances the social workers maintained a one-to-one relationship only at the level of closeness those patients could tolerate. In all instances, a continuing patient-social worker relationship rather than a crisis-oriented one was considered essential to meet the psychosocial needs of these young men at high risk.

The social workers' services to small groups of patients—four or five in a group—proved effective in helping patients to regain confidence in themselves and others and to strengthen their will and ability to attain greater self-fulfillment. The service to small groups started in the hospital with ward meetings to bring the patients' concerns into the open so that they could be discussed with staff. Up to that point, the patients had been sending complaints to Washington and to the press—avenues of communication within their rights at any time—but they had not been talking to the staff members about current and anticipated problems which might have been resolved with some dispatch by people within the boundaries of the facility. These problems were connected mainly with hospital structure, program, regulations, and so on.

Later, the small groups were instituted to supplement the continuing one-to-one mode of help provided by the social workers. The new operative element was the interaction among the patients in their respective small groups for the purpose of helping one another. The agreement was that each group would discuss specific concerns the members had in common, with the aim of finding solutions to problems.

The social workers assume active roles in this small group process: they try to keep a step ahead of the patients; they may deepen what the group talks about in order to make the self-help more effective; they may open up topics that are being smoothed over or make concrete matters that the patients are dismissing with vague generalities. The leadership role is complicated: it involves dealing with ideas coming from a number of patients, emotions and attitudes that crisscross among patients and between patients and the social worker-leader. The role also requires maintaining the confidentiality of data disclosed by an individual patient in his one-to-one relationship with the leader. These are among the components of service to groups that makes it an intricate process.

When a new group was formed, the pattern was for its members first to make numerous complaints and then to turn to discussing how they could improve things. Once they entered into the problem-solving phase, they were likely to start with the decision to break the monotony of their hospital-bound lives.

Arranging a trip to a sports event or a party for the ward were usual first efforts. Subtler problems—more difficult to explore and resolve—were apt to come up at later group sessions. The patients helped one another with their feelings about being disabled, with living through periods of depression, and with reestablishing old relationships and forming new ones. They learned how others managed specific situations similar to theirs and discovered better ways to manage their own. Mutual help centered frequently on such matters as going home for a weekend ("How do you get your mother off your back?") and sex and friendship (the first date in a wheelchair, how to "risk yourself" with women, how not to look on yourself as a "freak," how to get back to men friends). Some of the mutual help came out of one patient's recognition of another's self-defeating behavior. For example, a patient who described the details he gave an old friend about his disability was told by another patient that he was scaring his friend away. The group discussions are used to good advantage when patients prepare for discharge from the hospital. Again, they supplement the individual interviews the patients have with their respective social workers.

The physicians who attend such severely injured young men in a military hospital have a more than usual significance to these unusually helpless patients. As hospital staff members like the social workers, they have the opportunity from the day of the patient's admittance to contribute to the ultimate goal of maximum self-realization—the optimum social-health status each patient can achieve.

Strong one-to-one relationships between patients and their physicians are highly desirable. The patient-physician relationship can be the most potent force in the patient's achieving his potential for social functioning—that is, achieving the most he can within the limits of the irreversible elements of his disability.

Some social workers who are strong advocates of closer patient-physician relations offer the following suggestions to their medical colleagues, which can be summed up in the following brief sentence: "See the man lying on the bed."

- Reach for the patient's feelings.
- Do not rush on rounds; talk to the patients and listen to them.
- Take the initiative with patients so they know you want to hear.
- If you feel at ease doing it, sit on the bed to talk and put a hand on the patient's shoulder.
- If you can do it without seeming forced, use the patient's vocabulary.

Another way to reinforce the patient-physician relationship is through the physicians' active participation with groups of patients. As a rule, physicians respond with interest when patients invite them to join in small-group discussions about matters such as the patients' disabilities, bodily functions, and dysfunctions. Equally useful would be physicians' frequent attendance at ward meetings; it would heighten mutual trust and strengthen the physicians' understanding of patients' concerns and of how they and their relatives attempt to resolve their problems. The patients' need is for a strong, reliable patient-physician relationship, costly though it may be in time, effort, and self-discipline for the busy professional to establish and nourish.

Because the professional education of social workers requires that they become self-aware and self-appraising, they frequently voice their understanding of colleagues in other professions. In a truly collaborative, interprofessional effort such understanding would be the outcome of a free exchange of ideas. Since such communication is not universally fostered, many of the social workers' interpretations are speculative, though based on careful observation. They have been explicit at times about the stress-producing conditions that in their opinion make it difficult for physicians to acquire the detached concern that is the keystone of the professional's attitude toward the people he or she serves. The consequence of reaching for the patient's unexpressed feelings when he or she says that everything is fine can be a flood of angry frustration which has to be listened to, understood, and handled without irritation and impatience. A physician who consistently hopes to heal or cure may withdraw physically and psychologically from the severely disabled young adult. The surgeon who is making up his or her mind whether a second amputation is necessary may indeed avoid the patient while the patient's anxiety mounts because intuitively he or she knows that "something is up." Telling a patient what he or she needs to know when the patient is afraid to hear may make it as hard for the physician as it is for the patient to face reality. There is an implicit understanding in these comments that physicians, like all other givers of care in the hospital, need to protect themselves from feelings that overwhelm and demands that exceed the time and energy at their disposal. But social workers are saying also that a giver-of-service has to create coping—or defensive— mechanisms that are not as depriving to the patient as withdrawal and avoidance.

The nurses and their aides are indispensable givers of care around the clock every day of the week. They meet with many kinds of problematic patient behavior—the loud demands and complaints of the patient who "yells" when things don't go right; the passive, apathetic patient; the openly resistive, noncompliant patient. Staff members having to deal with these diverse behaviors often feel the need for more active support from physicians and others who function as administrators and teachers; the nurses and aides want to help in evaluating the delivery of services in their unit and in developing the competence of nurses and aides to deal with patients' difficult behavior. It is encouraging to note the desire for collaboration being expressed openly by the several professional and vocational groups on a hospital staff.

Nurses and aides have a fund of information about patients which is invaluable to physicians and social workers. They know who are buddies, who is drinking, and who is and is not eating well. Such information, which physicians and social workers have far less opportunity to acquire first-hand, contributes to the understanding and assessment of a young adult patient's life-and-illness situation and to the plans for his or her treatment and rehabilitation.

The demands for adaptation described for this specific patient population occurred with extraordinary force at a crucial point in the young men's lives. Outstanding were the demands to adapt to changes in self-image, self-regard, and the regard of others; to changes in status of freedom of choice; to changes in the ability to carry out an accustomed pattern of daily living; to the loss of bodily integrity; to the loss of control over one's environment; and to gross uncertainty about emotional fulfillment through intimate personal relationships.[1]

THE ELDERLY PATIENT: MAJOR THEMES AND SPECIAL RISKS [2, 3]

In our society, 65 years of age officially marks a person's entry into the group of the elderly. It is an arbitrary designation in that the process and symptoms of aging may start earlier or later than 65, proceed at different rates among members of the age group, and manifest themselves differently in respect to matters such as preservation or loss of energy and sensory acuity, quality of social functioning, and emotional responses to changes demanded by the aging process and by developments in society itself.

In other words, the approximately 10 percent of the population that is called "the elderly" is by no means monolithic, though its members do have characteristics in common that put them at special risk. In general, the elderly constitute three subgroups: 65 through 74, 75 through 84, and 85 and older. Usual expectations are that people experience more serious degenerative symptoms as they move from one subgroup to the next; that loss of relatives and friends increases as does the danger of isolation; and that the individual's status of social-health deteriorates as he or she enters successively older subgroups. These are characteristics to be alert to, but a given aging or aged person may differ from the expected, and it is important not to stereotype.

The elderly differ from one another as they did in their prime, in their adolescence, and in their childhood. Very frequently their earlier individual characteristics are exaggerated in old age. In the vernacular, "they are the same, only more so."

For the most part there is a strong impulse in the elderly to preserve their self-esteem. This impulse is compatible with the large numbers of elderly patients who need, want, and use the services provided by social workers. The services are needed by patients in ambulatory care clinics, in hospital beds, and in home care programs. The social worker's perspective is that elderly patients are living through the final phase of the human life cycle and that they are entitled to live it with the fullest possible realization of their potentials. It is a perspective that insists not on mere survival but on survival for a life of optimum quality; that recognizes the tasks, risks, and problems inherent in this developmental phase of life; and that perceives the social worker's professional task as helping elderly patients to master the developmental tasks, surmount the risks, and resolve the problems when help is needed.

Anyone who reaches the age of 65 has been through many changes in the circumstances of his or her life; has made many adaptations—some successful, some not so successful; has learned new facts; and has accumulated some wisdom from experiencing life. The official advent of old age at 65 and the onset of discernible signs of aging do not spell the end of significant life experience, nor of the capacity to learn, or of the ability to use and apply knowledge, exercise judgment, and make decisions. Except in instances of severe intellectual impairment which destroys the elderly person's awareness, understanding, and judgmental processes, the elderly person will cope with any number of stress-producing events and conditions though usually at a slower pace and with less physical endurance than formerly. Some of the more important ones are either loss or substantial reduction of occupational status, changes in the amount and kind of responsibility assumed as a parent or a spouse, a narrowing range of social relationships and activities concurrent with substantially increased amounts of leisure or free time, new living arrangements, and decreased incomes, limited in part by governmental law and regulation.

Not all of the changes are depriving in nature. The relatively recent recognition of the special needs of the elderly is manifested in the provision of human services such as Medicare and special health facilities, neighborhood centers with special programs for elderly residents, supplemental security income, special designs in housing, programs for continuing education, and special arrangements for transportation. No claim can be made that these programs and services and others like them are fully adequate in coverage, volume, quality, accessibility, coordination, or collaboration. They are, however, signs of hope for future developments.[4]

The shape of current society shows some changes that have particular relevance for the elderly. For one thing, they now approximate 10 percent of the population in this nation—a size that gives them visibility and a potential for influencing the society in which they live. Moreover, an exceedingly large percentage of the elderly live in the community—approximately 96 percent. Many need no special services; some get along well with the help of supportive services from time to time; others are able to remain in the community but only with continuous services such as those provided in comprehensive home care programs. (The fact that the subgroup of those 85 and over will be the fastest growing sector in the immediate future warns of predictable needs ahead.) Although not too long ago this was largely a two-generation society, the trend is clearly toward a three- and four-generation society; and the greatest burden is falling on the middle-aged, who have frequently to manage pressures from the older generations.

The existence of three or four living generations strongly supports belief in the continuing existence of the family. Despite pronouncements that the family is out of style, dead, or dying, it is in fact alive, although sometimes in unfamiliar forms; it is dynamic and influential; it is apparently indestructible as a social institution; and the elderly are in large numbers members of a functioning family. These members do not necessarily live under one roof in the same community—people are much more mobile geographically than they were three or four decades ago—but in general they are not alienated from, or lacking in interest and concern for, their kin in the family network.

The elderly ill in hospital-based care receive medical services in a variety of ways that reflect different perspectives and policies from institution to institution. A municipal hospital with a large annual population of elderly hospitalized patients gives them medical care in a special unit designated geriatric service. In several voluntary hospitals the elderly in-patients are assigned to beds in the traditional way by diagnosis and method of intervention.

Similarly, arrangements vary for patients receiving ambulatory care. For instance, a voluntary hospital established an outpatient clinic for elderly patients who are in need of specialized care. When their conditions become stabilized, the patients are transferred to the regular clinic for the comprehensive care of adults.

The patients for whom these provisions are made are, like their peers in the general population, predominantly women and tend to be living on small and frequently insufficient fixed incomes, although many had the security of middle-class status before they became old. Their illnesses are for the most part chronic, and the older they are, the greater the likelihood that a patient has more than one chronic disease or disability. Acute episodes in a chronic illness bring many of the elderly to the hospital for out-patient or in-patient care, and in large numbers they remain in, or return to, the community to live. Others need care that is available only in special facilities, and the patient's acknowledgment of this need can be one of life's hardest tasks.

Some elderly patients do come to the hospital with acute conditions, such as fractures, which are not connected with a chronic illness. But these patients usually have chronic conditions as well, and the acute and chronic conditions in combination may affect treatment, recovery, and social rehabilitation.

Elderly patients seem prone to experience a strong degree of anxiety in response to stress-producing aspects of illness and aging. It has been said that there might be "a greater *generality* of caution, i.e., less dependency upon specific situational factors, among the old than among the young"[5] and that "older individuals seem particularly susceptible to stress, and thus it is possible that under current 'normal' conditions they reflect more anxiety."[6] The precipitating factors of anxiety most frequently cited are the patients' apprehension about their recovery, lack of emotional support when relatives are not available, inadequate finances, and above all the possibility that they might not be able to remain in or return to their own homes.

Consequently, social workers perceive elderly patients as having a greater need for their services than patients in other age groups—a need that springs from the demands to adapt to changes that result not only from the processes and consequences of aging but also from the course of illness or injury; the processes and outcomes of diagnosis, treatment, and rehabilitation; and the impact of all these events and conditions on the personal relationships of the people involved. The social workers' interest and concern spring fundamentally from the belief that the emphasis should not be merely on the elderly patient's survival but on the quality of his or her remaining life. Social workers balance their awareness that the elderly patient's intertwined biopsychosocial problems are often of a serious nature with a hopeful outlook on the elderly patient's ability to cope with change. To quote one social worker, "Given time and stability in their surroundings, debilitated [elderly] people do respond. When staff has high expectations, the patients respond [with greater achievement], but the expectations of staff and patient must be related to reality." Another social worker emphasized that "patients need considerable support to reach their maximum potential in functioning because they are usually so fearful."

In addition to the essential resources of time, environmental stability, and support, social workers advocated programs for physical and social rehabilitation of the elderly patient and recommended frequent revaluation by hospital personnel of the elderly patient's total life-and-illness situation. Taken together, these are the general provisions that experienced social workers recommend for strengthening the elderly patient's ability to achieve his or her maximum status of social-health.

There are many elderly patients whose cultural heritage includes looking upon physicians and hospitals as people and places of last resort, and for them becoming a patient is a highly stress-producing experience when their usual home remedies have failed. The generalized fear these people feel upon turning to the conventional resources of our society is sometimes extreme; physicians and hospitals may forebode death rather than offer a chance for life.

Aspects of hospital-based care, even when the elderly patient considers modern Western medicine a boon, may impinge adversely upon the patient. For example, in large hospitals with many specialty clinics, the elderly ambulatory patient may attend a dozen or more different clinics. The lack of a physician who has primary responsibility for the patient's medical care may result in problems such as contradictory recommendations for the patient's regimen or medication being prescribed for one disease that is contraindicated for another disease the patient has. The amount of energy, time, and money exacted by attendance at so many clinics is excessive for many elderly patients and for those who accompany him or her to clinic; and the very task of keeping track of countless appointments and numerous prescriptions is beyond many elderly people's impaired intellectual ability. The establishment of a geriatric unit centralizes ambulatory care and permits adequate communication and coordination among the general and specialized services. It may also reduce substantially the cumulative cost of transportation between home and hospital.

Clinics often are scheduled for hours that are difficult for the elderly or for the friends and relatives who escort them; early morning travel by public transportation in a crowded urban community is a hardship for people of any age whose physical functioning is impaired. Relatives who must get children off to school before they escort elderly patients find that early morning clinic hours create a serious conflict in responsibility. One needs to be mindful in general whether administrative procedures facilitate service to patients. For example, in a hospital that did not register patients for clinic services until the day of the patient's first appointment, it took so long to register that at times the patient could not be seen by a physician at all that day.

A turnabout in hospital policies, regulations, or procedures from those that impede to those that facilitate the giving of services is sometimes easy to achieve, but more often it is exceedingly difficult for people to accept and put into effect. In general, procedural changes are the easy ones to effect because they seldom penetrate into fundamental beliefs and values. On the other hand, changes in policy and regulations disturb more deeply rooted convictions about the provision and delivery of services and are likely to engender stronger resistance. In any case, justification for change is always a preliminary condition. On occasion a simple survey over a short period of time proves the need for change and pinpoints the nature of the required change. An illustration of this kind of administrative change is the reordering of procedures to register new patients in ambulatory care which solves the problem for patients of all ages described in the preceding paragraph. In contrast, determining whether a central geriatric service for in-patients is more effective than the traditional distribution of elderly in-patients would call for an evaluative study of some magnitude and complexity and a well-planned period of preparation for the study.

Excessive anxiety felt by elderly in-patients seems most frequently connected with fear about their recovery—not necessarily a fear or premonition of death but perhaps more often an anticipatory fear about their ability to live with further impairments of their physical and social functioning. More specifically, the fear is that their customary living arrangements may no longer be suitable or even that they will have no voice in the plans made for their future.

On the whole, elderly in-patients have more problems, and more difficult times than younger in-patients that affect planning for discharge and postdischarge living. Planning for discharge in itself becomes a stress-producing event because it is inextricable from such factors as financial problems, psychosocial impacts of chronic illness on patients/families, and limited resources in the community. These are factors that influence planning for discharge regardless of the patient's age, but they assume unusual weight when they bear on being both elderly and ill. A substantial amount of social work service is required for the problem-solving tasks that are involved.

Financial strain continues to be an important source of stress for the elderly ill and their relatives despite the provision of resources described above. Many of these patients have always lived at or near the poverty level, and old age and illness add to their burdens. Other elderly patients are adjusting to the lowered standard of living that for so many elderly persons in this country marks the final phase of life.

Certain characteristics of our several systems of income maintenance and health care increase the severity of financial strain commonly felt by the elderly poor and their relatives. In particular, there are the fragmentation and incomplete coverage of these systems and the frequent changes in eligibility requirements, most commonly in the financial criterion. Patients and their relatives are frequently inaccurately informed about matters such as current eligibility requirements, the range of their benefits, or the amounts of so-called deductible or coinsurance items for which they are financially responsible. For example, premiums for Medicare may be increased and so may the costs of deductible items, while the amount of income that makes elderly people eligible for Medicaid (to supplement the coverage of Medicare) is frequently decreased. The psychological effect on the elderly patient who is referred to Medicaid as "medically indigent" is particularly traumatic when the patient has worked hard, practiced thrift all his or her life, and has never received public assistance. Examples of inadequate coverage are the failure of Medicare to pay for self-administered medicines and the failure of some programs for income maintenance to pay for telephones which are scarcely luxuries for the elderly, well or ill. There is a point at which quantitatively inadequate coverage creates distinctly qualitative consequences in patients/families' life-situations. Lack of adequate services and supports all too often leads to discouragement, depression, and finally apathy—a resignation to the status quo instead of a stimulus to fight for recovery and restoration.

The financial status of the elderly patient is apt to be a strong determinant when the patient requires institutional care following discharge from an acute care hospital.* Although the decision to obtain institutional care for the patient is at best a collaborative one in which members of several professions and the patient/family participate, finding the most suitable institutions is usually the task of a social worker, who has to be up to date on such matters as the kinds of

* See the sections on leaving the hospital, pp. 104–108 and hospital-based home care, pp. 116–121.

service being offered in various types of facilities, limitations of time, and the sources of payments available to the patient/family in question. Because details differ so widely within and among states, legislation and regulations vary so much among governmental levels, and changes occur frequently, students and practitioners will find it useful to have accurate general information about the programs and services available at a given time in their respective localities.

Some of the complicating factors in selecting an institution suitable for an elderly patient upon leaving the hospital are the existence of both institutions for the elderly only and voluntary and proprietary nursing homes not exclusively for the aged, the trend in psychiatric hospitals to exclude the elderly patient who is not demonstrably psychotic, a corollary trend in voluntary institutions to admit some mentally impaired elderly who are ineligible for care in psychiatric hospitals, the limits on time and scope of services written into the provisions of Medicare and the complex requirements for transferring elderly patients between hospitals and other health facilities, and the fragmentation and discontinuities in services and the uncertainties regarding payment for services which result from the incoordination of multiple systems of services such as Medicare, Medicaid, and voluntary insurance programs.

The availability of suitable institutions for an elderly patient changes constantly. Whether there will be a vacancy at the time the patient will be discharged from the hospital is only one problem. Other problems have to do with unpredictable changes in institutional policy and function which are often determined by the amount and promptness of payments made by public or voluntary sources of funding rather than by the prevailing need in a given community for a specific kind of institution or qualified staff. In consequence, some elderly patients are in facilities that provide less than the level of care they need or are unsuitable in some other way, such as accessibility. And as is only too well known, the shortage of adequate programs for home health care may result in a patient's living in an institution when his or her condition does not require it. Forced adaptation to unsuitable living arrangements endangers the social well-being and social functioning of patient and relatives alike. "The line that divides health problems from social problems inevitably grows thinner and thinner. . . . Society's limited tolerance for the dependency that chronic illness is likely to bring with it is the major source of the difficulties which confront society in dealing with illness."[7] This observation is peculiarly applicable to the elderly ill, since in large numbers they have one or more chronic conditions for which provisions are still inadequate ten years or more after these words were written.

Family attitudes and relationships have great significance for elderly patients, many of whom have natural human resources as do younger patients. In fact, there is an interesting array of spouses, siblings, adult children, grandchildren and great-grandchildren, grand-nieces and grand-nephews, and substitute family in the form of close friends, concerned neighbors, and the like.[8] These relationships have to be carefully assessed for strengths and weaknesses. There are almost always problematic aspects in human relationships, and the areas of high and low risk have to be determined.

For example, if an elderly patient has been dependent on family members for help and care over a long period, by the time the patient is hospitalized his or her relatives may have reached the limit of their ability to care for him or her again in the same way. Their emotions may be spent, and they care less; their physical strength may give out; or financial strain may prohibit further contribution of money. Positive elements in the relationship may remain, despite some erosion, stressful frustrations, and the like. As one social worker put it, "When it is no longer possible for relatives to give a patient physical care in their home, their psychological, emotional, and social support remains an important source of strength."

There are instances in which relatives will not consider any plan except the patient's return to their home, even if the strains amount to hardship. In other instances, relatives are fearful for the patient's safety if he or she returns home to live alone. Still others are fearful of what may happen if the patient, coming to live with them, is left alone for any length of time. Then there are those who resist encroachment on their time and do not want to get too involved. Some of these attitudes reflect environmental, social, and emotional circumstances which realistically prevent relatives from giving or continuing to give shelter, physical care, or financial aid to elderly patients.

What comes through clearly is that the elderly patient's need to change his or her accustomed patterns of coping and living and to adapt to the demands of being elderly and ill have a reciprocal effect on his or her relatives. They also as a rule have to adapt to the patient's changed circumstances and abilities, with the result that changes occur in their own patterns of living. Taken in its broadest context, patterns of living may be affected by such factors as physical living arrangements (e.g., space, equipment, supplies), the extent and kind of self-care for which the patient can take responsibility versus the medical and nursing care required by illnesses and disabilities, and the geographic distance between a patient in his or her own home (or in an institution) and his or her relatives.

Shifts in the balance of interdependence between the elderly patients and their relatives may be sources of fear and anxiety, but changes in tasks and responsibilities occurring in the lives of elderly patients and their concerned relatives are expected psychosocial developments. In assessing such changes it is good to remember that "there can be no true role reversal and no second childhood. . . . Half a century or more of adulthood cannot be wiped out; though some areas of memory and function may be eroded, there can be no consistent return to a previous level."[9] The reader may remember an earlier caution about the concept of role reversal when younger adults—spouses, usually—renounce accustomed tasks or assume new ones in consequence of the impaired functioning of one of them.*

Even when the decision that an elderly patient should enter an institution is made on a sound, realistic basis, old problems in relationships and long-discarded feelings of rejection, rivalry, or resentment are often reactivated during the ordeal of decision making. For the patient, the usual anticipated stresses stemming from the expected loss of privacy, curtailed freedom in one's daily regimen, separation from beloved people and cherished possessions, and the like are apt to be augmented by a not unreasonable fear that this will be his or her final home. Thus, in the making of the decision there is for everyone involved a constellation of emotionally charged considerations, many of them embedded in values that patients/families have lived by and do not wish to violate.

* See p. 85.

Because privacy and self-reliance are so treasured in our society, special mention should be made of the elderly patients who insist on returning to their familiar living arrangements despite risks to physical safety and health. It is astonishing how effective a patient's drive to carry out his or her preferred plan can be. Of course, the patient who acknowledges impairment and disabilities will have a healthy apprehension and try to protect himself or herself from harm. The patient who refuses to be cared for in an institution because he or she denies his or her limitations is apt to disregard ordinary precautions, take unwise chances, and in the end defeat himself or herself.

The active participation of the elderly patient and his or her relatives perhaps needs special mention in order to offset mistaken ideas about the patient's ability to question, to understand, and to exercise judgment. Elderly people should not be treated automatically as if they were incompetent; even with a mental syndrome many elderly patients know what they want. One then explores how realistic the plan is; it may be wise for the patient to try it out, or it may be necessary to consider an alternative immediately. One social worker said, "The underlying concept is to keep intact as far as possible the patient's ability to act for himself." And as another social worker put it, "We need to remember that the elderly patient has planned his or her life before and can still exert control over it." It is extremely helpful to elderly patients when they can maintain some of the structure of life to which they have long been accustomed. There is little as debilitating and depressing as enforced inactivity with nothing to put in its place.

The attitudes and behavior of givers-of-service in respect to elderly patients tend to reflect the way in which our society as a whole looks upon the elderly. This way is changing, but obviously the elderly continue to be stereotyped more than are patients in other phases of the lifecycle. Although this nation received due warning from social scientists and other experts several decades ago of the rising tide of older persons in the general population, action to provide for them has been slow and relatively slight. Professional schools, including schools of medicine, have recently begun to develop areas of knowledge in their curricula that concern the social and emotional aspects of aging relevant to health and disease.

A final point hinges on the human experience. Young people have difficulty understanding what it is like to be old. It is hard to project oneself into an experience set far into one's future; it is sometimes frightening to contemplate aging, illness, and death; it is self-protective to turn away from the ending phase of life. Undoubtedly, people's reactions to the elderly and the elderly ill are caused in part by the experiences they have had in formative years with older relatives. These have sometimes been happy experiences, and the outlook of professionals as well as laypersons can be colored for good or for ill by these early encounters. One must reckon also with the effects of certain biases and beliefs which arouse pejorative and unsympathetic attitudes.

To illustrate, it is true that many elderly people have slow reaction times, poor memory for recent events, and a tendency to reminisce at length and to tell long-winded stories of circumstantial events before getting to the point. But the physiological manifestations of the processes of aging and the psychosocial manifestations of a deeply rooted, well-remembered, and meaningful past do not automatically spell senility or alienation from the contemporary world. The elderly can tell tales of streets lit by gaslight and trolley cars drawn by horses and still know about the new math, communication by satellite, and instruments left on the moon by astronauts.

INTERRELATED FRAMES OF REFERENCE FOR UNDERSTANDING LIFE AND ILLNESS

The young adult and the elderly patients in hospital-based medical care can be understood within the framework of the course of specific diseases and disabilities and the framework of a particular developmental phase in the life cycle.

However, the most enlightening basis for understanding and for being of service to patients of any age or with any specified illness, deviance, or deficit is an analysis of the crisscrossing and interacting impacts of the biological, psychological/emotional, and social/environmental aspects of living with a disease or disability. The entire text of this book was written with this perspective in mind, but Chapters VI, VII, and VIII have focused most consistently on the interactions of the continuum and course of life with the course and history of disease and disability.

The descriptive passages are dynamically illustrative, pointing to future as well as current ways of understanding and performing in the health care field. These ways will stem from values which will change slowly and from knowledge, techniques, and social behavior which will change more rapidly. A fundamental pattern of values that directs human beings will thus become manifest in new forms and patterns of adaptive behavior in patients, their relatives, and significant others and to an even greater degree in the givers of multiprofessional services.

REFERENCES

1. Helen J. Lane, "Working with Problems of Assault to Self-Image and Lifestyle," *Social Work in Health Care*, vol. 1, no. 2 (winter 1975-1976), pp. 191-198.
2. Elaine M. Brody, "Aging," in *Encyclopedia of Social Work*, 17th ed. (Washington, D.C.: National Association of Social Workers, 1977), pp. 55-78.
3. Michael Lesparre, "An Interview with Robert N. Butler, M.D., Director, National Institute on Aging," *Hospitals*, vol. 50, no. 22 (November 1976), p. 50.
4. Jordan I. Kosberg, "Nursing Homes," in *Encyclopedia of Social Work*, op. cit., pp. 1010-1017.
5. Raymond G. Kuhlen, "Developmental Changes in Motivation During the Adult Years," in *Middle Age and Aging: A Reader in Social Psychology*, ed. Bernice L. Neugarten (Chicago: University of Chicago Press, 1968), p. 127.
6. Ibid., p. 130.
7. Bess Dana, "Health, Medical Care and Social Responsibility," in *Trends in Social Work Practice and Knowledge*, National Association of Social Workers Tenth Anniversary Symposium, New York, 1966, p. 58.
8. Bernice L. Neugarten, "Patterns of Aging: Past, Present and Future," *Social Service Review* (School of Social Service Administration, University of Chicago), vol. 47, no. 4 (December 1973), pp. 571-580.
9. Brody, op. cit., p. 56.

PART 3
CONCLUDING COMMENTS

Chapter 9
Concluding Comments
on the Practice of
Hospital-Based Social Work:

TODAY AND TOMORROW

The practice of social work from which the substance of this book derives is fashioned in part by the mission and functions of the hospitals in which it takes place. They are hospitals, both voluntary and public, established to provide secondary and tertiary medical care of high quality, to advance knowledge and skills in the practice of medicine, and to offer optimum learning opportunities to students at various levels of education for the health and health-related professions.

Over the years hospitals such as these have become in name and in fact the centers of the health industry in this country. In an evolutionary process, this nation has seen the hospital develop from an institution for the care of the sick poor—in the early days, primarily custodial care—through a period of many specialty hospitals—among them hospitals for patients with chronic diseases, infectious diseases, or diseases affecting specific organs or systems of the body—into a period that saw the development of different kinds of institutions, such as nursing homes, and of substantial growth in the number of facilities, hospitals and others, sponsored and subsidized in whole or in part by the federal government.

In this current era specialized hospitals have decreased in number, but specialized medical care in special service units has greatly increased in the acute general teaching hospitals. These are customarily affiliated with universities, the better to fulfill their missions in treatment, research, and education.[1]

Those voluntary hospitals that now excel in secondary and tertiary treatment are entering a new developmental phase. One of the important goals is to redress certain imbalances in the hospitals' services by making possible concerted attention to ambulatory patients and by meeting the urgent need for primary care. The lack of primary care has resulted in an accelerated rate of misuse and overuse of emergency services for nonemergency conditions as well as in too little attention being given to phenomena such as the absence of opportunities to provide preventive interventions.

It has been many years since voluntary hospitals have been able to rely on philanthropic contributions as a major source of support. The correction of imbalances, the introduction of new techniques, and the development of new programs are activities too costly for the hospitals to afford without subsidy from various levels of government. At best, the initial period of such innovations is very costly, although in the long run they may reduce the hospitals' expenses.

If, however, the fiscal problems are eased by the use of public monies, the voluntary hospitals are obligated to maintain professional accountability to governmental agencies, for example, for protecting the legal rights of patients receiving direct services or participating as subjects in research efforts, and to maintain administrative accountability for their use of money, for example, for construction of buildings and for equipment required by new techniques.

With acknowledgment of these probable developments, this final chapter will both assess current social work practice in a small, selected sample of hospitals offering secondary and tertiary care and look carefully at unrealized potentials. It is hoped that the assessment will facilitate the use of social work experience by students and educators in the health care field and that the look forward will be relevant to the continuing efforts of educators and practitioners to enable them and their students to meet the demands of the future.[2]

The very fact that social workers are viewing their professional experience as a source for multiprofessional learning and teaching in the health care field indicates a considerable historical development from their beginnings in 1905.[3] Their role then was perceived, and continued to be perceived for some time, as ancillary or subsidiary to the physician's. For the most part the subsidiary role was manifested in the hospital by the social worker's entry into a patient/family's situation only when the physician requested it and for the purpose requested. At first obtaining data on the patient's background was the social worker's major function; the data were intended to enhance understanding of the patient so that he or she could be helped to make maximum use of medical care.

Social workers began to appear in other health-related institutions, and in them and in the hospitals the utilization of the social workers' knowledge and skills began to spread. For example, the social worker's ability to inquire into, understand, and remove or reduce some burdensome impacts of illness on patients/families was recognized fairly early. The linkage between problems of income maintenance and problems of health was well enough understood so that the medical social workers, as they were then called, became important staff members in the programs established in 1935 and thereafter under the Social Security Act.[4]

In some hospitals as far back as 20 or 30 years ago or more medical rounds developed into medical-social rounds, and psychosocial factors became more important in the processes and procedures of hospital-based medical care. Slowly, changes at the administrative level of the hospital occurred in fuller recognition of the professional nature of social work in health care. In some hospitals directors of social service departments are now full voting members of the medical board. In other hospitals the social service department's director may be an ex officio member of the medical board, free to participate in discussions but without voting privileges. In still other hospitals the director of social services attends meetings of the medical board by invitation when his or her expertness is considered necessary. However, it is more common for the director or other members of a social service department to be regular voting members of both standing and ad hoc committees or subcommittees of a medical board.

From the ancillary role to the role of professional collaboration in administration and service is a far distance, and the full length has not yet been traveled in all health settings. It is now a goal that seems reasonable, attainable, desirable, and essential to a quality of excellence in the delivery of medical care. It is a goal that testifies to the "striking relationships of social opportunity, social provision, and social behavior to the cause, course, and outcome of . . . critical health problems" and to the belief that "the capacity to define and deal with health problems in social-health terms emerges as a professional necessity rather than an ideological nicety."[5]

While considering the assessment of current social work practice and the glance at the future which follow below, the reader may wish to keep in mind the value concepts and concepts of knowledge described in Chapter 1 and the major functions of direct service practitioners outlined in Chapter 2. Since these ideas were inductively arrived at from the practitioners' recounting of their professional performance and experience, there should be some illuminating relationships between them and the substance of the assessment. Ultimately, all aspects of direct services by the hospital-based social worker have to be assessed against the general purpose of these services—to assist people to achieve their maximum status of social-health.*

THE STRENGTHS IN SOCIAL WORK PRACTICE

Strengths at the plane of professional practice in direct service are manifested most obviously at the level where proficiency and competence in professional functioning emerge from the successful integration of values, knowledge, and technical skills. However, any one of these three elements may, under special conditions, appear to be a notable strength. In the listing that follows, the separate elements as well as the integrated end product are given recognition.

Exploring and assessing life-situations is an outstanding proficiency and a major area of the social worker's participation in the care of the patient/family. The social worker's awareness, understanding, and ability to make beneficial use of the interaction of mind, body, and social environment aid in directing the social worker's inquiry into individual situations and subsequently in estimating how the various aspects of a given life-and-illness-situation may combine to strengthen or impede the patient/family's capacity to cope.

A competent and accurate assessment draws on the social worker's strongly developed ability to be empathic; to observe, listen, and hear people's messages; to encourage and develop a two-way channel of communication with others; to know when to suggest a new direction of the other person's thoughts and when not to intrude. These are significant elements in the social worker's professional use of himself or herself in working with others—elements that contribute to the development and maintenance of a working relationship. This relationship is the dynamic, human medium for achieving openly agreed-upon, shared goals.

The social worker's first entry into a patient/family's life-and-illness-situation also marks his or her initial efforts to establish a working relationship

---

* See p. 27.

with them. At the point of entry these efforts usually center on the patient/family's need to make known, and the reciprocal need of the social worker to know and assess, their concerns and problems, their hopes and inner strengths, and the conditions that determine their way of life. The social worker's understanding of the working relationship as a means rather than an end, a constant self-awareness of the quality and intensity of relationships, and a sense of accountability for the use of relationships to achieve professional ends are professional attributes that are well developed. Since they are demonstrable attributes that can be discussed in intellectual as well as emotional terms, social workers can be enabling to students and members of the health professions who are similarly concerned with developing effective working relationships to reach those objectives that are compatible with their professions.

The ability to observe, explore, and understand relationships among family members or between family members and their significant others is as basic as are the similar steps in establishing and developing professional working relationships. Assessment of a life-and-illness-situation would be sterile if it were to omit or devalue the personal relationships that at their best constitute the supports and sources of human strength that people in problematic circumstances require.

Adequate exploration and assessment depend also on the ability to be empathic and compassionate with individual members of a family who may have conflicting points of view, who may not be consistently empathic with one another, and who may resent the social worker's commitment to consider everyone's right to maximum feasible self-realization and self-determination and everyone's right to be treated fairly and equitably.

Exploration and assessment of life-situations is usually a matter of reexploration and reassessment at times of known or suspected change. The expected course of illness and its treatment may undergo change; the material resources in the natural or organized social environment may change for better or worse; human resources may become either more or less available and accessible; new knowledge about medical or social conditions may induce positive change or create controversy and doubt. In other words, change may increase or decrease the burden of stress and influence the pastient/family's ability to grow and adapt. Being alert to the fluidity of life in our society requires the social worker's constant scrutiny and inquiry in order to keep abreast of the matching and mismatching of abilities and disabilities in a patient/family's situation on the one side and opportunities and deprivations in the sociocultural environment on the other.

Helping people identify and manage realities is one of the social worker's most important responsibilities that follows assessment of a patient/family's life-situation. The social worker's ability to identify the realities in a life-situation must be accompanied by the ability to distinguish between those that are unequivocal strengths to be exploited and those that are stress producing and need to be mastered. Social workers often have a "heal thyself" attitude which impels them to face as fully as possible the stressful realities in their patients/-families' lives before attempting to help them to cope.* In essence, the social worker's self-respect and regard for his or her own potential for growth and adaptation are prerequisites for respecting and facilitating this potential in others.

* See the social-medical history of Mrs. Riviera, p. 63.

Realities is a broadly conceived term which includes not only the facts of the physical, socioeconomic environment and the facts that describe an illness or disability and its consequences but the facts and significance of personal relationships, attitudes, and feelings.

The social worker often sees significant realities that others ignore and sometimes assesses as fantasy or distortion what others see as fact and reality. Social workers develop competence in seeking out the realities of the situations of others without denying the importance of the irrational and imagined ideas that so often increase the emotional burden of those involved in situations of illness. Providing information where there was ignorance, correcting misunderstandings, drawing on peoples' inner strengths and natural resources, making available the resources of the institution and community: these are among the most effective means of help at the social worker's disposal. The selection of resources is again one of his or her greatest strengths, and it takes many forms. It is just as crucial to know when the patient's physician is the proper resource for giving a patient/family needed information and explanations as it is to know the source and procedures for obtaining a prosthesis for an amputee.

Just as exploration and assessment of life-situations are recurrent functions that are not confined to a particular phase of illness or medical care, so is the responsibility for helping people sort out and deal with the realities of their life-and-illness-situations. It is a form of help that may be of great value, for example, to a patient/family having to make a decision about a recommended diagnostic or therapeutic procedure, to an elderly patient who has to choose between the risks of living alone and the risks of making his or her home with an adult married daughter, or to a young woman who is afraid to tell the man she loves that she is diabetic and is ashamed of not telling him.

These immediate purposes underscore a variety of values, such as the primacy of the individual, the importance of each family member in relation to the others, and the individual's right, within limits, to self-determination and to optimum self-fulfillment.

Thus, helping patients/families deal with realities may be at the same time a preparation for a "next step," a strengthening of patient/family participation, or the prelude to the constructive use of resources, the solution of medical-social problems, and the like.

The reduction of psychosocial stress, which is a potential hazard to the coping capacities of patients/families, is one of the social worker's most desirable end products. As a goal, it is compatible with the social worker's major functions, each of which serves social work's general purpose in the hospital setting. The reduction of a patient/family's excessive stress—the degree or kind of stress that is psychologically paralyzing or immobilizing—is not only enabling to patients and their relatives but facilitating to medical and medically related personnel.

Tension and anxiety greatly complicate matters for patients/families and, from the physician's point of view, may have effects such as increased risk, exacerbation of pain, and retarded recovery. It follows that a major professional asset lies in the social worker's knowledge of, and sensitivity to, the stress-producing elements in the course and treatment of illness and disability and during the process of rehabilitation.

Many stress-producing elements are either reduced in severity or eliminated by means of resources provided to meet social and health needs. The social worker is an expert in knowing what the resources are, who is eligible for them, and how they can be obtained. In the field of health care some resources are specific to specific diseases and disabilities; some are legislated and some are provided by voluntary organizations; some can be paid for by third-party providers and some cannot; some are time limited and some are available throughout the period of the patient/family's need; some are age specific and some are not. These are only a few of the many determinants that govern the selection of resources. Thus the use of resources hinges on a wealth of information and good judgment insofar as choices are possible in the scarce economy of our current programs and services.

Much of the anticipatory and preparatory process in which the social worker engages the patient/family is undertaken to remove or reduce the impacts of stress-producing factors which create crises and hardship if they become excessive in volume, scope, frequency, or intensity.

On the other hand, the social worker will exploit constructively a patient/-family's ability to use reasonable kinds and amounts of stress as stimuli and incentives to problem-solving responses. Building on patients/families' strengths and encouraging the development of their latent capacities to deal with stress-producing situations offer patients/families experiences in mastery and growth and the gratification of coping successfully.

The pursuit of maximum benefits by social workers in behalf of the patients/families they are serving is a professional attribute used in the face of challenge; it is as important as the patient/family's persistent efforts to meet the demands and make adaptations required by illness and disability. The social worker's determination to obtain maximum benefits for patients/families under-pins his or her extended efforts to overcome obstacles. In the social worker's lexicon, maximum benefits go beyond those essential to the patient's physical recovery and rehabilitation and extend into the realm of social rehabilitation in the sense of maximum social functioning and the highest achievable quality of living. Among the obstacles to the attainment of these goals are the scarcity and fragmentation of needed resources, the inadequacy of provisions for income maintenance and for payment for needed services, and the incoordination among the related systems of health and social welfare.

In addition, there are differences in values and philosophy among givers-of-service in the health care field which influence strongly their attitudes toward the use of scarce resources and can lead to heated debate in the decision-making process. Both the determination of policy and the consequences of policy manifested in practice incorporate these differences in beliefs and commitments.

Who can be the judge and how can it be judged whether one patient or another should be the beneficiary of resources that will provide the most likely opportunity for the patient's maximum self-realization—not merely the opportunity to survive, but to survive with gratification in living.[6]

But there is one more side to the issue of maximum benefits. The patient who decides that prolongation of life will afford him or her no gratifying experiences and nothing pleasurable that can be shared with others may make the decision that death will confer a greater benefit than life. The right of mentally competent adults to reject recommended procedures, to request with-drawal of life supports, and the like is a complicated issue medically, socially, morally, and legally. It is currently being fought out on all fronts by coalitions of concerned citizens, in legislatures, in the courts, and in professional organizations involved in the health care field.

The solution—if there is a final solution—is not in sight, but it is necessary to be aware that values sometimes are in conflict with one another and that derivative codes of behavior usually contain clauses that under certain conditions will clash and nullify one another. To make the right decisions under these conditions is the essence of ethical conduct and professional behavior.

Understanding the developmental nature of process is a highly valuable piece of the social worker's knowledge. During the course of an illness, the word *process* takes on great meaning for both the recipients and the givers of medical care. Social workers by and large have a good sense of process, that is, of steps and phases over time—a sense that supports their professional efforts to be helpful. They know that there is little that is instant, although there appears to be an expectation of the instantaneous action, result, and gratification in our current society. To the contrary, it is natural for people to test each other out for trustworthiness and sincerity, so that normally relationships develop rather than spring full-blown. This is an important fact to be considered in crises and crisis intervention, as well as in planned long-term treatment procedures. In Chapter III it was made clear that diagnosis and diagnostic procedures, which so often extend over time in a sequence of events, constitute a process in the spectrum of medical care rather than an instant result. Most people recognize that treatment and rehabilitation also involve steps, stages, and phases. The social worker has a keen awareness of the significance of the flow and course of these phenomena—in essence, that the persons involved have constantly to make adaptations and adjustments, not only or even primarily physical but psychosocial in nature, and these can be very demanding indeed. The understanding of process, coupled with the realization that each human being has his or her own limits of tolerance for anxiety and struggle, underlies the social worker's technique of partializing—that is, of helping people to cope by taking a first-things-first, one-step-at-a-time approach to the complex problems of life-and-illness.

The social worker's understanding of the meanings of process in the context of life-and-illness should be seen in connection with several aspects of his or her work: It helps to determine the points of entry and reentry into a patient's situation; it keeps the social worker aware that anticipatory and preparatory work, assessment of a situation, and efforts to help people perceive and contend with burdensome realities are continual for each patient/family. Since a life-situation and an illness-situation are always in flux, their interaction changes too; change demands psychosocial adjustment and adaptation, which can be facilitated by the social worker's intervention.

The concept of process, like other good ideas, is liable to misuse. At worst, it can become an interminable substitute for decisive action and for coming to terms with realities. Fortunately, the limits that are built into or inherent in many conditions and circumstances of life can serve as pivotal points for precipitating the end of a process and the attainment of a goal.

UNREALIZED POTENTIALITIES
IN CURRENT SOCIAL WORK PRACTICE

An examination of a professional practice is expected to disclose shortcomings as well as strengths. In fact, the advancement of a profession depends in no small part on the identification of the gaps, flaws, and deficiencies about which remedial action can be taken in professional education and in the world of work.

Social work practice is broadly conceived here to include the various functions and kinds of responsibility that social workers assume in general teaching hospitals—in particular, giving direct service, supervising, providing and using consultation, participating in research, administering departments and units of social service, and both formally and informally teaching students at various educational levels who have a major interest in the health care field. Preventive social work is not listed as one of the profession's missions—a situation akin to the relatively minor practice of preventive medicine.[7]

In this field, intraprofessional and interprofessional collaboration as a way of working may occur in each of the functions and specific tasks that social workers undertake. Collaboration is, in these terms, not a function but an instrumentality in the performance of a function.

Formulating and using concepts of practice are behaviors that characterize professions generally. Concepts are abstractions drawn from specifics and particulars. Concepts are a form of generalization that bind and give meaning to a constellation of particulars that have attributes in common, though at first glance they may seem to be disparate. Because concepts help to classify and unify experience and can serve as organizing themes, they are valuable aids in the learning process, in research, in building knowledge, and in applying knowledge by consciously translating it into concrete skills or techniques.

Both the formulation and the utilization of concepts are, so to speak, conservators. Concepts, once tested and found true, eliminate the necessity for starting each specific experience anew. Although intuition certainly plays a part, formulating, testing, and applying concepts are activities that are largely intellectual in nature. Social workers as a group of professionals do not excel in these activities, but there is every reason to expect that in the future large numbers will acquire much greater proficiency in them. It will be rewarding in all of their professional efforts.

The social worker tends to illustrate and demonstrate through the use of individual case histories or descriptions of professional performance case-by-case, and he or she uses such specific experiences with skill and considerable effectiveness. It is a skill to be valued; it makes people and situations come alive and makes matters human and psychologically palpable that would otherwise be remote and depersonalized phenomena.

However, a professionally useful understanding of patients/families' experiences in illness or of the decisions and actions of givers-of-service requires going behind or beyond empirical data to generalizations in the forms of principles and concepts which explain, elucidate, and interpret people's actions and reactions as well as the ebb and flow of life-situations.

This discussion, which began with the importance of concepts, must now be expanded into a statement on intellectual effort as a disciplining, productive, and creative way of working in a profession concerned with human services. Social workers must constantly ask questions such as "Why?" "Under what circumstances?" "What is the evidence?" "How do the needs and resources balance out?" "What interventions are suitable?" "What are the probable outcomes?" Hunches, intuitions, emotions, and observations must be put to the test.

It is by means of the intellect that logical conclusions can be drawn from empirical data, individual and social problems can be identified, priorities for professional attention can be determined, suitable interventions can be selected, hypotheses can be formulated for research, and research can be designed, executed, and concluded. Principles and concepts emerge from such rigorous intellectual activity and can then be applied as needed to specific situations. The solution of human problems that are psychosocial in nature requires constant movement from inductive to deductive processes and back again—from the synthesis of data into generalizations to their analysis into constituent elements.

An expanded base of knowledge is a recommendation consistent with the formulation and use of generalizations. Urging an expanded base of knowledge stems, first, from the immediate need of social workers to understand and use currently available information, truths, and perceptions that they do not now command and, second, from the long-term need to keep abreast of newly learned substance from their own and their allied fields of interest.[8]

Such short-term and long-term objectives are usually attained in a variety of ways, for example, through programs of staff development and continuing education; well-ordered, small, and informal searches; highly organized and controlled formal research designs; and, always and endlessly, reading the professional literature in the multiprofessional and multidisciplinary health care field. New learnings from the biomedical sciences, new observations from direct service practitioners in allied fields as well as from researchers, findings that result from social workers' applying new knowledge from allied fields to their own understanding and skills—these are but a few of the resources that social workers can tap to expand their base of knowledge.

What new light is being thrown on the natural history of both the cause and course of disease? On the physical growth and development of human beings? On the fetus' protection from, and vulnerability to, damaging forces such as infectious diseases, drug and alcohol addiction, and abnormal genetic materials?[9] On the institution of the family as a unit, which in the midst of change has identifiable characteristics (cohesiveness or disunity, mutual support or mutual sabotage, mutual respect or mutual disregard) which can be described in regard to ideals, values, goals, ambitions, mores, patterns of behavior, place in the community, and even at times patterns of illness? A dimension of this broadened concept of family—one not yet well enough explored—is the growth of the family in developmental stages that correspond to changes in life-situations induced both by demands made by society and by the developmental changes occurring in the lives of family members. Considerable material about the family as a unit is available in the literature of the behavioral and social sciences and needs to be assessed and adapted by social workers for use in their professional fields—health care, family and child welfare, income maintenance, corrections, among others. A literal transposition of ideas from a contributing discipline to a practicing profession is seldom feasible; distillation and adaptation by members of the profession are essential intermediate steps.

It is necessary to be aware of and to understand the interacting relationships of individual family members and to recognize when one person among them needs help in his or her own right. However, unless the family is conceived of also as a unit, even when ill-functioning, the social worker may fail to identify and use inherent strengths, or at worst may further fragment an already disintegrating group. Until recently the idea of the family as a unit and the practice of family therapy and other forms of family intervention has been more familiar to, and more frequently used by, practitioners in the field of mental health than by those involved in physical health care. As the term *social-health* acquires more meaning for those involved in physical health care and the interdependence of systems of care is better understood, they are placing greater weight than formerly on knowing and working with family members, individually and in groups. Sometimes it is the chief of medical service whose humanistic interests make him or her peculiarly sensitive to the idea of family. Sometimes the fact that a disease or deficiency is genetic in nature has a part in promoting a more rounded notion of the family as a unit. In addition, the practice of social workers in hospital-based home care programs reflects a perception of family that closely approximates the idea of the family as a unit.

The hospital setting itself rarely organizes clinical services in such a way as to promote the concept of the family as a unit and the practices of family intervention. When comprehensive medical care units have been established for ambulatory patients, separation of family members into age groups still occurs. As one knowledgeable social worker said, "If it is necessary to work with the family as a whole, it will be the social worker who does it." One suspects that putting greater weight on the family as a unit would be closer to a social model than to the classical medical model. In the hospital setting certainly, the deployment of social workers has usually conformed in this and other ways to the organization of medical and surgical services.

The tendency to overlook the family as a unit may also have been seen in relation to the social workers' hospital-bound practice. It gives rise to a number of questions: How might the concept of the family as a unit help to extend the social worker's activities beyond the hospital walls? How might the concept, put into operation, affect knowledge about, and services to, patients/families in the postdischarge period? Are there valid differences in the way the concept of the family as a unit should be operative in medical/surgical as compared to psychiatric services? Is an early assessment of the family as a unit essential to good medical care? The process of making an assessment of this kind does not lead inevitably to family intervention as the social worker's method of choice; this distinction should be kept clearly in mind.

But commitment to the concept of the family as a unit by multiprofessional personnel in a hospital setting could influence policy, regulations, procedures, and selected aspects of structure and organization.

The idea of the family as a unit also needs to be more fully developed in programs of education for social work. Traditionally, graduate schools of social work organized their teaching of practice into separate sequences for social work with individuals (social casework) and social work with groups (social group work). It was and still is also common in education and in work experience to refer to social work intervention with "individuals, families, and small groups"[11]—a manner of speaking that seems to place the family (unit or group) apart from small groups. There are great differences between kinship groups and nonkinship groups, but perhaps something valuable gets lost when no connections between the two are identified.

The more recent emphasis in educational programs for social workers on social problems and how to solve them has highlighted the need for students to acquire knowledge and skill in both social casework and social group work. This recognition may foster more widespread conviction about the concept of the family as a unit.

Collaboration might be designated as the most sought-after and perhaps the most elusive instrumentality in professional performance. As a rule, team-work now evokes the picture of a group that "works with a leader to whom every other member is subordinate. He therefore has jurisdiction over everyone else."[12] Although some persons use *team* also in another sense, it is becoming usual to think of this other sense as collaborative work or simply collaboration. Collaboration implies a group

> of people with different sets of skills and knowledge [which]
> constitute a cluster of skills and knowledge appropriate to the
> needs of a particular patient or groups of patients or clients. The
> connotation is that the determination of the appropriateness of a
> particular individual professional person must be made largely by
> that person but with the knowledge of the other members of the
> team. In such a team, subordination and hierarchy are replaced
> by equal opportunity for the participating professionals to contrib-
> ute to the welfare of the human beings at and with whom they
> are directing their efforts—as a team.[13]

In the following comments the distinction will be preserved by using *collaboration* to denote the second meaning of *team*. The very substance of the definition above makes it easy to understand why collaboration is not easy to achieve. No one professional is "more equal," as we say cynically, than any other. Competitiveness for power and rank is out. Learning from one another is in, and so is working together, while differences in knowledge and skill are not only respected but utilized for the benefit of the patients/families under care.

There has to be congruity—or at least an empathic understanding—concerning significant values and ethical behaviors, and there has to be agreement about the ultimate goals to be reached, although members of the professional group will have diverse immediate and intermediate goals in accordance with their professional fields and specialties and the expected outcomes of their professional efforts.

There is probably no absolute autonomy that can be exercised by the members of any profession working either individually or collectively in an institutional setting. Certainly professional collaboration in a hospital requires renouncing the idea of autonomy in a pure sense; but on the other hand it requires of each member of a unit a strong sense of belonging to one's profession, self-reliance coupled with interdependence, willingness among personnel to learn from one another, and the ability to work together with respect for the differences in knowledge, skills, and specific objectives that characterize different professions or functions within a profession.

Intraprofessional collaboration has not received much attention in the literature. Perhaps the most significant references have been to the problematic situations that exist between social work educators in schools of social work and social work practitioners at various levels of the hierarchies in social agencies.[14] A few of the most controversial issues have concerned the undergraduate and graduate schools' end product. What should the social worker with a baccalaure-ate or a master's degree from an accredited school be able to do at the point of entry into professional practice? What are the most desirable areas of knowledge the beginning social worker should have? What are the optimal conditions for a social work student's field work experience—the practicum—including the qualifications of the field work instructor? Does education or practice have the leading edge? It may be surprising that professional social workers, all of whom share the ultimate goal of improving the general social welfare, have difficulty working collaboratively. Yet there are tensions between administrators and middle management personnel and between each of these groups and the givers of direct service. There is also a lingering tension between social workers assigned to medical and surgical services on the one hand and psychiatric services on the other, even in hospitals in which all social workers are members of one department.

As in any group of professionals, there is diversity among individuals in respect to such matters as preferred policies, attitudes toward change, priorities in goals, the most desirable methods for achieving agreed-upon goals and the like. Some tensions are therefore inevitable; some are even useful insofar as advancement is often the consequence of resolved issues.

In contrast to the relative silence concerning the problems of intraprofessional collaboration, there is a clamor about the desirability of improving the quality of interprofessional collaboration, of making it a more pervasive instrument throughout the health care field, and of initiating the concept and the practice of collaborative efforts in programs of education for the health professions.[15, 16, 17] These are concerns openly expressed by members of several health and health-related professions, and the candor with which they have explored this aspect of practice testifies to their wish to master the problems.[18]

The social worker's efforts to develop effective collaborative relationships with physicians have usually been on a one-by-one, one-to-one basis. The social workers have used what they know about individuals, their characteristics, and their patterns of behavior to observe a physician's predilections and dislikes, ways of working, demonstrated responsiveness or lack of it to social work activities, and most cherished professional values, and how they compare with those of the social worker. Essentially, the social worker has endeavored to encourage the physician's interest in the psychosocial components of the patient/family's situation and his or her understanding of the relation between these components and the biomedical aspects of the patient's condition. The social worker has hoped that with an individual physician's enriched understanding, the two professionals could work together more effectively and that successful collaboration on behalf of a number of patients/families would act cumulatively to achieve a more permanent and stable collaborative relationship between the social worker and the physician.

The one-to-one approach is often gratifyingly successful, and there may be also an encouraging ripple effect that reaches other social workers and other physicians. However, it is an approach that by nature cannot institutionalize belief in or competent use of collaboration. To speed progress and to incorporate collaboration as an integral component of professional competence, more extensive underpinnings and supports are needed to create a broader strategy.

First, social workers need a broader base from which to work, and it is hoped that the fundamentals will be provided in their programs of professional education. Social workers in all fields of practice have to work with members of other professions. Although the field of health and medical care probably makes the greatest demand in this regard, one has to look at the frequency with which social workers must work with schoolteachers, lawyers, judges, and correctional officers, as well as with people in industry, government, experimental laboratories, and the like.[19]

The notion that interprofessional collaboration is a way of working that can be analyzed, conceptualized, taught, and learned—by doing—should do much to reduce the current level of frustration expressed by so many who are engaged in the human services. It does take at least two to collaborate, and, among many factors, gaps in the physician's professional education, similar to those found in the social worker's, as well as society's perception of the physician as a person of awesome knowledge and authority, play their part in making collaboration difficult.

Since many who wish to develop their skill in collaboration have long since completed their basic professional education, the potentials residing in programs for staff development and for continuing education must also be considered in the quest for new and broader supports.

The excerpt that follows is from the report of a social worker who was a participant in a seminar for staff development concerned with interprofessional collaboration. The leader of the seminar used a conceptual approach which is clearly reflected in the participant's report on the effectiveness of a disciplined learning experience.

> I have become more cautious and more objective in the analysis
> of some difficulties. I have become more aware of the variables
> which influence the collaborative process. I am less prone to put
> the blame [for] our difficulties on differences in ideology.... I
> tend now to look more for a common ground, shared values and
> goals, encouraging a better knowledge, understanding and respect
> of each discipline. I am trying to avoid ... the social worker's
> "messiah-type" approach which ... generally evokes negative re-
> sponse in others[20]

Another underpinning that facilitates successful collaboration is the mutual understanding that members of the various professions can gain of the objectives, content, organization, and expected product of one another's programs of professional education. Identifying the similarities and differences among these programs facilitates the understanding of what working together will mean.

The active, vigorous support of administrators in the hospital or other institutional setting is essential to promote the efforts of those at the operational level to work collaboratively. Interprofessional collaboration has to be wanted and fostered as an institution-wide policy by the leaders and administrators of the facility. Although it is widely conceded that health care is not and cannot be the responsibility of any one profession, we are still in the early stages of developing a truly collective approach to problems in the field, whether in a single institution or in the larger systems of delivering services.

The involvement of social workers in social work research[21] has continued to be restricted despite the increase in doctoral programs over the past 20 years and the inclusion of research in the master's degree programs for many years more than that.

> *Medical social work has long had empirical knowledge in the*
> *health field concerning different categories of individuals. . . . How-*
> *ever, the profession has shown little inclination to use the*
> *knowledge in creating new approaches to problem-solving for*
> *these groups. Social workers in health and medical care must not*
> *only become involved in research but must be more articulate*
> *regarding their findings if their contribution to the health field is*
> *to be identified and used."* [22]

The comparative lack of research activity is accompanied by few planned attempts to apply or test the research findings that are available.

The orientation of social work to social problems, whether it occurs in educational programs, in professional practice, or in social work research, makes it imperative for social workers to understand the significance of epidemiology, the principles and concepts that constitute its base of operations, and the applicability of this scientific method of research to social work. [23, 24]

Epidemiology won formal recognition at the turn of this century when the search for the causal agents of, effective treatment modalities for, and preventive measures against infectious diseases expanded and intensified. Although infectious diseases are currently of lesser urgency in the United States, medicine continues to find this science indispensable for the study of chronic diseases and other medical problems affecting individuals, families, and populations, small and large.

The knowledge and application of epidemiology in social work research are now overdue. The independent and dependent variables that are suitable for the study of social problems will differ from those identified for medical problems. However, the principles and concepts on which social work studies will be based will not differ, and the final yield from such inquiries will be as relevant to the advancement of social work and the general welfare as comparable inquiries are to medicine and public health.

Social workers have professional responsibility for identifying the problems to be investigated, selecting the appropriate variables, applying their knowledge of statistics, thinking logically about the relationships among variables, and noting patterns in the qualitative and quantitative data they obtain. It is by means of epidemiological studies that social workers will discover the facts about social problems under investigation, such as their incidence and prevalence, their characteristics, the conditions associated with them, the conditions that may have cause-and-effect relationships to a specified problem, and the questions that have been generated for further study.

In essence, risk factors may be positively or tentatively identified, as may the loci in which the social problems occur, the people who have to cope with the problems, and so on. Findings of this sort will spur ideas about the entry of social workers into problem situations, their reasons and objectives, ideas about the deployment of social workers in the case of both small and large populations, and similar issues.

Considering that epidemiological studies have traditionally been concerned with populations of considerable size, it is understandable that their appropriateness in regard to smaller populations has been overlooked. In the field of health care, social workers should not only participate in such studies of populations but should also initiate their own inquiries in the facility in which they work—inquiries that may be institution-wide or confined to a selected population, such as the patients in a single service unit or in a particular risk category.

The studies may be motivated by a variety of professional problems which call for better understanding by social workers in both direct and indirect (implementing) services. The important point is that social workers recognize how fundamental the application of epidemiology is to the solution of some of their unanswered questions.

Social workers in the health care field are—or, it is hoped, will soon be— in a particularly good position to promote the idea of interdisciplinary and interprofessional studies in epidemiology. For example, child abuse is a social and medical problem that engages the interest of social and behavioral scientists as well as professional practitioners.[25]

The unrealized potentials concerning research in social work raise questions such as the following: Do the graduate schools of social work fail to connect research activity for the advancement of knowledge with examining the day-by-day, bread-and-butter problems of social work practice? Is the discomfort of social workers with generalizations, principles, and concepts associated with their sparse involvement in research? Has research become so identified with large grants and complicated designs that the application of an orderly method of study to small, clearly defined, and highly focused problem areas is not recognized as research activity?

Coming closer to research in the health care field, under what circumstances can research be confined to one profession or discipline? The concept of biopsychosocial integrity leads one more and more to believe that multiprofessional and multidisciplinary involvement should become more the rule and less the exception.

It is cause for concern that social workers are so seldom participants in the planning and conduct of research projects that are originated by physicians in hospital settings. When the social worker does come into the picture, it is more often as a person outside the research design who is asked to help patients cope with the consequences of being the subjects of research. Physicians are sometimes startled to hear from the administrator of the social services department that without prior planning and budgetary arrangements a staff member cannot be made available to the research project. Although these may be unhappy occasions, in the long run they often have excellent results in that they precipitate clarifying exchanges about the multiprofessional aspects of health care. One fruitful outcome may be agreement to consider from the beginning whether interprofessional activity is an essential component of a projected undertaking. This is collaborative preparatory work as important in research (and in teaching, administration, and so on) as it is in giving direct service to patients/families.

The increasing development of programs for peer review within and among the several health and health-related professions is an added stimulus for social workers to develop greater interest and skill in research oriented to their professional practice. Unless peer review is based as far as possible on the planned study of relevant, substantiated facts, peer review could be capricious and unjust, regardless of the intent to be fair and unbiased.

Effecting institutional change is usually a long and challenging process at any level of operations. Many people are affected by even small changes; several departments of an organization may be involved; and in the field of health and medical care institutional change tends to disturb the accustomed ways and status of persons who belong to different professional, technical, and vocational groups. What is of concern here is how some of the inherent difficulties might be made less severe and less frustrating to social workers who believe that change in a given situation will ultimately effect improvement in the quality and delivery of services.

A certain amount of inertia—a disinclination to move or to "make waves"—is to be expected in individuals and in groups. Except for the few already convinced of the need for change and who lead the struggle for change, there will be some resistance. While some resistive persons yield to emotional appeals or philosophical arguments, hard-nosed evidence is most persuasive.

Unilateral action directed toward achieving change is occasionally successful. However, more and more, planned change is achieved by coalitions of concerned individuals and groups whose concerted action is made possible by virtue of similar or compatible motives, goals, and methods of operation.

Social workers and their colleagues in other professions in the field of health care do not yet have the opportunities they need to learn the guiding concepts and principles and the methods and processes involved in making institutional (or systemic) change. They need to perceive more accurately and fully the relationship between the research method and the process of effecting institutional change. They would be helped greatly by making the dynamic connections that exist between the principles and concepts underlying collaboration and those that are basic to achieving institutional change.

By no means will all social workers have the taste and temperament for making large-scale institutional or systemic change their area of expertness. On the other hand, one can justify their being knowledgeable about ways and means because minimal expectations of the professional social worker should include (1) understanding the implications of policy, law, and programs in the human services; forming opinions of support or opposition; and, at the least, exercising one's right to take a position and (2) participating in effecting small-scale improvements to which there is little opposition and which promise immediate benefits to a circumscribed population of patients/families.

Thus the potential range of institutional change in which social workers may be involved is very wide—from a decision to make a social worker available immediately to every patient in the hospital for whom a laryngectomy is recommended or to make public telephones easily available to relatives waiting outside intensive care units, to a decision to work toward redistributing social work services throughout a given hospital for the purpose of increasing the coverage of ambulatory patients but without increasing the size of the social work staff or to work toward reducing the statewide costs of medical care while retaining essential services.[26]

The first two illustrations of change are quite limited in scope, in the numbers of patients/families affected, and in the number and range of personnel who would have to agree and provide for the changes. The second two illustrations are far-flung. The first within the boundaries of one institution will affect the total patient population and professional staff in the long run and requires highly sophisticated and creative efforts to establish criteria for selection of patients/families and probably some preparation of staff for new roles and patterns of work. The second spills over the boundaries of one institution to several systems of care related to the human services and to the deliberations of governmental bodies and the wishes and opinions of consumers of health care.

LOOKING AHEAD TO TOMORROW

It is an axiom that members of the professions have to be educated for the future. It is true that the exact shape of the profession's future is not predictable; nor can it be known with accuracy what technologies, instruments, knowledge, and new truths will be revealed or when they may be available. There will also be changes in society which we can speculate about with our usual human imprecision. The fact that the two kinds of change act upon each other is certain to compound the problems of preparing for the future.[27, 28]

These unknowns are part of living in a dynamic world, and for one thing they imply that being educated for the future means being prepared to handle and cope with uncertainty, doubt, frustration, gratification, failure, success, change, and adaptation. The preparation is not all attitudinal and emotional. It has its concrete, pragmatic aspects: knowing the optimum conditions for one's own learning and being aware of one's own learning patterns, identifying one's strongest motivations for learning, continuously determining one's own learning needs; and having a working knowledge of the best resources for learning and how to use them (the professional literature and the publications of allied sciences, programs of continuing education, professional consultants, and the like). Lastly, there are the stimuli imposed from without, such as required recertification or relicensing and peer review, which are instruments for control of the quality of services and the protection of the consumer-public.

Furthermore, though the image of the future is always blurred, trends and tendencies are identifiable and can be used as guide lines in the never-ending processes of improving professional practice; advancing the content, quality, and effectiveness of educational programs directed toward the human services; and making more adequate provision of resources needed by the various consumer groups in our society.

The trends and tendencies in health care have a number of inherent contradictions due largely to the choices that have to be made between the desirable and the possible. There seems to be no place to hide from the dilemmas created by an economy of scarcity. Social workers in or entering the field of health care and concerned about the future of their profession and its individual members will be considering what their purposes and functions may be in the vast and varied arena of health care. The trends and tendencies can be thought of as clustering around goals and institutions. If a perfect logic were achievable, projected or probable changes in institutions and systems would be compatible with goals, and they in turn would be compatible with society's needs. In the real world there is much illogic and compromise, vested interests play for power, and a rationale may be a rationalization. These are hazards in a democracy—partial costs of the unequaled benefits that accrue from an open society.

Some of the trends and tendencies are as yet only strongly held views, but even without supporting action they are influential ideas to be discussed and evaluated. Under the rubric of goals are the following: to extend more, and more adequate, health and medical care to patients who are ambulatory; to make more appropriate utilization of hospital beds; to enable more persons with chronic diseases or disabilities to live and function socially in their natural environments; to develop professionally sound and effective programs of consumer education which will help members of a community take both increased and appropriate responsibility for their own health; to encourage the formation of responsible organizations for self-help and make available to them the knowledge and skills of professionals in the health care field in order to enhance the competence and effectiveness of such groups of concerned laypersons; to strengthen greatly the causes of promoting and maintaining health and preventing disease, disability, and social dysfunctioning; to provide primary medical care, which is one of the greatest needs for the greatest numbers of people; to lower the costs of health care; to resolve or minimize the ethical dilemmas that are created by a range of dynamic forces, from the dissension about basic research into "gene splicing" or recombinant DNA to the conflicts between the patient's right to choose death and the physician's professional obligation to heal and to save, to factors such as the burdens of rising costs which affect individual givers-of-service, to the increasing pressure on groups of professionals to unionize.[29, 30]

Under the rubric of institutional/systemic trends are the following: an increase in the number of Health Maintenance Organizations, an increase in facilities and programs that will meet more adequately the need for progressive and other kinds of differentiated care, and increased provision of programs for genetic counseling. It is fairly safe to expect vigorous pursuit in research programs (established in industrial plants, in government-sponsored research organizations, in medical centers, and so on) on the effects of industrial materials and industrial waste matter on the health of individuals, families, and populations and similar problems connected with ecology that lend themselves to study and experimentation by the experts in environmental medicine and allied disciplines and professions. In some research projects now underway, there is encouraging evidence of coalitions among physicians, scientists, industrial management, and labor unions whose joint support in manpower and finances is producing valuable findings for the better protection and social functioning of our human resources.

The almost overpowering need to reduce the costs of health care and increase the efficiency of administration and the effectiveness of programs and services is being recognized at various governmental levels in actions that sometimes promise eventual benefits and sometimes threaten near disaster.

At the same time, at every governmental level medical and medically related services are being eliminated or drastically reduced, patients' copayments and deductibles are being increased, available services are being made less accessible through the closing of facilities, and the size of staffs is being controlled by attrition and dismissal. These measures are taken largely in response to fiscal crises and to the uncovering of fraudulent practices (some by patients but a large number by givers-of-service and institutional providers) and as a means of redressing old or preventing new forms of wrongdoing. Insofar as many of these and similar measures will not serve as correctives but will increase suffering and hardship, they are indicators of where future efforts by social workers and their colleagues in the related professions should be directed.[31]

Forecasting the fate of the many contemporary proposals for national health insurance is impossible, but the necessity for keeping abreast of developments, understanding the arguments for and against the respective proposals, and making valid judgments to support, modify, or reject them is indisputable.[32] National health insurance is a funding mechanism, not a system of delivering services. The experience of the last eight or nine years will have indicated to many consumers that money appropriated in the absence of sound medical-social policy and of coordinated, comprehensive programs which assure continuity of services is a means without an end.

Where, how, and in what roles social workers in health care will assume responsibility in the years immediately ahead cannot be foretold with precision. The answers will be shaped in part by developments in the professionalism of social work; by successful nurturing of social workers' currently unrealized potentials; by advancement toward socially desirable goals for health care agreed upon by coalitions of multiprofessional groups; by priorities established by governmental bodies and a democratic society for the education, allocation, and recompense of manpower needed in the health care field; and by other unforeseen ways in which political and professional powers influence the form, functions, and substance of health care. The differentiations among the related professions encourage a process of sharing with and contributing to one another that in the end can reach the persons served in the form of more enlightened and greatly enriched health and medical care. Perhaps it is reasonable to hope that the ultimate result of such collaboration will be a contribution to the enhancement of the human condition.

Social workers, as one group among many, should take a distinctive leadership role in the coming era of the health care field. Health care has become a major concern in this nation of over 200 million people. Concerns about the extent of coverage, financial and social costs, funding mechanisms, methods of delivering services, and assurance of high quality of service and of professional and financial accountability is expressed by the general public at all socioeconomic levels, by officials at all levels of government, by individual practitioners and institutional providers in our systems of health care, and by members of business, commerce, and industry.[33, 34]

Although the concerns are shared by these diverse groups, there are significant differences among them in perspectives and social philosophy, in priorities, in preferred methods of solving problems in the health care field, and in immediate and long-term objectives. An authentic democracy nourishes diversity but at the same time requires progress in the name of growth and advancement of the common good, so that persons with differing backgrounds, functions, and tasks will be able to work together toward the ultimate goals of individual fulfillment and the betterment of society.

Another kind of diversity which is becoming more and more widespread in the health care field is within the profession. Within the respective organizations of physicians, nurses, and social workers there are subgroups differentiated by kind and level of education, by function, and by the nature of their competence. From these differences result the allocation of those responsibilities best suited to people's highest qualifications. In general, the expectation is that such differentiated use of manpower will enhance the quality of direct services, reduce the fragmentation and interruption of health and medical services, lessen the cost of services in the long run, and improve patient education. Paramedics, physicians' assistants, licensed and unlicensed practical nurses, nurse-clinicians, nurse-practitioners, unit managers, social work assistants, social work aides, and social work advocates are among the now familiar titles. There is not yet full acceptance of these relatively new personnel or sufficient evaluative data regarding the efficiency and effectiveness of their performance and of the controls and safeguards maintained in behalf of patients. This is an enormous area calling for evaluative research.

Looking back at the recorded history of social welfare and social betterment in this country, there were the great pioneers and reformers of the nineteenth century who worked with one another, learned from one another, and enlisted the support of liberal-minded private citizens, philanthropists, and legislators, and achieved some remarkable results.[35] Their efforts in behalf of the poor, the disabled, and the physically and mentally ill began before the existence of schools of social work, organizations of social workers or indeed the title of social worker. We inherit from them a great legacy of commitment and conviction, as we do also from our immediate predecessors whose accomplishments were directed toward the issues of their day and, as is fitting, reflect the society in which they lived and worked.

As a social worker whose professional experience goes back over 50 years and among whose contemporaries numbered a few of the pioneers, many of the most creative of their immediate successors, as well as the luminaries of the current era, I am looking now at the past in order to hope for the future.

It is my personal assessment that as might be expected of members of any profession, social workers have made some notable mistakes that need not be repeated. We have frequently adopted rather than adapted knowledge and techniques from related professions and disciplines. This kind of behavior on our part has often looked faddish, especially when we have discarded what we knew and did instead of going through the process of modification and integration. Sometimes we have abdicated, allowing members of other professions or disciplines to take over when we should have worked with them in ways to use their knowledge and skills for the advancement of our own. During the decade or so of the urban crisis (although no crisis lasts ten years; the misnomer may have been part of our problem) there was a split in the organized profession of social work that was in itself a misfortune. It was the period when social activism reached a high point at the expense of advancing the development of direct services. There is no question but that both areas are essential, and both will continue to need our professional attention. Should we fail again to realize that the large-scale results of social activism are for the benefit of people here and now and in the future, we will lose an outstanding opportunity for leadership.[36]

Errors like these have served to distort our functions and objectives. Perhaps it is fundamental to those errors that we have insufficiently assured ourselves of our worth to society and the validity of our purpose and overall mission. Socialization into our own profession, in other words, is less than complete.[37, 38] The results are confusing, especially when social workers attempt to find professional stability and individual assurance by means of partial assimilation into a profession or discipline with greater status.

Although our unsureness reflects in part the attitudes of colleagues in other fields, the time has come for us to meet the challenge with both our tested and potential strengths.

Social workers possess some solid advantages for sharing leadership in the further development of health care. With few exceptions social workers are accustomed to practice collectively and to be aware of their influence on other people. They have extensive knowledge about human relationships, and in an age that puts a premium on ecology and the importance of the environment, their focal point is the interface between human beings and the outside world.

One of the greatest advantages that social workers have lies in their ability to be empathic with individuals very different from themselves in social philosophy and values, education, ethnic background, economic and occupational status, and the like. It is not that empathy is an attribute unique to social workers. It is rather that the demand on them is heavy and constant to develop the attribute fully and use it effectively. It is an essential quality for those whose professional focus is on the interaction between human beings with all their diversities and society with all the diverse impacts of its social and not-so-social institutions.

The expertness in empathic relationships is most often manifested in the giving of direct services to persons who are bound by a condition or interest held in common, as are patients and their relatives, but who are in disagreement or controversy with one another—over decisions that have to be made, plans that have to be formulated, options that have to be weighed and measured, behavioral changes that should take place.

It is expected that social workers in direct service learn to understand each individual locked in such psychological and emotional combat and to use their skills for the benefit of each individual in the group, kinship or other, to which that person may belong.

One of the few safe predictions is that the demand will increase for interprofessional and interdisciplinary collaboration and for consumer participation in making public policy and improving systems of delivering human services. These and similar administrative functions will afford social workers an unusual opportunity to put their talents for empathic relationships to the test. This is a transparent plea for social workers to develop to the fullest the capacity to advocate a cause, defend a principle, and uphold an opinion without becoming hostile opponents or turning dissenters into adversaries.

At bottom this is conduct that persuades and convinces and that eschews destroying or damaging others, but one that has a place for anger against injustice and the violation of human rights.

REFERENCES

1. John D. Thompson, "Health Care System: General Hospital," in *Encyclopedia of Social Work*, 16th ed. (New York: National Association of Social Workers, 1971) pp. 530-538.
2. Henry J. Meyer and Sheldon Siegel, "Profession of Social Work: Contemporary Characteristics," in *Encyclopedia of Social Work*, 17th ed. (Washington, D.C.: National Association of Social Workers, 1977) pp. 1067-1081.
3. Beatrice Phillips, "Social Workers in Health Services," in *Encyclopedia of Social Work*, 16th ed., op. cit., pp. 565-575.
4. Ibid.
5. Bess Dana, H. David Banta, and Kurt W. Deuschle, "An Agenda for the Future of Interprofessionalism," in *Medicine and Social Work*, ed. Helen Rehr (New York: Prodist, 1974), p. 79.
6. Victor R. Fuchs, *Who Shall Live?* (New York: Basic Books, 1974).

7. Milton Wittman, "Preventive Social Work," in *Encyclopedia of Social Work*, 17th ed., op. cit., pp. 1049-1054.

8. Øystein Sakala LaBianca and Gerald E. Cubelli, "A New Approach to Building Social Work Knowledge," *Social Work in Health Care*, vol. 2, no. 2 (winter 1976-1977), pp. 139-152.

9. Sylvia Schild, "Health Services: Genetic Counseling," in *Encyclopedia of Social Work*, op. cit., pp. 590-595.

10. L. Diane Bernard, "Education for Social Work," in *Encyclopedia of Social Work*, op. cit., pp. 290-300.

11. Scott Briar, "Social Casework and Social Group Work: Historical and Social Science Foundations," in *Encyclopedia of Social Work*, 16th ed., op. cit., p. 1244.

12. Cecil G. Sheps, "Developmental Perspectives in Interprofessional Education," in Rehr, op. cit., p. 3.

13. Ibid.

14. Jerome Cohen, "Selected Constraints in the Relationship Between Social Work Education and Practice," *Journal of Education for Social Work*, vol. 13, no. 1 (winter 1977), pp. 3-7.

15. Rosalie A. Kane, "Interprofessional Education and Social Work: A Survey," *Social Work in Health Care*, vol. 2, no. 2 (winter 1976-1977), pp. 229-238.

16. Betty Zippin Bassoff, "Interdisciplinary Education for Health Professions: Issues and Directions," *Social Work in Health Care*, vol. 2, no. 2 (winter 1976-1977), pp. 219-228.

17. Frances Nason and Thomas L. Delbanco, "Soft Services: A Major Cost-Effective Component of Primary Medical Care," *Social Work in Health Care*, vol. 1, no. 3 (spring 1976), pp. 297-308.

18. Jeanette Regensburg, "A Venture in Interprofessional Discussion," in Rehr, op. cit., pp. 35-73.

19. Betty Rusnack, "Planned Change: Interdisciplinary Education for Health Care," *Journal of Education for Social Work*, vol. 13, no. 1 (winter 1977), pp. 104-111.

20. *Skills in Interdisciplinary Collaboration*, mimeographed (Papers by participants in a seminar conducted by Dr. Hyman J. Weiner at the Mount Sinai Hospital Services, City Hospital Center at Elmhurst, Social Service Department, June 1974), p. 10.

21. Henry S. Maas, "Research in Social Work," in *Encyclopedia of Social Work*, 17th ed., op. cit., pp. 1183-1193.

22. Beatrice Phillips, "Social Workers in Health Services," in *Encyclopedia of Social Work*, 16th ed., op. cit., p. 571.

23. Brian M. MacMahon and Thomas F. Pugh, *Epidemiology: Principles and Methods* (Boston: Little, Brown, 1970).

24. Gary Friedman, *Primer of Epidemiology* (New York: McGraw-Hill, 1974).

25. B. Simons et al., "Child Abuse: Epidemiologic Study of Medically Reported Cases," *New York State Journal of Medicine*, vol. 66, no. 21 (November 1966), pp. 2783-2788.

26. Abraham Lurie, "Staffing Patterns: Issues and Program Implications for Health Care Agencies," *Social Work in Health Care*, vol. 2, no. 1 (fall 1976), pp. 85-94.

27. Bess S. Dana, "Health Care: Social Components," in *Encyclopedia of Social Work*, 17th ed., op. cit., pp. 544-550.

28. George L. Engel, "The Need for a New Medical Model: A Challenge for Biomedicine," *Science*, vol. 196, no. 4286 (April 1977), pp. 129-136.

29. Bess Dana, "Consumer Health Education," in *Health Services: The Local Perspective*, ed. Arthur Levin (*Proceedings of the Academy of Political Science*, vol. 32, no. 3 [1977]), pp. 182-192.

30. Bernard Ross, "Professional Dilemmas," in *Social Work Practice and Social Justice*, ed. Bernard Ross and Charles Shireman (Washington, D.C.: National Association of Social Workers, 1973), pp. 147-152.

31. Dorothy P. Rice, "Financial Social Welfare: Health Care," in *Encyclopedia of Social Work*, 17th ed., op. cit., pp. 468-478.

32. Jules H. Berman, "Medical Care in the United States: A Background for Health Insurance," *Washington Bulletin* (Social Legislation Information Service, January 24, 1977, vol. 25, issue 2.)

33. Sumner J. Hoisington, "Accountability in Social Welfare," in *Encyclopedia of Social Work*, 17th ed., op. cit., pp. 2-7.

34. Patricia Volland, "Social Work Information and Accountability Systems in a Hospital Setting," *Social Work in Health Care*, vol. 1, no. 3 (spring 1976), pp. 277-285.

35. Blanche D. Call, "Social Welfare: History," in *Encyclopedia of Social Work*, 17th ed., op. cit., pp. 1503-1512.

36. Katherine A. Kendall, "Signals from an Illustrious Past," *Social Casework*, vol. 58, no. 6 (June 1977), pp. 328-336.

37. Arthur G. Cryns, "Social Work Education and Student Ideology: A Multivariate Study of Professional Socialization," *Journal of Education for Social Work*, vol. 13, no. 1 (winter 1977), pp. 44-51.

38. Sidney M. Clearfield, "Professional Self-Image of the Social Workers: Implications for Social Work Education," *Journal of Education for Social Work*, vol. 13, no. 1 (winter 1977), pp. 23-30.

Appendix A

Appendix A

Appendix A
The Course of Illness:

CONSEQUENCES IN CHILDHOOD AND ADOLESCENCE

A general description of the effects of chronic illness and disability upon pediatric and adolescent patients, their relatives, significant others, and health care personnel needs the illumination of more precise and specific data. By tracing the natural course of two conditions through childhood and adolescence the continuum of their effects on the continuum of life will become apparent.

The illustrations that follow are reported from the perspective of social workers whose central focus is on psychosocial issues. They are issues that also have meaning for members of related professions and vocations in the field of health care. They are not issues unique to the conditions of diabetes in childhood and the congenital anomaly of cleft palate. Rather, they are examples that point up patterns of reactions and of cause-and-effect relationships which can be adapted for the better understanding of disorders with comparable characteristics.

DIABETES OF CHILDHOOD

Diabetes of childhood starts within the first 18 to 20 years of life, that is, anywhere from infancy and early childhood through adolescence. The general characteristics are its known familial and its possible genetic nature, and its chronicity and irreversibility. Since its origins are unknown, measures of primary prevention are unknown, although secondary measures can be taken, such as controlling the body weight of family members who are vulnerable to the disease and helping the family in other appropriate ways to maintain general good health. The fact that the disease is controllable in most instances is of great importance psychologically and socially to the patient/family, since they are faced with the fact that the condition is incurable.

Because the injection of insulin as well as dietary restrictions are essential to the medical treatment of the childhood diabetic, and since these interventions have special psychosocial implications for the patient/family, the course of treatment itself becomes a major condition of life. Of special importance are the need for continuity of care and of personnel, for a collaborative interprofessional approach by givers-of-service, and for the indispensable active participation by the patient and the caretaking adults in his or her natural milieu in the processes of diagnosis and treatment.

Impacts on the life-situation of the patient/family are continuous when there is a diabetic member of any age, and for this reason there should be constant reassessment by professional personnel of the family's life-situation. What goes on within the family constellation has special meaning. An emotional upset can send a patient's diabetes out of control or precipitate the onset of the disease. Therefore, helping a family to maintain as stable a climate as possible becomes an important task for all personnel involved in the family's care when it is known that a member is diabetic or the likelihood is clear that diabetes may develop in a member of the family. Since it is impossible to eliminate all upsets and strains, the availability of psychiatric consultation and treatment has unusual significance for these patients/families.

The familial nature of diabetes is one of its most stress-producing aspects. If the parents did not know it before, they learn it when a child's diabetes is diagnosed; the inquiry into the family's health and medical history always includes questions about diabetes in other family members. The child's parents may recall memories of a grandparent or aunt and his or her loss of a limb or serious vascular disturbance or visual difficulty. These memories are upsetting, and the parents' anxiety for their child is heightened and affects their way of relating to and caring for the young patient.

It is unusual for parents not to place blame, perhaps on each other, on ancestors, or on themselves, as they begin to cope with the idea of a familial, lifetime illness in the family. The marital relationship can withstand this stressful period when it is fundamentally sound to start with and when the partners have inner resources to draw on, as they probably have had in the past, to meet critical situations. It is a time when a social worker can be actively supportive and helpful; if the strain threatens disintegration more than it promises increased cohesion between parents, they may need psychiatric help as well.

A diabetic child's siblings may find the care and attention given to the young patient a source of considerable distress. The younger the patient, the more direct care and protection he or she gets from his or her parents. It is usual for the mother to be giving most of this care; a specially close tie may develop between her and the patient that arouses jealousy, competitiveness, and frustration in the child's siblings. The parents' attention is also apt to be drawn away from the nondiabetic children when the patient is hospitalized. He or she is prone to infections which do not clear up easily and therefore is admitted to the hospital for treatment far more than nondiabetic children. Commitment of the social worker to the inherent values of a nurturing family, as well as interest in serving the patient per se, lead the social worker to include the patient's siblings in plans for enhancing the well-being of the family group. The social worker is likely to be helpful to the patient's siblings via counseling with their parents on problems connected with the patient's condition. Such counseling rests on the premise that it is more desirable to enable parents to work problems out with their children than for the social worker to take over, though at times it is necessary to work directly with the children.

The injection of insulin, necessary throughout life when diabetes starts in childhood, is observed to be a source of conflict at some point in almost every family. A child under eight or nine years of age has to be given injections, and it is usually his or her mother who takes the responsibility. Sometimes she fears being responsible for something so important to her child's life; sometimes she can't stick a needle into her child; sometimes she and others in the family associate injection of insulin with the socially unacceptable use of drugs. In most instances, the mother masters her reluctance with the help of the physician, the nurse (who teaches her how to measure the dose and make the injection), and the social worker. At times, however, she cannot learn to cope with her problem, and her husband takes the responsibility. In any case, at least two adults should be thoroughly informed and prepared to do what is necessary for the care of a diabetic child; one must anticipate that a parent's illness, occasional absence from the home, and the like make a back-up indispensable.

The child himself or herself may resist the injections; he or she doesn't want the constant reminder that his or her body doesn't work as other children's bodies work; he or she doesn't want to be different; he or she doesn't want to be "stuck."

The next point of conflict is apt to be when the child is determined by the doctor to be mature and intelligent enough to self-administer the injection. In general, it is considered wise to avoid a child's becoming unnecessarily dependent on adults for the insulin. However, a strong interdependence often has to be reckoned with, and a change in its balance may raise objections in both patient and parent. Plainly, some patients do not want to do for themselves but prefer counting on the ministering parent for continued care and attention. The patient's reluctance to become more self-reliant may be reinforced by a mother who wants to continue with her familiar task. She may be fearful that the child will not follow the prescribed dosage and regimen; this is a risk everyone has to take and test out when the child is judged ready to do more for himself or herself. It is more difficult to break the old routine if the mother's reluctance is rooted in an emotional bond that exists between her and her particularly needy child. The tie may be markedly ambivalent, with her guilt about the child's disease a strong element; and in this case the mother may need help to give up an old source of gratification and replace it with satisfaction in the child's developing maturity. One social worker cited the sad tale of an unbroken bond which held a mother and her grown married daughter in a kind of thralldom. The mother traveled every day from one city borough to another and back in order to give her daughter her insulin—a task the younger woman should normally have taken over a good 15 years earlier.

The next incidence of a major problem within the family group is likely to occur when the young diabetic patient enters adolescence. The combination of physiological change and emotional upsets may send a diabetic child's previously well-regulated disease out of control, or it may precipitate the onset of diabetes in a hitherto symptom-free adolescent. The adolescent's tendencies to fight authority and to wish to be like his or her peers identify this phase of his or her life-and-illness-situation as peculiarly threatening to his or her status of social-health. If the adolescent's behavior becomes deviant in regard to medication, diet, limitations on exercise, and so on, his or her parents' anxiety will mount and so will their efforts to reinstate the prescribed regimen.

An adolescent's anxiety about his or her body is a normal reaction, but for the diabetic it may be augmented. With a fuller realization of what diabetes is like, the adolescent may become discouraged and then depressed. A serious attempt to disregard or deny the disease may precipitate real threats to survival; in other words, the patient may become self-destructive. Parents, siblings, and the climate of the family unit may be upset by the patient's turmoil at the very time when his or her close relatives and givers-of-service need to work together to enable the adolescent patient to cope with his or her complex of medical, emotional, and social problems. Insofar as the family's difficulties may be aroused by and affect the patient's mental condition, it is often the physician who starts to explore with the adolescent and his or her close relatives what is taking place and for what reasons.

The reliability of individual informants is important. The accuracy of facts about their day-by-day living and behavior has great significance. For instance, when her child's diabetes goes out of control, what does the mother do? Pray? Call in the neighbors? Or give the child orange juice? A simple question like "What did you do?" will usually uncover more about emotions and attitudes than the question "How did you feel?"

In exploring the why's and wherefore's of an acute episode in the adolescent's condition, it is often a good idea to review, and perhaps add to, the patient/family's understanding of diabetes, its treatment, and the measures that will help to control the disease. Minor problems call for exploration in the hope of preventing escalation into major problems. Assessment of strengths and resources as well as of problems should lead to suitable steps toward resolution or diminution of problematic situations. For the most part, a matter-of-fact approach by professionals to the realities of the medical, psychological, and socioenvironmental aspects of the disease is anxiety reducing and effective in stimulating the patient/family's coping and adaptive mechanisms.

In the hospital setting, the physician's basic exploration and handling of the situation may lead to the patient/family's planned, continuous contact with a social worker. The social worker can strengthen the patient/family's understanding of the physician's explanations and recommendations, can help resolve conflict inherent in psychosocial problems, and can make available community resources suitable to the patient/family's needs.

The financial costs of insulin, of attending clinic, of transportation between home and hospital, of providing certain dietary items—that is, the money costs of the illness—cannot be ignored. If they create a strain on the family's budget, as they often do, they are likely to precipitate emotional strains as well. The social worker's knowledge of community resources is used to remove or diminish as many stress-producing factors in the socioeconomic arena as possible. This kind of help has value as a secondary preventive measure, but also it frees more of the patient/family's energies to cope with those pressures that cannot be removed by external means.

In many families the diabetic adolescent's special diet does not create major housekeeping problems. People seem to find ways to accommodate the diet within their habitual eating patterns. However, at the first point at which the physician's recommendations must be translated into portions, substitute foods are initially introduced, or the family homemaker immediately needs practical suggestions about marketing, the services of a dietitian are invaluable.

*Demands on the patient for adaptation** range far beyond those that occur within the family circle. However, within or outside the family unit the demands

* See introduction to Part II, pp. 45

are all connected and interacting, stemming as they do from the impacts of the same stress-producing disease. Looking at the demands made outside the family unit will help to understand how widespread the effects of the illness are. It must be emphasized that no matter where the impacts originate and how they impinge on the patient, their ripple effect touches relatives, significant others, and givers-of-service. So many adaptations have to be made by the patient that one social worker called the childhood diabetic a social deviant, though, to be sure, the deviance is imposed by a metabolic dysfunctioning for which the patient has no responsibility.

Changes in the patient's accustomed pattern of living come first to mind: the injection of insulin which must become an integral part of his or her regimen if he or she is to survive; the testing of urine; the regular medical examinations; the elimination of sweets from his or her diet; limits on the amount of food he or she should eat and of exercise he or she can engage in; carrying food in his or her pocket, not for a pleasurable snack but as a measure against insulin shock.

If the diagnosis of diabetes is made after the child has entered school, there will be changes in his or her pattern of school life. If the child enters school after the known onset of the illness, he or she will also have to adapt to differences in reactions from peers which affect his or her self-regard and the way in which others perceive the patient. The child's teacher must know that he or she is diabetic, must be informed about such symptoms as sleepiness or sweating, must allow the child to leave the room frequently to urinate, and must know that he or she takes insulin and what effects there may be. The teacher must also know that foods like ice cream and candy are forbidden and that this restriction is one of the child's most severe deprivations. In other words, the teacher has to keep an eye on the young patients and help them live within medical recommendations while at the same time allowing them to be as much as possible like their classmates.

The diabetic child's school life is apt to suffer more frequent interruptions than other children's. If the patient is not receiving adequate care at home or acquires an infection, he or she may be hospitalized recurrently. If he or she has overanxious parents, they may keep the child at home unnecessarily each day he or she is not feeling well. An underprotective parent, on the other hand, may ignore a child's infection too long and send him or her to school when the patient should be seen by a physician. One can expect then that the patient, family members, teachers, and schoolmates will influence one another, as not only the patient but all of them feel the impact from some aspect of the disease. These changes in everyday living are inseparable from changes in the patient's self-image and self-regard insofar as he or she develops understanding that a deficiency in bodily functioning makes him or her different from others.

Another demand inherent in the young diabetic's condition is adapting to a change in the amount and kind of responsibility he or she has to take increasingly to maintain his or her maximum status of social-health. Depending on the age of onset, the diabetic child is faced when quite young with restrictions on his or her freedom of choice in regard to food, games, and pace of exercise. As the patient grows into puberty and adolescence, he or she will wonder about other different and more difficult choices—about dating, a career, marrying, and having children.

The threat of curtailed freedom of choice that the patient feels should be recognized with him or her. The medical and social realities have to be openly discussed, unnecessary fears allayed, and risks frankly acknowledged. Anticipation of experiences such as staying overnight with friends, going on camping trips, or leaving home for boarding school or college raises a host of questions: "Do I tell them?" "Do I hide my insulin kit?" "What if they see a needle?" Although technical advances have made it relatively easy for a well-controlled adolescent diabetic to have a satisfying social life, there are still marks of difference from his or her peers and fears about their attitudes and feelings.

When the adolescent diabetic thinks about a career, he or she may again fear for his or her freedom of choice, and this fear will be based on certain realities. It is difficult, for example, for a diabetic to gain admission to a school of nursing; some employers are reluctant to hire diabetics because their schedules for mealtimes have to be relatively inflexible; or there may be a problem about obtaining a driver's license. Thus, a diabetic of any age may be in a dilemma about informing prospective employers of his or her condition. If the information is concealed and the patient one day goes into shock, he or she may lose the job and have great difficulty obtaining another. If the patient is frank about his or her diabetes, he or she may not get the job at all.

Lastly, there are many uncertainties with which a diabetic has to live, though some will become less acute and burdensome as time goes on. For example, as the patient learns to regulate and control the disease, modify the dosage of insulin to compensate for going off his or her diet and indulging in too much hard exercise, and so on, he or she is likely to endure less apprehension about going into shock and to feel more in control of his or her life. On the other hand, there are uncertainties that will be constants throughout life, even though not always in the forefront of consciousness. For the most part these are the uncertainties about the possible consequences of diabetes; the young patient learns more about them from contacts with older diabetics, from popular sources of information, and from scientific publications. The uncertainties will be about such unknowns as whether his or her bodily integrity will be further violated, by how much his or her life span may be shortened, or how difficult pregnancy may be and what risks the baby will run. Well before adulthood, the young diabetic may know that obtaining various kinds of insurance and compensation, including coverage for hospitalization, poses problems for him or her that other people do not have.

This account of demands for adaptation to stress-producing circumstances should not distort the realities of the young diabetic's opportunities for achieving a more satisfactory status of social-health than was true even ten years ago. He or she can attend regular classes at school and can learn to keep the disease under control even when he or she occasionally goes beyond prescribed bounds. A school-aged child can go to a camp that provides adequate care and when older can take trips, go away to college, choose among a number of vocations and professions, date, marry, and have children. Although these activities are in some degree limited and some carry definite risks to the patient and others, the overall gains are remarkable. Strong influence on the patient's well-being is exercised by the psychological support of family members; by available resources in medical care, education, and recreation; by the enlightened attitudes and technical competence of professional personnel; and, by no means last, by the continued expansion of biomedical knowledge.

CLEFT PALATE

Cleft palate was selected to illustrate the psychosocial impacts of a congenital anomaly because this defect has psychological and social effects comparable to other congenital conditions, such as spinal bifida and hydrocephalus, and some chromosomal defects such as microcephaly. The existence of the defect from the time of the infant's birth seems to call forth the guilt and anger of the baby's parents. Even though there is no certainty about the familial nature of the anomaly, this is the baby the parents made, and their first response is fairly universal. If the infant has a cleft lip as well, the child's appearance heightens the parents' emotions. They are further beset by stares, comments, and questions from the people who see the baby before the lip is repaired and often afterward; the shape of the baby's nose and lips makes his or her defect immediately visible to people in the patient/family's environment.

A significant characteristic of cleft palate is the extremely long period of treatment required. It starts during the newborn's first two months of life if he or she has a cleft lip; it includes surgery to repair the cleft palate when the child is between one-and-a-half and two years of age; it involves considerable dental care, often including use of a prosthesis; and during adolescence treatment in the form of surgery may be desirable to improve the appearance of the young person's nose. This is not only long but also arduous treatment which is stress producing for the entire patient/family unit. Speech therapy is included among the general features of treatment. The child's ability to talk clearly enough for others to understand is impaired by the deformity of his or her mouth. Speech therapy is therefore essential for adequate social communication and functioning; it too may require a long and hard period of persistent work.

In the instance of this defect, as in the case of diabetes of childhood, the chronicity of the condition and the prolonged period of treatment make the givers of care of great personal significance to the patient/family. One social worker said, "The hospital becomes personified and takes on personal characteristics because of . . . the dependence of patient/family on the hospital and personnel."

Impacts on the patient/family are discernible immediately in the parents' emotional reactions to the newborn with cleft palate. They are not restricted to guilt and anger. They may also feel fear, pity, disgust, and at times rejection; their attitudes may range from perceiving the child's defect as a curse to declaring him or her "as good as anyone else." The parents need time and opportunity to express their feelings, especially those they think are wrong and shameful, to people who can listen without condemning and be empathic without sentimentality. The practical help received from physicians, nurses, and social workers to meet the unusual strains of feeding and caring for these babies serves also to reduce the parents' fears and anxieties. The parents have to adjust to such phenomena as the unusually long time it takes to feed a baby with a cleft palate, the baby's need for a special nipple, and the baby's burping through his nose and mouth. Over the long haul, they must be prepared for the child's vulnerability to respiratory problems which will need medical care. Knowing about these possibilities may add for a time to the parents' burden of guilt, but in the end it is relieving in that they can exercise extra precautions, and they are not totally surprised and shocked by the child's frequent need for medical care.

There are special interventions on behalf of the infant with a cleft lip.

When the baby is about six weeks old, he or she returns to the hospital to have the lip closed. The procedure ordinarily so improves the baby's appearance that the parents feel marked relief, less anger, less guilt and shame, and at times pride in the infant's appearance.

The improved appearance has an unfortunate effect on some parents in that they try to forget the cleft palate is still there. Yet until the palate is closed, the child's vulnerability to infections continues, and he or she is often hospitalized for pneumonia.

Then the parents have to be prepared for other problems, which are largely dental but are as burdensome as were the earlier difficulties. The child's teeth do not develop normally, orthodontia is often needed, and this may also be the time for a prosthesis. Most of these children suffer from an excessive number of caries. All in all the children and their parents have to be prepared to follow through on medical and dental care at least through adolescence. It is hard to distinguish when parents seek medical care because of a real physical threat to the child and when they seek it out of excessive fear and overprotectiveness. Because the child is at special risk, the physicians tend to encourage the parents to bring the child to clinic when in their judgment they detect symptoms.

The parents need repeated explanations and encouragement, repeated instructions, and renewal of hope that each next step is worthwhile. The value to the patient and parents of frequent communication with the physicians and other givers of care cannot be overemphasized. The seeming endlessness of the treatment is hard indeed for both child and adult, and there may be episodes of wanting to give it all up. The patient/family's dependence upon the hospital and personnel may be both prized and resented. So many procedures have to be followed over so long a period of time; so many different professionals become involved as therapists and consultants; pain and separation have to be endured during intervals of hospitalization—these are among the significant events and conditions that cause resentment from time to time. It is true that these are experiences that directly affect the patient; but from their child's infancy through adolescence the parents have to take responsibility for decision making and giving informed consent, for bringing the pediatric patient to clinic innumerable times, for relating to specialists in several different fields, and for many other prescribed activities over the years. Thus, there are disruptions of day-by-day routines, distractions from other parental responsibilities, and restraints on parents' leisure time, to identify a few of the impacts upon the family's life-situation. What affects patients and parents influences siblings and may alter the climate and functioning of the family unit.

When the patient enters adolescence, there is usually an encouraging burst of self-interest and self-reliance. The patient begins to take some initiative, such as raising his or her own questions and making his or her desires known. For example, the adolescent may ask for surgery that will improve his or her appearance. The resentment that younger patients show because of the demands imposed by treatment decreases when adolescents begin consciously to value medical and surgical measures that might enhance their self-perception and the perceptions that others have of them. These changes in the patient's attitudes and behavior often help to relax the tensions in the families' situations. When the adolescent becomes a more active and willing participant in treatment, the burdens the parents have been carrying are reduced.

The patient/family suffer certain stress-producing events that stem from people's lack of information or misinformation about cleft palate. Relatives, neighbors, and schoolteachers are among those who may not understand how such an anomaly occurs and fall back on superstitions and old wives' tales. Those who give direct medical and related services to the patient perform a useful act when they inquire into what patients, parents, and others think they know about the defect so that they can dispel fantasies and ease anxieties.

One can understand why social workers and other personnel in health care facilities need to be prepared to work with handicapped children, their close relatives, and significant others such as teachers. In this context, preparation is a complex process of education and self-discipline by means of which professional givers-of-service develop the ability to apply the information and knowledge they have acquired with good judgment, compassion, and detached concern.

Some parents of children with cleft palate have established self-help groups. No doubt, competent professionals can provide consultation and leadership upon request without detracting from the efficacy of self-help but in fact enhancing it.

These parents have to contend not only with their and others' strong personal feelings but often with socioeconomic factors which are potential sources of stress and distress. The unusually frequent visits to a variety of clinics make proximity to the medical facility of special importance. Accessibility to, and time and money for, transportation are significant in facilitating or impeding continuous compliance with prescribed remedial measures. Financial strain during the many years of required medical and dental care may exacerbate resentment and provoke interruptions in treatment. Social workers know better than most what the resources in their community are for resolving such problems; they also know better than most whether provisions for paying the costs of a child's treatment when the family's income is low or moderate are comprehensive or fragmented and partial in coverage.

In New York City, for example, if a family's income is so low as to meet eligibility requirements for Medicaid, all costs of the patient's care are covered. Families with slightly higher but still limited incomes are eligible for help from the New York City Bureau for Handicapped Children. This is where the fragmentation begins to hurt; the bureau pays for treatment directly connected with the child's cleft palate, but it does not pay for treatment of serious secondary problems such as the unusual number of caries these children develop. Worst off are the families with just too much income to be eligible for aid from the city's bureau and without private insurance.

Even families with prepaid group insurance may suffer from financial strain. One such plan used widely in the New York metropolitan area does not cover clinic fees, although many members have to attend hospital-based specialty clinics, among them children with cleft palate.

The demands for adaptation made on the young patient with cleft palate are associated with the many ways in which he or she is different from his or her peers: in appearance, in carrying out developmental tasks such as feeding and talking, in experiencing frequent periods of illness and hospitalization, and in requiring special care and protection from birth throughout most of adolescence.

Even before the children are conscious of differences such as these, they will have to be separated from their parents at least once for surgical procedures.

As the children grow older and are aware of the constant need for medical and dental care and speech therapy, the consciousness of difference becomes more acute, and their attitudes toward themselves and others begin the crystallize. A range of reactions can be observed, from low self-esteem coupled with a feeling of isolation from the world to realistic self-acceptance leading to socially effective self-confidence.

Outstanding among the child's frustrations is what he or she experiences when his or her speech is not understood. The failure to convey verbal messages successfully to other human beings can be devastating, isolating, and depressing in its effects or infuriating and enraging. Imagine an eighth-grader, incapable of clear speech, who in exasperation throws a book at the teacher and for punishment is suspended from classes. It is this kind of reaction on the part of adults that convinces one of people's need to be better informed about handicapped children and better prepared to relate to them.

The adolescent's behavior and attitudes regarding his or her defect, the treatment, and the hospital staff are related to new strivings for a life and place of his or her own. The patient is now concerned about the significance the defect has for his or her choice of career and for the kind of person he or she wants to be. Socially, he or she becomes increasingly conscious of the impairment at a time when conformity with peers is as important as is pulling away from adults in authority. The adolescent patient becomes aware of physicians in ways that reflect his or her own developing maturity. The patient begins to have expectations and reacts with anger or hurt when they are not fulfilled. For example, the adolescent may think that the physician has failed to impart information the patient should have, and he or she freely expresses resentment. Or in another kind of situation, the patient may feel that the medical staff is insufficiently interested, and he or she finds a way to let them know. In one such instance, the chain of communication was from an adolescent patient to her mother to the social worker to the physicians. The physicians acknowledged that they had been neglectful and revised their treatment plan as well as their attitudes. It is worth describing the young girl's perceptions of the physicians and of herself when the atmosphere was cleared. She saw the change in the physicians as evidence of their caring about her but also—and this seems of major importance—as a sign that they were optimistic about the outcome of treatment. "When I felt the doctors didn't care about me, I lost my enthusiasm about myself," the patient told her social worker, "but now I'm curling my hair again, and I've shortened some dresses, and I've made some dates." This young patient's response to her restoration of hope is both moving and instructive.

On the other hand, the adolescent's expressions of anger and rebellion may be extensions of conflicts with parents rather than actual dissatisfaction with givers-of-service. These behaviors are usually acts of noncompliance, calling not for punishment but for understanding of what lies behind them. For example, the patient fails to keep an appointment not because he or she doesn't care about his or her treatment but because he or she is discouraged, because money for transportation ran low that week, or because at age 15 there are times when the track team meet or basketball practice has to take precedence. It is better, a social worker suggested, not to write the patient off and not to leave it to him or her but to make another appointment and then try to learn what is going on.

When the patient is in the middle teens, surgery on his or her nose will often improve facial appearance. The patient's self-awareness and self-consciousness about others' perceptions of him or her may lead the patient to ask for the surgery. In the patient's preparation for the procedure, there has to be an emphasis on reducing fantasies and heightening understanding of the probable outcomes of the surgery. The adolescent patient is likely to have a series of magical thoughts. This is the time more than ever when the patient asks, "When is it going to be over?" "When will the last treatment be?" He or she has to know that this surgical procedure is not the last treatment; it will improve his or her appearance, but there will be continuing need for dental work, and if he or she wears a prosthesis it may have to be altered from time to time.

The patient's expectations may be wide of the mark. In preparatory conversations with the plastic surgeon and the social worker, the adolescent patient describes what kind of nose he or she wants, and then they discuss how the nose will probably look. The patient is told about the discomfort he or she will experience, how he or she will look immediately after the operation (swollen and bruised), and how long it will probably be before he or she can see the real results.

When these patients are fearful and doubtful about their vocational and social future, their fantasies about the effects of surgery will require special consideration. If discussions of vocational plans and of the patient's aspirations and problems connected with his or her social life are begun in advance of discussions of surgery, it may be somewhat easier for the patients to give up the most improbable expectations. A good example is the situation of a 17-year-old girl whose dissatisfaction with her social life centered on "not being asked out" and whose solution to the problem focused on the surgery she had requested ("Everything will be all right after the operation.") But her talks with the social worker stimulated her to make some new friends and to initiate some social activities with them. Though she still hoped for the surgery, she knew now that not everything depended on it. When her request was approved and the operation completed, she was happy with the results and hopeful about her future.

In respect to vocational choice, the patient may err in either direction: he or she may think the defect will be an obstacle when it will not, or think it will be no obstacle when experience shows otherwise. Available information and the opinion of experts in the field of employment are useful realistic guide lines to which the patients should have access. They should also have ample opportunity to discuss their wishes, other choices, the satisfactions and dissatisfactions these choices may offer, and the time, effort, and money it will take to reach their goals. Here again the social worker's command of community resources and ability to make them available to patients/families in accordance with their needs and capabilities are valuable aids to the patients' attainment of maximum social functioning.

It is natural that adolescents born with cleft palate should ask whether their children will have the defect. There is no firm evidence, but physicians can give the patients the few available facts. In general the patients can be told that their children will probably not have cleft palate, but that the risk is greater than for parents who do not have the defect. This information confronts the patients with still another reality and an uncertainty that is indeed difficult to cope with at any age.

In tracing the course of childhood diabetes and the congenital anomaly of cleft palate, it becomes clear that patients with either condition must struggle to master or accommodate to many of the same stress-producing characteristics: chronicity, since in each instance both the deviant condition and its treatment and management are coterminous with life; impairment in bodily functioning; restraints on social functioning; a threatened self-image and self-regard which, among other things, affects social relationships; a heavy involvement of the child's parents in the patient's health care; and an influence on the patient's siblings and on the shape and functioning of the family unit.

There are significant differentiations to be noted, too: a diabetic's expectation of a shortened life span and of physiological complications, the proven familial nature of diabetes, the visibility of a cleft lip, and the instant recognition by others of the patient's difficulty in speech.

How patients/families deal with these potential sources of stress and demands for adaptation is the end result of their inner strengths being brought to bear upon their deprivations through successful use of health care, the psychological and social support of personnel in the human services, the utilization of appropriate resources in the community, and their response to the warmth and caring of the people in their natural milieu.

INDEX

78 79 80 7 6 5 4 3 2 1